Informed Treatment

Informed Treatment

Milieu Management in Psychiatric Hospitals and Residential Treatment Centers

Nancy Britton Soth

Medical Library Association
and
The Scarecrow Press
Lanham, Md. & London

SCARECROW PRESS, INC.

Published in the United States of America
by Scarecrow Press, Inc.
4720 Boston Way
Lanham, Maryland 20706

4 Pleydell Gardens, Folkestone
Kent CT20 2DN, England

British Library Cataloguing in Publication Information Available

Library of Congress Cataloging-in-Publication Data

Soth, Nancy Britton.
Informed treatment : milieu management in psychiatric hospitals and residential treatment centers / Nancy Britton Soth.
p. cm.
Includes bibliographical references and index.
ISBN 0–8108–3202–X (cloth : alk. paper)
1. Milieu therapy. 2. Therapeutic communitites. 3. Psychiatry—Differential therapeutics. I. Title.
[DNLM: 1. Milieu therapy—organization & administration. 2. Informed Consent. 3. Hospitals, Psychiatric—organization & administration. WM 440 S7171 1996]
RC489.M5S68 1996
362.2'1—dc21 96—49627

ISBN 0–8108–3202–X (cloth : alk. paper)

™ The paper used in this publication meets the minimum requirements of American National Standard for Information Sciences—Permanence of Paper for Printed Library Materials, ANSI Z39.48–1984.
Manufactured in the United States of America.

To:

Laura Burns-Levison, 1951–1994

Contents

Preface

This book is written for those who design inpatient psychiatric treatment and those who carry it out and for the librarians who inform this effort. It began with questions about diagnosis. If the staff knows that the patient has a schizophrenic disorder, what does it reveal about the patient's treatment on the psychiatric unit? Does diagnosis make a difference in milieu treatment? The psychiatric hospital or residential treatment center usually treats patients of varying diagnoses within a single unit, so that milieu treatment itself cannot be tailored to the diagnosis. Instead, those who work in the milieu must share a body of knowledge about what the patient's diagnosis tells them about treatment. This will enable the milieu staff to better understand the patient and develop diagnostic-specific techniques for milieu management.

There were also questions about how to organize the treatment environment, how to solve the many problems that arise in the milieu, and what techniques are available. Bringing this literature together in one volume should help the treatment staff from continuously needing to reinvent solutions for each new problem. The book is for all who work in the psychiatric milieu but is not addressed to any single specialty. There is no specific information about family therapy, medical treatment, psychopharmacology, or individual psychotherapy. Those who practice these special professions still belong to the psychiatric milieu and cannot afford disinterest in the design of its programs and techniques or solutions to its problems.

The book brings together a body of literature that is scattered and segregated throughout many disciplines: psychiatry, psychology, sociology, and nursing. It collects literature in English from many countries, other than the United States: from Canada, Germany, the Scandinavian countries, Israel, Australia, and the United Kingdom. It combines literature from many inpatient settings: hospitals, residential treatment centers, substance abuse programs, and day treatment centers. The book concentrates on providing information that can be used immediately, recognizing that those who work directly with patients don't always have the luxury of long study and that literature searches do not always give the answers. It might be called a narrative bibliography that not only provides immediate assistance but can lead the reader to further information. It should be of help to hospital staff development directors and serve as a basis for further study. *Informed Treatment* cumulates milieu wisdom from many sources, but primarily from the periodical literature, the best source of information for the busy professional. Books cited in the text are classical or cumulative works that extend the coverage of topics in the periodical literature.

Few of the periodical articles cited represent controlled, empirical studies, since this is difficult to accomplish in the psychiatric milieu. A truly informed treatment would be represented by a synthesis of work with adequate controls, meaningful outcome criteria, well-designed methodology, statistical analyses and comprehensive conclusions. Since interpersonal relations and interpersonal techniques do not lend themselves to exact study, this will never be accomplished. Few of us can lead our daily lives guided by empirical findings. *Informed Treatment* refers instead to the clinical wisdom of those who have worked in the psychiatric milieu and have attempted to create a beneficial therapeutic environment for the mentally ill. They have also been generous enough to share this wisdom. It is heartening to know that even now in very competitive times, treatment methods have not become a business secret. Not all of this literature is of high quality. Some of it is of the "We had a problem and here's what we did" variety. But in the middle of such writing comes one good idea that makes sense. Case histories of individual patients are not presented. Descriptions of treatment programs are presented from time to time as examples of programs in action, to illustrate what might be attempted, not to certify their success. In this work, the names of institutions are usually not given. Psychiatric institutions thrive on change, so there is good reason to believe that no matter how impressive the program described, it is no longer there. One should telephone before making a pilgrimage.

A few words about language in this book are necessary. Substituting the preferred term "clients" for "patients" proved unwieldy. It did not fit with the term "inpatient". It was difficult to write about children or adolescents and envision them as "clients". Moreover, many persons in psychiatric hospitals do not seem to be clients, because they have not chosen to be there. Changing the words in the older literature and replacing "patients" with "clients" seemed artificial, while replacing the word "client" with "patient" brought only temporary pangs of political embarrassment. This work is a synthesis from a rich body of literature. My attempts to change the language and make it my own were often frustrating; much of this material is too close to the original text. There was always the risk of changing the meaning, a fear that the writers would reappear to say: "That's not what I meant at all." The writing seemed sacred, forged from painful and triumphant experiences. Every word seemed to be *le mot juste.* I might have strayed further from the original text, but it never seemed to work. It seemed artificial, sometimes arbitrary, and in no way exact. Sometimes by trying to say it another way, I felt that I was draining it of impact and meaning. I can only state that nothing in this book is my original thought. It was tempting at times to insert my own ideas, to give some good advice here and there, but I am the librarian, not the clinician. I hope that the original authors of these works will understand. The risk of changing their meaning and losing the full impact of the way they said it was stronger than my fear of being accused of borrowing their words.

This book represents a rich heritage of writing on inpatient treatment that should be both used and preserved, for it may not be produced again. These techniques were developed in long-term treatment. Short-term treatment will not provide the opportunity for experimentation, reflection, and an analysis of results. There will be fewer sources for guidance. There is some hope that future literature may come from new applications of family or cognitive therapy techniques or methods that have been successful in educational settings. The articles collected here represent the century's most useful writing on the milieu and serve as a tender farewell to the hope of milieu therapy. This may be the last work touching on milieu therapy to be published in the United States, a final summing up of what is known about milieu management.

It is only fair to confess my own bias, or at least to describe my own favorites in this literature. I am comforted by work that strives to be exact, that confidently states that there is indeed an informed way to do things. The American Psychiatric Association's 3-volume *Treatments of Mental Disorders,* practice guidelines in the *American Journal of Psychiatry* and practice parameters in the *Journal of the American Academy of Child and Adolescent Psychiatry* that scrutinize and synthesize all that is known about the treatment of specific disorders are welcome examples of this kind of writing. I find hope in the phrase "cognitive milieu," even though its methods have not yet been thoroughly tested. The success of Linehan's cognitive-dialectal therapy in inpatient treatment of borderline personality disorder is an exciting breakthrough. I receive a similar satisfaction when reading Kiser's or Harper's or Nurcombe's articles on treatment planning. I am deeply satisfied by writers who can capture the symbolic meanings of milieu treatment and take us beyond the day-to-day reality to provide vision and emotional meaning to the work. The writing of Melvyn Rose is an example. I am excited by those writers who can fight their way through the interpersonal blizzards of patient and staff relations and tell us why it's happening—writers like Gabbard, Ogden, Kernberg or Kets de Vries. I am pleased by the many writers in psychiatric nursing journals who can translate difficult concepts into practical milieu applications and those like Gallop or Morrison who proceed further with valuable research. I am thrilled when I find writers who can simply turn treatment upside down and make us examine what we're doing and start again. Those who write about systemic or contextual or cybernetic treatment models are doing that now.

The book begins with an examination of the heritage of milieu therapy, the concepts, treatment models and organization, and environments that provide a foundation for this work. It then reviews what is known about milieu treatment specific to diagnosis, and examines milieu problems and techniques. For ease of consultation, entries on treatment models, populations, problems, and techniques are arranged in alphabetical order under each chapter.

It has been a pleasure to follow some of these good writers from their early days, to imagine them still working together at places like Timberlawn or at Menninger or White Plains. Certain places become a kind of imagined paradise. Those who create a therapeutic milieu must contemplate Utopia. They must dream about creating a perfect society where everyone can thrive. Much of the writing on milieu therapy is inspiring and relevant to everyday life because it examines what makes a good society, how to create an environment that promotes both sanity and happiness. This book is a tribute to such special places. I found the psychiatric environment a most rewarding to place to live, work, and strive for honesty, a place where one can be constantly immersed in the drama of human life and yet feel so released and so free. I will always treasure the strong bonds I had with patients, amazing and mystifying in their depth and intensity, resembling no other relationship before or after, and the pure pleasure of working with people who were good with people.

I could not have written this book without the help I received from the Association of Mental Health Librarians. This exceptional group gave me a research grant many years ago and continued to advise and support me. I would like to express my gratitude to the many libraries where I worked on this manuscript: the University of North Carolina, University of Iowa, Howard University, and the University of Washington. I will always be grateful to the University of Minnesota, not only for the Biomedical Library but also for the MINITEX interlibrary loan system that makes it possible for scholars to continue to thrive in any small town in Minnesota. I am especially grateful for the warm hospitality of my home libraries at Carleton College and St. Olaf College, and to all the librarians who helped: Ann Niles, Richard E. Miller, Carolyn Sanford, Lisa Brusseau, Sandy Allen, and Robert Bruce. I was very fortunate to work with editors J. Michael Homan and David Biesel. Special appreciation goes to my friends and colleagues who advised and supported me, particularly David Bly, Christina Colwell, Loris Damaron, Lulu Fierst, Jackie Gimse, Ann Hodgson, Annalee Larson, Joyce Lindquist, Sue Lloyd, Judy Mason, Anne Mullinax-Jones, Martha Pierce, Linda Rue, and Jo Zimmerman. M. Robert Wilson deserves a special tribute for many reasons, one of which is for bringing all these magnificent people together in Old Main.

Informed Treatment

CHAPTER

I

Milieu Therapy and Management

The fundamental difference between inpatient and outpatient treatment is that inpatient treatment occurs in a controlled environment. The environment can be modified to give the patient new and significant life experiences not provided in individual psychotherapy. Milieu management rests upon the heritage of writing about milieu therapy. The use of the word milieu to describe a carefully arranged therapeutic environment began to appear in the psychiatric literature of the 1940s. It extended the boundaries of therapy beyond the therapist to include the patient's total environment [1–3].

Milieu therapy refers to the organization of the entire social system of the hospital as a therapeutic instrument, a planned environment exerting an independent force. The total setting in which the patient lives, including the activities and interactions within it, can be structured to meet treatment goals and respond to changing internal and external dynamics. The patients themselves can become a therapeutic force in the milieu. Milieu therapy provides a method for assuring that various interactions experienced by the patient do not occur in isolation from each other. It systematically uses every available technique to help the patient control symptomatic behaviors and learn appropriate social skills [4–7].

Dysfunctional behavior is affected by the environment and can be altered by its conscious modification. The environment can produce specific changes in a patient's behavior and thereby stimulate changes in personality. Behavior can improve because the milieu provides human relationships that will satisfy emotional needs and strengthen impaired ego functions. Some patients will need milieu management and therapy more than others. When the external environment (family or peer relationships, for example) is disturbed or the equilibrium between internal dynamics and the external environment disrupted, milieu therapy can be a corrective force. Gralnick describes the therapeutic milieu as a healthy environment to which the patient comes for repair from an unhealthy milieu [8–10].

There is a basic assumption in milieu therapy that a healthy environment discourages pathology. The milieu program can provide patients with planned group activities with a therapeutic goal. Patients can learn new skills, practice problem solving, and establish new norms and values. A group of people with shared values forms a potent social teaching device since patients can quickly learn how they interact and how their behavior affects others. The treatment center provides a realistic ground for relationships and experiences that will provide insight into the patient's recurring difficulties and help to develop more adaptive patterns. These difficulties can also be explored in group sessions and in community meetings [10–11].

These social interactions in the milieu give the patient the opportunity to work out in real life what has merely been talked about in psychotherapy. The patient can practice trying to change. In addition, the milieu also generates problems to be brought to psychotherapy, in that this known environment imposes appropriate and realistic demands. The patient's own struggles and successes in mastering them provide current material for psychotherapy sessions. Milieu therapy can be more "relevant" than psychotherapy since it gives control to the patient's primary group, as in real life, rather than exclusively in the psychotherapy relationship. Therapeutic interventions occur in the "here and now" of the patient's life rather than in the psychotherapy hour. Part of the therapeutic work therefore takes place in the social field, with direction from the professional staff. The patient learns about the effects and reasons for behavior. This in turn helps the psychotherapist to increase the patient's insight, and the daily interactive process provides the patient with further insight, usually acquired in individual therapy [10–12].

The milieu expresses certain values, many of which are conscious and explicit. Redl describes the "value system that oozes out of our pores." Treatment can often stress values and question the unhealthy values of patients with the goal of eventually changing them. Values are important, not only to help in treating the patient's symptoms but also to help to create a healthier, more human person. Tuck and Keels mention some predominant values in milieu therapy, many of which have to do with individual responsibility. Some predominant values are that openness is good; dependency is not; responsibility for one's self is good, and for another person is better; and the responsibility for the group is even better [12–13].

The Descent of Milieu Therapy

Advances in pharmacotherapy have made the psychiatric milieu easier to manage. The shorter hospital stay diluted the milieu's potential influence. Milieu therapy still provides the conceptual underpinning for inpatient practice and the activities that occur during the patient's stay, but it is no longer an independent treatment. The medical model alone, without attention to the milieu, can neglect the group dynamic forces that often operate antitherapeutically. Active management of such forces improves the therapeutic climate. The literature of milieu therapy will continue to inform even those who deny its importance. Milieu therapy lost some of its clinical usefulness because it was not easy to connect treatment philosophy with actual patient outcomes, nor its individual components with success. It could not always be demonstrated that milieu therapy did what it was designed to do [14].

Gunderson's Therapeutic Milieu Processes

Although milieu therapy is an ideology that often lacks a technology, Gunderson provided a framework by delineating the functions of a therapeutic milieu. He identified five therapeutic functions that a psychiatric milieu can provide: containment, support, structure, involvement and validation [14–16].

Containment refers to the structures that sustain and protect the patient and prevent violence and dangerous actions. It provides external controls when the patient lacks inner controls. Holding and containment can give a feeling of safety and help patients tolerate anxiety. This security will later allow them to open up to understanding the thoughts and feelings that have affected their behaviors. A reliable staff that keeps patients aware of the realities of their world also provides containment and holding. Containment helps patients who are out of control get control of themselves. The staff and the hospital function temporarily as an auxiliary ego for the patients and provide for them what they can't provide for themselves. Patients know that the staff is predictable, what to expect from them, and what the consequences are for positive and negative behavior [16–18].

Support describes the provision of nurturance in the treatment setting, the attempts to help patients feel secure, to reassure them, and to improve their self-esteem. It is particularly valuable for patients with depression. Support may include designing activities and experiences that will give patients confidence. It makes patients feel better and gives them sufficient comfort and security to modulate their distress. Verbal reassurance, directions or advice, or even back-rubs, give support. When not reassured, patients may secretly fear that their situation is hopeless. However, routine statements or reassurance given in authoritative or condescending manner does not provide genuine support. Providing information can give support. Stanton and Schwartz write that there are times when patients report that a repeated explanation was one of the most helpful factors in their improvement [16–21].

Structure refers to the stable organization of the milieu, the organization of time, space, and persons. Staff has definite roles and responsibilities. Scheduled patient and staff activities provide a framework for living. Redl, discussing the therapeutic benefits of structure for children, feels that it significantly increases the child's feelings of security. A time schedule for the day, the repetition of the same routines at morning, evening, and bedtime and clear expectations have a relaxing and soothing effect on the children and therefore become an ego-strengthening factor. Privilege systems, token economies, contracts, and defined consequences also establish structure. Treatment centers using a medical or behavioral model place great emphasis on structure. Structure helps patients to think before acting and to consider the consequences of their behavior. The final purpose of structure is to effect changes in the patient's symptoms and behavior. Structure can replace the patient's inner self, filling a void until recovery can occur. As treatment progresses, the patient will develop internal ego structures. Gunderson notes that staff on units where structure is primary must be comfortable with firmly setting limits and tolerating anger. He believes that when both patients and staff agree on what behaviors are maladaptive and together create a structure to modify them, structure then becomes a therapeutic modality. He cautions, however, that too much structure may conceal pathology and changes that the patient makes in a highly structured setting may be lost quickly after discharge. Structure must be titrated according to the patient's situation. Tight controls can smother interaction between staff and patients. Novotny warns that structure can become rigid and its deadening effect can become antitherapeutic. Too much structure leaves patients unprepared to function in the unstructured world to which they are discharged [16–23].

Involvement describes those processes that encourage patients to interact with their environment. Involvement helps to modify maladaptive interpersonal patterns and improve social skills and competence, decreasing the patient's isolation and passivity. The milieu staff encourages open discussion of problems. Therapeutic processes include mandatory milieu groups, patient-led groups and many community activities. Treatment settings that emphasize involvement have a distribution of power and decision-making and feature group processes of "cooperation, compromise, confrontation, and conformity." Involvement can also include the belief that patients can and should care for each other and that this, too, can be a source of growth. Involvement decreases passivity and thus can be helpful for the withdrawn and depressed, but it is not therapeutic for all patients [24].

Validation refers to the affirmation of individuality in the psychiatric setting. Individual treatment programming, private talks, and good relationships build validation. Validation helps patients develop intimacy and restores identity. The most characteristic feature of validation is the initial acceptance of the patient's illness. In a setting that stresses validation, the patient can express symptoms without bringing about serious consequences. Validation allows the patient to try and fail but provides encouragement to reach full potential. It provides an antidote to hopelessness and helplessness. Wright and colleagues report that a cognitive milieu builds validation by identifying and using the patient's assets and developing an individualized treatment plan specifically for the patient's problems, and respecting the patient's rights [24–25].

Although the psychiatric milieu provides all of these functions, a single function may be primary and others supplementary. Characterizing the predominant function of the psychiatric milieu can be helpful in selecting staff since various functions will require certain personality traits. Staff in a setting where containment is important will need self-control, reliability and physical strength. While older staff members comfortably give support, younger staff can become more easily involved. If structure is primary, the staff member should be well-organized and punctual, be able to set limits and be firm and not frightened by aggression. Staff members who are comfortable with introspection, who are empathic and sensitive, will flourish in a milieu that stresses validation [24–25].

These therapeutic functions don't just happen in the milieu. An informed and experienced staff engineers them. The staff that provides containment and structure for the aggressive, conduct-disordered adolescent must also involve and validate the experience of the depressed and withdrawn person. Gunderson's therapeutic functions can characterize and differentiate various treatment milieus and are valuable in designing treatment units for specific disorders. The staff on short-term units with mixed populations will usually work to provide a flexible milieu to provide all of these functions [25].

The Foundations of Milieu Therapy

Milieu therapy in America was developed from psychoanalytic theory by Europeans and European émigrés who worked with children in residential treatment. August Aichhorn (1878–1949) was one of the first to apply psychoanalytic theory to residential treatment. Aichhorn was concerned with combining children and children and adults to create optimal therapeutic relationships. Not only did he intuitively pair untrained workers with children who could benefit psychologically through their care, he composed groups in such a way that group life could influence behavior difficulties (26–27).

Bruno Bettelheim

Bruno Bettelheim's work is discussed throughout this book. For Bettelheim, milieu therapy meant endowing every detail of the child's life with meaning. Bettelheim's therapeutic milieu provided almost unconditional gratification of the child's needs with appropriate doses of reality. He created an environment of freedom and abundance and full approval of infantile pleasures even when they were below the child's chronological age. Bettelheim believed that the therapeutic milieu helped children develop mastery over inner and outer forces because gratification of their basic needs was available at all times. He described the Orthogenic School as an all-embracing society that joined beneficial effects for children with the same effects for staff [28–30].

FRITZ REDL

Fritz Redl conceived of the milieu as "total group therapy," with the emotional currents that can be turned on and off for therapeutic purposes. Redl believed that with children, most of the therapy occurred in daily life situations—getting up, going to bed, working and playing. Redl based much of his work on ego psychology, which dominated psychoanalytic thinking during the 1950s and 1960s. Redl described the ego as a negotiator at the border between outside and inside reality [31–32].

Redl described the weak ego as not having sufficient strength to contain impulses. He observed various ego disturbances in residential treatment, such as inability to cope with frustration and aggression or a loss of ego control through "group psychological intoxication." Redl felt that children with disturbed egos could not retain memories of previous satisfaction or anticipation of future contentment sufficient to carry them through periods of crises or boredom. He writes of the many "collapses" of ego functioning in the lives of children in residential treatment. Redl found that residential group life provided a number of ego supports which did not depend completely on individual rapport or verbal communication. Something as simple as traditional routine provided great ego support. Redl describes many ego-supportive techniques, such as "manipulation of hang-over effects," "preventive signal interference," "interpretation through reshuffled reality," and "exploration of group psychological securities" [33–34].

Redl made milieu concepts and techniques a pleasure to learn and difficult to forget by a unique use of language. He seems able to zoom directly into what happens in the milieu and help everyone to experience it with great immediacy. Consider the chapter titles in *Controls from Within*, which virtually outline the ingredients of the therapeutic milieu: "a house which smiles, props which invite, space which allows, routines which occupy." Many of Redl's other terms dramatically convey what should be done in the residential milieu: hygienic behavior control, antiseptic handling of surface behavior, impulse drainage, hypodermic affection. Redl's legacy remains alive, not as much through his writings as through the number of leaders in residential treatment who worked and studied with him and who continue to quote his many lessons [34].

Maxwell Jones and Thomas Main

In the 1950s in England, Maxwell Jones and Thomas Main created therapeutic communities that gave patients the major role in the therapeutic process. Jones and Main believed that a community with a shared value system could unify and empower the patients, so they would no longer need to be dishonest or manipulative to combat their helplessness. The milieu's work was carried out in the community meeting, which still continues to be an effective therapeutic process in inpatient treatment [35–36].

Albert Stanton and Morris Schwartz

Psychoanalytic thinkers on milieu therapy were followed by sociologists who used participant observation to study the inner workings of the psychiatric hospital. Albert Stanton, a psychiatrist and Morris Schwartz, a sociologist, in the study of a private psychoanalytic hospital, found that the functioning of the institution influenced the patients' disturbances. Increased agitation and patient disturbances were linked to covert staff disagreements about how their cases should be handled. When these disagreements were uncovered and resolved, the patients quickly improved [37].

Erving Goffman and D. L. Rosenhan

The foundation of milieu therapy is incomplete without consideration of the valid criticism from sociologists and psychologists. In *Asylums*, Erving Goffman, a sociologist, examines the social environment of "total institutions." The total institution is a place of residence and work removed from the outside world, which completely circumscribes the lives of its inhabitants. Goffman found that total institutions, such as mental hospitals, prisons, boarding schools, or convents, strongly resembled each other and created remarkably similar social conditions for their inhabitants, whom he called "inmates." He described them as "forcing houses" for changing persons. The total institution is essentially a closed environment that controls the time and space of those who live there [38].

Goffman's most significant contribution to the work of the psychiatric hospital was to show what happens to the person who lives there. Goffman lived there, too, at St. Elizabeth's Hospital in Washington, D.C., where he assumed the role of the inmate and was able to describe institutional life from the inmate's point of view. His work helped mental health professionals to scrutinize those hospital practices that erode the patient's identity as well as the various ways in which mental illness can be institutionally created. Goffman demonstrated how admission procedures in total institutions can become rituals of degradation. The person comes to the mental hospital from a social world that provided a fixed definition of self but must discard these stable arrangements upon admission. The barrier that the total institution places between the person and the outer world begins an erosion of the self. The institution strips the person of any worldly role other than patienthood, with a series of degradations and humiliations. Total institutions erode identity by restricting the person's privacy and by making personal information public. The self becomes a continuously invaded "open city." This leaves the person without any feeling of importance or individuality. Moreover, there is no escape from these mortifying situations [38].

Goffman asks the mental health profession to be skeptical of what is considers pathological. When an institution operates to correct abnormal behavior, it expects abnormality. Even normal behavior or behavior in response to hospitalization may then be re-interpreted as subtle signs of pathology. Biographical information, when translated into a case summary, may be written in such a way as to confirm pathology. Pathology may be more the result of the person's current situation (i.e., hospitalization), rather than the person's individual characteristics [38].

Goffman did not offer solutions for these problems; nor was that his stated task. Nevertheless, his work had a significant impact on mental hospitals and is not irrelevant today. While staff members continue to congratulate themselves upon the benign healing communities they have established, they probably enjoy them much more than the patients. Goffman's ability to relate the subjective experience of the patient can bring every hospital procedure into serious question. Recent works, such as Kaysen's *Girl, Interrupted* question the basic assumptions of hospitalization, the behavior of the staff, and the kind of writing that goes into medical records. No matter how much the staff feels it knows the patients, it will always need this view from the other side [38–39].

D. L. Rosenhan, in his 1973 article "On being sane in insane places" effectively challenged the validity of the diagnosis of mental illness in psychiatric hospitals. He engaged a number of sane persons (pseudopatients) who got themselves admitted with little difficulty to 12 different psychiatric hospitals in 5 different states. Their only psychiatric problem was that they heard voices that commented on the meaninglessness of their lives. After admission the pseudopatients behaved normally and displayed no further symptoms. Rosenhan found that facts from the patients' histories were often distorted to fit psychodynamic formulations. None of these pseudopatients, however, were found to be sane despite their sane behavior during their hospitalization. Rosenhan concludes from this that in the context of the psychiatric hospital the normal cannot be detected as sane. The failure to detect sanity in the hospital may be due to the physician's professional caution, since in medicine it is dangerous to overlook illness and pronounce the patient healthy [40].

Rosenhan then tried another experiment. The hospital staff was told that at some time during the following three months one or more pseudopatients would be admitted to the hospital. Each staff member was asked to rate the likelihood of a person's being a pseudopatient. After three months, 41 patients had been alleged by at least one staff member to be a pseudopatient. The alert had been false. No genuine pseudopatients had been admitted during that time [40].

Both of these experiences prove that illnesses are given meaning by their context. Rosenhan was challenging the accuracy of diagnosis, but was also demonstrating how quickly the normal can be seen as pathological in the psychiatric hospital—that everyone who has a hammer is looking for a nail. In addition, behaviors that may be stimulated by the environment are misattributed to the patient's disorder. Rosenhan's findings should not be foreign to anyone who has worked or lived in a psychiatric institution [40].

References

1. Leeman CP. The therapeutic milieu. In: Sederer LI, ed. Inpatient psychiatry: Diagnosis and Treatment. Baltimore: Williams & Wilkins, 1983, 222–34.
2. Schlesinger HJ, Holzman PS. The therapeutic aspects of the hospital milieu. Bulletin Menninger Clinic 1970;34(1):1–11.
3. Bettelheim B, Sylvester E. A therapeutic milieu. American Journal of Orthopsychiatry 1948 Apr;18(2):191–206.
4. Menninger K, Pruyser PW, Mayman M, Houston M. The prescription of treatment. Bulletin Menninger Clinic 1960 Sep;24(5):217–49.
5. Kopolow LE, Cohen GD. Milieu therapy: toward a definition for reimbursement. American Journal of Psychiatry 1976 Sep;133(9):1060–3.
6. Van Putten T. Milieu therapy: Contraindications? Archives of General Psychiatry 1973 Nov;29:640–3.
7. Abroms GM. Defining milieu therapy. Archives of General Psychiatry 1969;21:553–60.
8. Melville PH. The rights of the person to be sick: a critique of milieu therapy. Journal Canadian Psychiatric Association 1965; 10:502–10.
9. Stainbrook E. Milieu therapy. In: Freedman AM, Kaplan HI, eds. A comprehensive textbook of psychiatry. Baltimore: Williams and Wilkins, 1978, 1296–1300.
10. Gralnick A. The socially-oriented psychiatric hospital. International Journal of Social Psychiatry 1987;33(3):218–55.
11. See reference 2.
12. Tuck I, Keels MC. Milieu therapy: a review of development of this concept and its implications for psychiatric nursing. Issues in Mental Health Nursing 1992;13:52–58.
13. Redl F. The concept of a "therapeutic milieu." American Journal of Orthopsychiatry 1959;29:721–36.
14. Delaney KR. Nursing in child psychiatric milieus. Part II. Mapping conceptual footholds. Journal of Child & Adolescent Psychiatric Nursing 1992;5(1):15–9.
15. Perrow C. Hospitals: technology, structures and goals. In: Marsh J, ed. Handbook of organizations. New York: Rand McNally, 1965.
16. Gunderson JG. Defining the therapeutic processes in psychiatric milieus. Psychiatry 1978;41(4):327–35.
17. James O. Role of the nurse-therapist relationship in the therapeutic community. International Review of Psychoanalysis 1984;11:151–9.

18. Stamm I. A psychoanalytic model. In: Lyman RD, Prentice-Dunn S, Gabel S. eds. Residential and inpatient treatment of children and adolescents. New York: Plenum Press, 1989.
19. Lewis J. The changing face of adolescent inpatient psychiatric treatment. Psychiatric Hospital 1991;22(4):161–3.
20. Stanton AM, Schwartz M. The Mental hospital: Study of institutional participation in psychiatric illness and treatment. New York: Basic Books, 1954.
21. Redl F. The concept of ego disturbance and ego support. American Journal of Orthosychiatry 1951;21(2):273–84.
22. Denber HCB. Analysis of the operation after two years. In: Denber HCB, ed. Research conference on the therapeutic xommunity. Springfield IL: Charles C. Thomas, 1960, 57–79.
23. Novotny PC. The pseudopsychoanalytic hospital. Bulletin Menninger Clinic 1973 (May);37(3):193–210.
24. See reference 16.
25. Wright JH, Thase ME, Ludgate JW, Beck AT. Cognitive therapy with inpatients. In: Wright JH, Thase ME, Beck AT, Ludgate JW, eds. The Cognitive milieu: structure and process. New York: Plenum Press, 1993, 61–90.
26. Swartz MS, Harget AB, Fraker WW, Noll BK, et al. The inpatient milieu: organizational and functional principles. Psychiatric Annals 1988 Feb;18(2): 80–4.
27. Aichhorn A. The wayward child. New York: Viking Press, 1965.
28. Rosen JL. Personality factors in reactions of child care workers to emotionally disturbed children. Psychiatry 1963;26(3):257–65.
29. Bettelheim B. Home for the heart. New York: Knopf, 1974.
30. Bettelheim B. Love is not enough: The treatment of emotionally disturbed children. Glencoe IL: Free Press, 1950.
31. Zimmerman DP. The clinical thought of Bruno Bettelheim: A critical historical review. Residential Treatment for Children & Youth 1993;10(3):3–36
32. Redl F. When we deal with children. New York: Free Press, 1966.
33. Redl F. The concept of ego disturbance and ego support. American Journal of Orthopsychiatry 1951 Apr;21(2):273–84.
34. Redl F, Wineman D. Controls from within: Techniques for the treatment of the aggressive child. New York: Free Press, 1952.
35. Jones M. The treatment of personality disorders in a therapeutic community. Psychiatry 1957;20:211–20.
36. Main TF. The hospital as a therapeutic community. Bulletin Menninger Clinic 1946; 10:66–70.
37. See reference 20.
38. Goffman E. Asylums: Essays on the social situation of mental patients and other inmates. Chicago: Aldine, 1962.
39. Kaysen S. Girl, interrupted. New York: Random, 1993.
40. Rosenhan DL. On being sane in insane places. Science 1973 Jan 19; 179 (4070):250–8.

CHAPTER

II

Concepts and their Application in Milieu Treatment.

Many of the concepts discussed in this chapter originated in psychoanalysis. They are significant in inpatient treatment since the staff's therapeutic responses, rather than the therapist's, may constitute the basic healing ingredient in the milieu. The attempt to present these concepts clearly may make them seem less complex than they are. Further reading is recommended for full understanding. Other concepts, such as manipulation, splitting, or reframing will be discussed in the chapters on Addressing Special Problems in the Milieu (Chapter VII) and Techniques in Milieu Therapy and Management (Chapter VIII).

Transference

Patients enter treatment with established patterns of relationships and behaviors toward others. Transference reactions are the unconscious emotions transferred from parents and others, updated editions of old relationships. The patient transfers these earlier relationships to the new setting with a script that will be re-enacted with a new cast of characters. Although not all of the person's behavior is transference, staff members will recognize it when they find themselves the recipient of thoughts, feelings or conflicts they could not have caused. These transference behaviors should be recorded and scrutinized rather than prevented, for they will help to provide a narrative of the person's early life. Treatment may focus on a revision of the script, an unlocking of the earlier mutually reinforcing pathology between child and parents [1].

COUNTERTRANSFERENCE

Countertransference refers to the feelings that patients arouse in those who treat them. Although the term referred originally to the feelings that the patient's transference evoked in the therapist, it has been extended to describe feelings evoked by patients in the milieu. The patient brings earlier modes of relating to the new setting, as if directing a play, bringing a familiar script, using staff members to play the parts and feel the feelings assigned. The familiar script provides security, but if staff members continue to play these predetermined roles, the patient will never change. When staff members act on the basis of countertransference they play a part in reinforcing and preserving the patient's maladaptive behavior [2].

Countertransference is either concordant or complementary. When the transference is concordant, the staff member identifies strongly with the patient and often begins to experience some of the patient's emotions. Stamm notes that often a doctor or nurse will identify so strongly with a patient that they will not allow negative reactions from other staff members. The treatment team's hostility will then explode sporadically and destructively. When experiencing complementary countertransference, the staff member is pulled in to replay a role in the patient's life, often that of the parent. Bonier notes that staff responses to adolescent patients are similar, if not identical to those of their parents. Complementary countertransference may lead to romantic involvements, as patients become as seductive with staff members as they have been with others in their past. A much less visible form of complementary countertransference is the deep attachment that staff members can develop toward patients. Both forms of transference, if identified and shared with the treatment team, can help the staff understand patients and help rather than hinder treatment [3–6].

Countertransference acting out in hospital treatment occurs when staff members take a specific action based on feelings, attitudes or fantasies that either should not be expressed at all or expressed only verbally. Stamm, for example, notes that countertransference can express itself in benign neglect in the treatment of a patient with schizophrenia or in overprotectiveness toward patients who are close to discharge. He describes this overprotectiveness as complementary transference. These patients make the staff feel that they are too fragile to make it on their own outside the hospital. Lerner describes a similar staff behavior as an "excessive need to treat," an overzealous, infantilizing attitude toward patients. Lerner believes that when a staff member assumes excessive responsibility for patients and is all-providing, such feelings continually reaffirm the patient's helplessness. Wesselius notes that when staff members give in to patients' spoken or behavioral demands in order to make peace, placate them or have problem-free relationships, this countertransferential response will merely "shape the environment to suit the illness." Pollack and Battle report that the staff member's empathy with the patient can intensify into "symbiotic confusion" and leave staff members isolated and unable to cooperate with colleagues. Countertransference feelings, if not brought into awareness, can result in the patient's premature discharge, the staff's inappropriate expression of anger toward the patient, and even staff romantic involvement with the patient. Lakovics suggests that it is often the staff's behavior that requires control, not the patient's [7–11].

Certain patient behaviors or diagnoses elicit a predictable countertransference in the milieu. Patients with character pathology, who are demanding, manipulative or hostile can evoke anger in the staff. These angry reactions result from the staff's expecting more than patients can give, considering the severity of their ego deficits. Countertransference anger toward these patients will mask their need for nurturance. Withdrawn and psychotic patients evoke staff confusion and helplessness. Staff usually responds with kind interest and protectiveness to patients who are depressed and suicidal. However, Maltsberger who restricts his examination of countertransference evoked by suicidal patient to the therapist (not milieu staff) reports that the suicidal person can elicit countertransference feelings of malice and aversion. The therapist may experience hopelessness and self-hatred and may eventually project this countertransference hatred upon the patients. All of these feelings increase the likelihood of suicide. Gabbard and Coyne name disbelief and collusion as two common countertransference reactions to antisocial patients. Staff members refuse to believe that the patient is capable of antisocial behaviors. They may see the patient as deprived of love and then begin to make exceptions to the rules, thinking this will build a therapeutic alliance. They don't enforce the rules, fearing that firmly enforcing them is punitive [12–14].

The increase of patients with borderline personality disorder has made attention to countertransference mandatory. Bauer and colleagues believe that these patients lack an integrated sense of self and others and thus develop dissociated, contradictory relationships with staff. Staff members hold opposing views of the patient—some in response to the patients' own idealization or devaluation of them. Book and colleagues regard these differing views of the patient as a result of the patient's projecting varying parts of the self, with the internal drama of the patient becoming the staff's battleground. Another common countertransference reaction to borderline patients is a feeling of hopelessness, a concordant response to the patient's abandonment depression [15–17].

Perkins believes the appropriate use of countertransference engagements is the core of the therapeutic process. By not making the response that the patient powerfully evokes, the staff member does not reinforce the patient's behavior. This asocial response jolts and disrupts the patient's maladaptive pattern of interaction and begins a change toward healthier interpersonal behavior. Shapiro recommends that staff members, faced with countertransference, ask: What is happening to me and why?" and then share feelings in an appropriate forum by first examining the patient's history and how it is replayed in present interactions. This enables them to investigate their concordant and complementary identifications and adjust their emotional stance accordingly. Staff members should not automatically believe their emotional reactions to patients are harmful to the treatment alliance. Instead, staff education should teach how specific forms of patient difficulty can cause division within the team. Processing this stress is critical to building a therapeutic milieu. Colson suggests that sometimes the team should make no decisions when it meets but should simply examine each member's interactions and reactions to each patient. With such sharing, Stamm feels that the team becomes the "emotional repository or container of the patient's projections, fantasies and illness." Stamm believes that an environment that provides security, containment and staff consistency has the capacity to absorb the patient's severe emotional illness. When staff members don't respond as expected to patient behaviors, they can begin to change because they sense "a calm steady, seasoned therapeutic presence in all staff members." Boundaries and limits are clear and firm. The investigation of countertransference enables the staff to critically evaluate its reactions to patients. The goal is to stop providing "more of the same" in response to the patient's repertoire in order to create a corrective emotional experience [18–21].

HOLDING ENVIRONMENT

The psychiatric milieu is often referred to as a holding environment. The term was borrowed from Donald Winnicott who described its use in "good-enough" mothering and in psychoanalysis. In psychoanalysis, the analyst takes on a parental function, "holding" the patient, and conveying in words a deep understanding of the patient's anxiety, thus providing a background of safety. The patient's experience of the milieu may be compared to the maternal holding environment, which provides empathy and satisfies emotional needs. A consistent, trustworthy environment can provide a constant object and can allow ego consolidation and maturation to take place. The concept of the holding environment includes both the nurturant and restraining functions of the milieu. Bleiberg describes the nurturant aspect as "attuning" and describes the holding environment as competent, nurturing and supporting, setting limits to destructive behavior, responding to and affirming the real person. The holding environment establishes boundaries for the patient, boundaries between self and others, between impulse and action, and between reality and fantasy. It protects the patient from both outside and inner turmoil and from overwhelming, destructive emotions [22–25].

The patient not only develops security and good feelings toward the holding environment but also directs hateful feelings toward it. To provide a holding environment, staff members must be firm when necessary, empathize and help to contain the patient's overwhelming emotions, as well as absorb the patient's anger without retaliating. Quaytman describes the holding environment as a structure that will hold the patient who is fragmented and unstructured. Quaytman believes that in order to provide a holding environment staff members must care enough to say "no" over and over again. If staff members give in because it is easier, the patient will not really trust their care [26–29]. Then Stamm describes the treatment team as psychologically and symbolically "holding" the patient. The team communicates this holding not only by responding empathically but also doing what will in the long term be the most beneficial for the patient, regardless of the need to gain the patient's love and approval.

The concept of the holding environment has been helpful in the treatment of the person with borderline personality disorder. It requires setting limits, analogous to holding a child with a temper tantrum. It is also a catalyst than can help the person resume normal development. It is not really a technique, but more an ambiance or climate that the staff strives to maintain. The staff creates a holding environment through warmth, kindness, and empathy with proper attention to structure and clearly defined limits and boundaries. The patient may gradually internalize the holding environment [30].

Object Relations

Object relations theory has made a strong contribution to milieu therapy. It provides an explanation for the disturbed relationships that come into play in the psychiatric milieu and helps to conceptualize treatment. The person's internal world is built by an accretion of experiences of self and others. From experiences that begin in infancy the person develops a nucleus of self-representations and internalized interpersonal relationships. These internalized representations of self and others are called object relations. The average person may not be aware of his or her own "object relations." One way to think about the concept is to remember how often one is affected by "internal" parents or their attitudes. A mother may find herself talking to her child in the same voice as her own mother, or a father may find that he is talking to "himself" at certain private moments of the day. These early relationships are described as being "introjected" or incorporated into the personality. The object may be called an "introject," which in turn may be called a "maternal" or "paternal" introject [31].

Object relations become a frame of reference for future experience. In the hospital, the patient's internal world of object relations is revealed by transference and countertransference. Gabbard believes that transference and countertransference are best understood as an "interpersonal externalization" of an internal object relationship. He describes the milieu as a "fertile field for the externalization of the patient's internal object world" [32].

The concept of object relationships is helpful in understanding treatment.

The person who has internalized early relationships is capable of new relationships in the hospital that can later be internalized as part of the self. Gabbard believes that when staff members resist responding like internal object representations, they can offer the patient new objects and models. Successful hospital treatment may rely on the staff's ability to process what is happening with the patient and avoid identification with projected object representations. Kernberg believes that through the work of a "neutral" hospital team, the patient's object relationships can be clarified and confronted, with the goal of modifying the primitive object-relationships activated in the interpersonal field. Although patients may try to re-create an earlier internal world in the hospital, they will also try out more gratifying ways of relating. These new experiences of self and others can form the nucleus for further personality development. Rinsley describes this process as the definitive stage in the hospitalization of adolescents and refers to it as "introject work" [32–34].

PROJECTIVE IDENTIFICATION

Projective identification is a defense mechanism. An understanding of projective identification helps to explain why some forms of countertransference occur. In interaction with others, patients unconsciously attempt to elicit thoughts, feelings and impulses within another person that originally belonged to them. They symbolically place a part of themselves in another person and then act toward that person in a way that brings about a response confirming the projection. Although this usually happens with the patient and the analyst, other treatment figures can be recipients of the patient's projections. For example, the patient (projecting an internal rage) may begin to act as if the nurse were a sadistic person. The nurse, in turn, will begin to feel rageful toward the patient without understanding why. Marcus believes that strong emotions are projected simply because they can't be contained within the person and are more easily containable by staff members if they are completely aware of what is happening [35].

Projective identification resembles an emotional transfusion and the staff member has the experience of these projected emotions being mobilized within. Somehow the patient pressures the staff member to feel and behave as if the staff member now owned the feelings the patient has projected. Levine and Wilson discuss Ogden's view that projective identification occurs in three stages. The first stage is the projection by the patient into the staff member of some "unwanted aspects of the self." The second stage is the pressuring toward the recipient to begin to act on these emotions. The third stage can occur when the recipient "metabolizes" this projected content and renders it less harmful by modulating it and then "makes it available for reintrojection by the projector" [36–37].

Bion's concept of the "container" and the contained is helpful here. The treatment figure becomes a container of the patient's projective identifications. The emotional transfusion should not enter the bloodstream (that is, the staff member's own personality) but remains in the container to be neutralized and even metabolized for the patient. Hamilton describes the analyst as being able to modify these projections and give them meaning so that the patient can "reintroject" them [38–39].

Kernberg clarifies the use of projective identification in hospital treatment by employing Racker's distinction between concordant and complementary identification, which precede concordant and complementary countertransference. Concordant identification occurs when the therapist empathizes with the patient's subjective experience. When complementary identification occurs, it is often a result of projective identification, and the hospital therapist begins to act as a figure in the patient's past. The result is that the patient's family pathology, which is projected in parts among the hospital staff creates an emotional storm. Gabbard describes the intensity of projective identification and finds that staff members are unconsciously "bullied" into taking up the role that has been assigned to them [40–42].

The concept of countertransference is perhaps easier to understand but projective identification helps to explain how some types of countertransference occur—particularly the intense countertransference that originates in an unconscious identification with the projected parts of the patient's internal world.

Boundaries

Boundaries refer to lines of demarcation. Ego boundaries refer to the line of demarcation between what is within the person and what is outside. Severely ill patients may often not be able to distinguish between their inner thoughts and outer reality or they may not realize where they end and another person begins. Brown notes that boundary disturbances are pervasive in the psychiatric milieu and are often evident in a patient's inability to distinguish between the varying roles of staff members. Brown describes some patients who conceive of themselves as perforated or sieve-like. They may feel transparent as if others can see inside them or they may feel that they cannot hold themselves within their own boundaries, that their feelings and impulses are simply "leaking" out of them [43].

Many of the concepts described above have to do with boundaries and boundary disturbances. Transference transcends the boundary between past and present. Countertransference and projective identification are caused by blurred boundaries between the self and others. The establishment of the holding environment enables the staff to set boundaries for the patient. Staff members, too, must also think of appropriate boundaries and constantly be aware of where they end and the patient begins. Although empathy with the patient is extremely desirable for good treatment, Pollack and Battle caution that it can intensify into "symbiotic confusion." Levine and Wilson characterize some forms of staff overinvolvement with a patient as a boundary disturbance, at the same time pointing out that involvement itself is healthy and may be a developmental necessity. One example of overinvolvement occurs when a patient becomes involved almost exclusively with one staff member and is deprived of influences from others [44–45].

Oskarrson and Klein use the concept in another way, stressing that boundaries must be clearly defined on the inpatient unit. Their use of boundaries refer to the roles and tasks of staff members and to the professions to which they belong [46].

CORRECTIVE EMOTIONAL EXPERIENCE

The corrective emotional experience is a term that was first used by Franz Alexander to describe a curative factor in psychoanalytic treatment. The clinical staff provides a corrective emotional experience when it responds in new ways to the patient and resists reacting in ways that parents had previously responded. This then makes the patient's behavior a kind of "one-sided shadow boxing." The patient reexperiences conflicts that were once too difficult to bear, faces them successfully and writes a new ending to the story. The corrective emotional experience often does not require interpretation or insight but is a repetition of life experiences with new results [47].

The staff can't simply decide to provide a corrective emotional experience. It usually develops slowly and may have very little to do with the therapy itself. A corrective emotional experience cannot be designed by simply perceiving what the patient needs. It pertains much more to unacknowledged, unconscious needs that are far more real and pressing [48].

References

1. Newman CJ. The application of psychodynamic principles to day treatment. In: Zimet SG, Farley GK, eds. Day treatment for children with emotional disorders. v. 2. Models across the country. New York: Plenum Press, 1991, 117–138.
2. Perkins MJ, Hornsby LG. Common countertransference issues related to inpatient/residential treatment of children. Psychiatric Hospital 1984;15(2):65–74.
3. Racker H. Transference and countertransference. New York: International Universities Press, 1968.
4. Stamm I. Countertransference in hospital treatment: Basic concepts and paradigms. Bulletin Menninger Clinic 1985;49(5):432–50.
5. Bonier RJ. Staff countertransference in an adolescent milieu treatment setting. Adolescent Psychiatry 1982;9:382–90.
6. Witherspoon V. Using Lakovics' countertransference classifications. Journal of Psychosocial Nursing & Mental Health Services 1985;23(4):30–34.
7. See reference 4.
8. Lerner S. The excessive need to treat: a countertherapeutic force in psychiatric hospital treatment. Bulletin Menninger Clinic 1979;43(5):463–71.
9. Wesselius LF. Countertransference in milieu treatment. Bulletin Menninger Clinic 1968;18(1):47–52.
10. Pollack IW, Battle WC. Studies of the special patient. Archives of General Psychiatry 1963;9(4):344–50.

11. Lakovics M. A classification of countertransference phenomena and its application to inpatient psychiatry. Psychiatric Journal University of Ottawa 1985;10(3):132–138.
12. Colson DB, Allen JG, Coyne L, Jehl N, et al. An anatomy of countertransference: staff reactions to difficult psychiatric hospital patients. Hospital & Community Psychiatry 1986 Sep;37(9):923–28.
13. Maltsberger JT. Countertransference hate in the treatment of suicidal patients. Archives of General Psychiatry 1974;30(5):625–33.
14. Gabbard G, Coyne L. Predictors of response of antisocial patients to hospital treatment. Hospital & Community Psychiatry 1987 Jan; 36(1):1181–5.
15. Bauer SF, Goldstein EG, Haran K, Flye B. The role of the hospital milieu in structural diagnosis. Hospital & Community Psychiatry 1960 Mar;3(3):187–92.
16. Book HE, Sadavoy J, Silver D. Staff countertransference to borderline patients on an inpatient unit. American Journal of Psychotherapy 1978;32(4):521–32.
17. Book HE. Soft clinical research on an inpatient unit: Effects of findings on treatment. Psychotherapy & Psychosomatics 1986;46:209–13.
18. See reference 2.
19. Shapiro ER, Carr AW. Disguised countertransference in institutions. Psychiatry 1987;50(1):72–82.
20. Colson DB. Difficult patients in extended psychiatric hospitalization: a research perspective on the patient, staff, and team. Psychiatry 1990; 53(4):369–382
21. See reference 4.
22. Winnicott DW. Transitional objects and transitional phenomena. International Journal of Psychoanalysis 1953;34:89–97.
23. Wasylenki D A. Psychotherapy of schizophrenia revisited. Hospital & Community Psychiatry 1992 Feb;43(2):123–7.
24. Snyder S. Comprehensive inpatient treatment for the young adult patient. Occupational Therapy in Mental Health 1985;5(3):47–58.
25. Bleiberg E. Stages of residential treatment: Application of a developmental model. Residential Treatment for Children & Youth 1989;6(4):7–38.
26. Brown LJ. A short-term hospital program preparing borderline and schizophrenic patients for intensive psychotherapy. Psychiatry 1981;44(4):327–36.
27. Schulz CG. The struggle toward ambivalence. Psychiatry 1984;47(1):28–36.
28. Quaytman M. Developing a holding environment during the treatment of the borderline patient. Psychiatric Annals 1987;17(5):344–51.
29. Stamm I. The hospital as a holding environment. International Journal of Therapeutic Communities 1985;6(4):319–39.
30. Gabbard GO. A contemporary perspective on psychoanalytically-informed hospital treatment. Hospital & Community Psychiatry 1988 Dec;39(12):1291–5.
31. Bauer SF. Intrapsychic structure, object relations, and interpersonal interaction: Treatment process and change in the psychiatric hospital. Journal American Academy of Psychoanalysis 1990;18(4):566–86.
32. Gabbard GO. Therapeutic relationship in psychiatric hospital treatment. Bulletin Menninger Clinic 1992; 56(1):4–19.
33. Kernberg OF. Psychoanalytic object-relations theory, group processes and administration: Toward an integrative theory of hospital treatment. Annual of Psychoanalysis 1973;1:363–8.

34. Rinsley DB. Intensive psychiatric hospital treatment of adolescents: an object-relations view. Psychiatric Quarterly 1965;39(3):405–29.
35. Marcus E. Relationship of illness and intensive hospital treatment to length of stay. Psychiatric Clinics of North America 1987;10(2):247–55.
36. Levine I, Wilson A. Dynamic interpersonal processes and the inpatient holding environment. Psychiatry 1985;48(4):341–357.
37. Ogden TH. Projective identification in psychiatric hospital treatment. Bulletin Menninger Clinic 1981;45(4):317–33.
38. Bion WR. Second thoughts: Selected Papers on Psycho-Analysis. London: Heinemann, 1967.
39. Hamilton NG. Positive projective identification. International Journal of Psychoanalysis 1986;67(4):489–95.
40. Kernberg O. Projective identification, countertransference and hospital treatment. Psychiatric Clinics of North America 1987;10(2):257–92.
41. See reference 3.
42. See reference 32.
43. See reference 26.
44. See reference 10.
45. See reference 36.
46. Oskarrson H, Klein RF. Leadership and organizational regression. International Journal of Group Psychotherapy 1982;32(2):145–62.
47. Alexander FG, French TM. Psychoanalytic therapy: Principles and application. New York: Ronald Press, 1946.
48. Wells DM. Relationships with patients. In: Wells LA, ed. A handbook of psychiatric nursing. St.Louis: Warren H. Green, 1989, 139–47.

CHAPTER

III

Treatment Models in the Psychiatric Milieu

This chapter examines the predominant models used in psychiatric hospitals and in residential treatment. Most of these models have contributed to therapeutic management of the milieu, but not all of them continue to exist in pure form. The psychoanalytic model remains as the infrastructure of treatment, the distant music that remains when the words to the song are changed. It provides a mode of analysis for group processes, transference and countertransference, and difficult problems in the milieu. The medical model will remain as the standard model, with others being variations of it or revisions to change it. Some treatment models, such as the behavioral therapy model, are an integrated system of techniques, many of which can be lent successfully to other programs without changing the philosophy of treatment. The token economy and time-out from reinforcement are frequently used in inpatient settings that have adopted other models. The therapeutic community model remains strong in European settings and in substance abuse programs. This model established the foundation for group psychotherapy and the community meeting, and permanently extended the patient's role in treatment.

Historically, these models seem to develop in the direction of giving the patients more active roles in their own treatment. The substitution of the word "client" for "patient" reflects this direction. The therapeutic community model and the positive peer culture model center the entire program on the therapeutic influences that patients can exert upon each other. The peer culture model adopted what was already there (and not beneficial) and turned it into a therapeutic advantage. Not only did patients form helping relationships but they were also helped by helping each other. The Wilderness Challenge model carries this further by creating complete dependence on the group as its members carry out difficult and dangerous physical tasks. The rehabilitation model emphasizes the patients' active part in their own change. Although efforts at patient government have not always been successful, self-government has continued to be an effective component of the Teaching Family model. Residents make and change rules and consistently review their behavior.

Many of these models reflect an effort to eliminate dependency. The staff's surrogate parenting role for children and adolescents continues to change, as parents enter the treatment center and take increased responsibility. The systemic model reframes treatment so that residents know that they are responsible for initiating their own change. The contextual model gives back responsibility to the adolescent and family at the moment of admission, framing placement as the opportunity for everyone to try out a new direction. The staff tells the adolescent and parents that coming to the treatment center gives them the opportunity to take control over being together again and practice fitting together in new ways. When rules are introduced, they convey that the staff is not responsible for the adolescent; rules are simply provided as information, as to what will happen if the adolescent stops training.

The patient will need education in order to be autonomous, not only psychoeducation about the illness but also social skills, relaxation training, and learning new ways to cope. Education has always been a component of programs for children and adolescents. The Teaching Family model interprets delinquent behavior as a result of inadequate social learning and a deficit in essential skills. Teaching includes instruction, modeling, feedback and support. Every interaction becomes an opportunity for teaching. Professional educators serve as front-line staff in the Re-ED model.

The contextual model frames treatment as information gathering, experiment and practice. Staff members define their role as one of education, not one of caring or control. Discipline is framed as a way to give information rather than a way to modify behavior, using natural consequences whenever possible. If other consequences are imposed they are designed so that they provide information about responsibility.

Many models not only extend work to the family, but treat the child's "ecosystem." The Re-ED model formulates objectives not for the child, but for the child's ecosystem, and places a staff member specifically in charge of the ecosystem, while others work with the patient. Symptoms in the Re-ED model are seen not as individual pathology but as part of the child's ecosystem. Systemic therapy goes beyond the patient to treat the system. The teaching parent in the Teaching Family model is an advocate for the student in community and forms working relationships with school, juvenile court, social welfare, police, and the mental health center.

In the United States, treatment models have changed in response to the virtual disappearance of long-term treatment and the need for effective short-term treatment. Other models, such as crisis intervention models or the intensive care unit, have developed in response to this change. A more significant change, however, has been the honest recognition that inpatient treatment is only a beginning and not a definitive cure. The response, however, seems upbeat and optimistic, with little taste of defeat. Models that work toward permanent treatment must be ecological models that will analyze the patient's ecological system and community with the hope of changing it or systemic models that include the family. Treatment models have become more realistic and have few pretensions. The contextual model frames treatment as practice. The rehabilitation model focuses on restoring or developing the skills that permit the person to live outside the hospital. Cognitive milieu therapy is described as a coping model, not a mastery model.

Kazdin has suggested that it finally may be helpful to employ the chronic disease model in defining treatment. Treatment would be based on the assumption that the condition will need continued care and management. The traditional model for a chronic disease is to administer an intervention for a specified time period and to hope for change to last as long as possible. Kazdin specifically discusses conduct disorder and its resemblance to a chronic condition in its development and course [1]. (See the Conduct-Disordered, Antisocial and Delinquent Population in Chapter VI).

Short-term treatment does not preclude the development of treatment models. Successful techniques from outpatient psychotherapy efforts have now been retranslated for the milieu. Cognitive-behavioral techniques have revitalized behavioral treatment. Cognitive-dialectal therapy for borderline patients has been reformulated for inpatient therapy. The idea of a cognitive milieu, based on cognitive therapy, holds promise. Object relations theory has helped to revitalize the psychoanalytic model, explaining how patients reestablish their internal world in the hospital. Family therapy and systemic and strategic therapies promise exciting breakthroughs in milieu treatment.

The real breakthrough is that treatment models can no longer rely on "more of the same." The systemic model, for example, avoids a situation where more-of-the same kind of consequences is applied to deal with misbehavior, and therefore avoids power struggles. The patient's problem may no longer be attacked directly, but other conditions can be targeted for change. Since the patient's symptoms are often the least responsive to change, focus on another part of the system may unlock the symptom's grip. Even the Wilderness Challenge model has a relation to systemic therapy, in that it does not focus on a pathological behavior, but rather attempts to challenge some other aspect of the personality that will unlock a habitual way of acting to produce new results. Those who work in the psychoanalytic model help the patient get well by not providing the expected "more-of-the-same" kind of response, and therefore resist countertransference pulls.

Short-term treatment has sharpened the focus of the treatment models. Treatment itself can be reframed. A change in the context of treatment can change its meaning and effectiveness. Treatment models seem to have more clarity, with cognitive milieu therapy as a notable example. Treatment models seem less murky because they are no longer so concerned with motivation or etiology. The technique of externalizing the problem seems an example of this clarity. It removes speculation about the cause of the problem and simply puts it out there to be handled, creating a sort of "let's get down to business" mentality, removing it from emotional complexity. Externalizing takes away the pathologizing of negative labeling that defines the person having the problem as the problem itself. When the problem becomes part of a person's identity, it is much more difficult to remove. New treatment models begin to view the patient's problems more as an everyday matter to be dealt with rather than charged with powerful affect.

This represents a progression of models from a "hot" medium to a "cool" one, and creates a more active stance. Once the problem is externalized, everyone can then begin to take action against it. When the problem is framed as external, family members can see the possibility of doing something to act upon it or control it. One can target the eco-system without waiting to completely analyze the patient.

References

1. Kazdin AE. Hospitalization of antisocial children: clinical course, follow-up status, and prediction of outcome. Advances in Behavioral Research & Therapy 1989;2:1–67.

1. The Behavioral Model

Behaviorally oriented treatment programs focus on overt behavior rather than inner psychological states. Maladaptive behaviors, believed to be the result of previous learning, can be altered by systematic management of positive and negative consequences. The goal of inpatient behavior therapy is to provide new learning to increase adaptive behaviors and decrease maladaptive behaviors. Behavioral techniques concentrate on specific, objective and measurable behaviors to alter the patient's primary problems rather than making major changes in personality. All staff members must then be aware of the specifics of the behavioral program designed for each patient [1].

Operant conditioning, central to behavior therapy, is based on the belief that behavior is a function of its consequences and that it can be changed by the use of reinforcement or punishment. A reinforcer that follows a behavior increases the possibility of its repetition. Presenting the reinforcer is called positive reinforcement. Taking the reinforcers away is called extinction. Reinforcements may be highly individualized. If a behavior is reinforced positively, it is likely to be repeated again. This principle provides a theoretical foundation for the token economy [2].

Social learning theory and social skills training expand the behavioral model, acknowledging that learning and therefore behavior can also occur through vicarious, symbolic, and self-regulatory processes. Thus a person's behavior is not always the direct result of reinforcement, but may be learned through observation. The most prominent behavioral treatment founded on the theory is modeling. Modeling is often used to teach social skills. Social skills training involves 1) providing instructions and a rationale for the behavior being taught; 2) modeling or demonstration of the desired response; 3) rehearsal or repetition of the target behavior; 4) Praise or tangible reinforcement for correct responses, and 5) corrective feedback [2–3].

Cognitive-behavioral techniques are particularly effective for persons with anxiety or depression. Cognitive-behavioral approaches stress that the patients' beliefs about their environment affect emotions and behavior. Staff using a cognitive behavioral approach must be able to identify the patient's maladaptive styles, beliefs, and misperceptions of their environment [2–4].

Treatment centers that do not completely adopt the behavioral model use behavioral techniques. Predominant techniques include "time-out," the token economy, performance feedback and behavioral contracting. Time-out is more properly called "time-out from reinforcement." This means that inappropriate behaviors are followed by the removal of the person to another setting and from attention by others. The person usually goes to a hallway, nearby room, or special time-out room until appropriate behavior is restored. The token economy has become an integral part of many treatment programs. It gives participants immediate, concrete and nonthreatening feedback about their progress in the program. The token economy may also include response cost, monetary or behavioral penalties for inappropriate behaviors [5]. (For more information, see discussion of time-out and the token economy in Chapter VIII.)

Performance feedback is another way to present information that will influence the future occurrence of a specified behavior. Posting the results of a patient's performance in a public area can help to make clinical and educational changes in treatment settings. McMorrow and colleagues describe a program that assessed eight areas of patient performance: personal room care, program attendance, contributions to treatment contracts, contract completion, compliance with rules, mood and a personal/therapeutic evaluation. Performance feedback clarified behavioral expectations of both staff and patients and prevented the decline in expectations that often occurs as treatment continues. It helped patients to participate not only in their own treatment but also in the treatment of others [6].

Paul and Lentz demonstrated the superior effectiveness of the behavioral model for chronic schizophrenia, positively reinforcing prosocial skills while providing a response cost for inappropriate behavior. Although they did not measure the exact relationship, Paul and Lentz found that when the patients' interpersonal and self-care skills improved, their hallucinations and delusions decreased. One might then ask if an improvement of functional behaviors might lead to a decrease in psychotic behaviors. Behavioral techniques can also directly address psychotic behaviors. Token reinforcement can decrease delusional speech and reported hallucinations. However, it may be harmful to teach patients to not express symptoms, since it may prevent them from attending to the warning signs of their illness. "Self-talk" is an effective behavioral technique that improves functioning. Baenninger and Tang describe a program that taught chronic patients to use differential attention to change each other's behaviors. Differential attention is a process of providing immediate attention to desirable behaviors and withdrawing attention following undesirable behaviors [7–11].

Behavioral techniques are powerful tools that must be used carefully and usually require extensive staff training. The model has been integrated into many residential programs as well as specially designed behavioral therapy units and has been helpful for chronic patients and for a wide range of problem behaviors, such as phobias, enuresis or encopresis. The model works best when feelings and thoughts are also considered. It is more effective than psychoanalytic programs for patients with poor verbal and intellectual abilities and particularly effective when targeting specific disorders. The staff who works with this model must not forget that behavior is only a small part of the patient's being and that there is much more to treatment than control. The behavioral approach is most successful when it is a collaborative partnership between the patient and the staff [12–13].

References

1. Lyman RD, Prentice-Dunn S, Wilson DR, Taylor GE. Issues in residential and inpatient treatment. In: Lyman RD, Prentice-Dunn S, Gabel S, eds. Residential and inpatient treatment of children and adolescents. New York: Plenum Press, 1989,1–22.
2. Black JL, Bruce BK. Behavior therapy: a clinical update. Hospital & Community Psychiatry 1989 Nov;40(11):1152–62.
3. Wong SE, Wolsey JE, Innocent AJ, Liberman RP. Behavioral treatment of violent psychiatric patients. Psychiatric Clinics of North America 1988;11(4):569–80.
4. Pang J. Partial hospitalization: an alternative to inpatient care. Psychiatric Clinics of North America 1985;8(3):587–95.
5. Luber RF. Behavioral treatment in partial hospitalization. New Directions for Mental Health Services 1988 Sum;38:59–76.

6. McMorrow MJ, Sheeley ML, Meedke J, Treworgy S, et al. The use of publicly-posted performance feedback in an inpatient psychiatric setting. Behavioral Residential Treatment 1991;6(3):165–81.
7. Paul GJ, Lentz R. Psychosocial treatment of the chronic mental patient. Cambridge, MA: Harvard University Press, 1977.
8. Corrigan PW, Storzbach DM. Behavioral interventions for alleviating psychotic symptoms. Hospital & Community Psychiatry 1993 Apr;44(4):341–7.
9. Wincze JF, Leitenberg H, Agras WS. The effects of token reinforcement and feedback on delusional verbal behavior of chronic paranoid schizophrenics. Journal of Applied Behavioral Analysis 1972;5:247–62.
10. Meichenbaum DH, Cameron R. Training schizophrenics to talk to themselves: a means of developing attentional controls. Behavior Therapy 1973;4:515–34.
11. Baenninger LP, Tang W. Teaching chronic patients to use differential attention to change each other's behaviors. Hospital & Community Psychiatry 1990 Apr;41(4):425–9.
12. Pollard CA, Merkel WT, Obermeier HJ. Inpatient behavior therapy: the St. Louis University Model. Journal of Behavior Therapy & Experimental Psychiatry 1986;17(4):233–43.
13. Maxey JT. Behavioral treatment in partial hospitalization. New Directions for Mental Health Services 1989;38:77–84.

2. The Cognitive Model

Cognitive therapy, first developed by A. S. Beck in the 1960s and 1970s for depressed outpatients, can provide an effective ideological framework for inpatient treatment. The model highlights the primary role of cognition in affecting emotions and behavior. Underlying cognitive beliefs about the self, called cognitive schemas, affect the way the person interprets events and posits cause and effect. Cognitive therapy focuses upon the cognitive process that occurs between the perception of environmental information and the behavioral response to it. Although reality is subjective, the person seems to respond to events in a consistent pattern. These cognitive schemas, formed early in life, may lead to maladjustment or depression, conditions which can be changed if new experiences can challenge them [1].

Davis and Casey describe many examples of cognitive errors such as:

1. Arbitrary inference—making a conclusion without complete evidence.
2. Overgeneralization—drawing a rule or conclusion from a single incident.
3. Selective abstraction—focusing only on one detail and not seeing the total situation.
4. Minimizing or magnifying.
5. Black or white thinking—for example, seeing another person or the self as all good or all bad.

6. Reasoning only from feelings—"I feel ugly today. Therefore I am."
7. Personalization—relating events to the self without any reason to do so [2].

Although it may not be the responsibility of milieu staff members to point out these errors, they may be asked to gather examples of this thinking, to help design experiences that will challenge it, and introduce the person into activities that will stimulate new beliefs. Perris reexamines Gunderson's milieu therapy principles for their relevance in a cognitive milieu and finds some more relevant than others. Containment in the cognitive milieu would focus on reinforcing the patient's internal controls. Support in the cognitive milieu would often involve encouraging patients to engage in activities that could lead to success. Support should be titrated so as not to add to the patient's feeling of inadequacy [2–3].

A comprehensive model of cognitive milieu therapy is still in an early stage of formulation, but cognitive therapy, just as psychoanalytic therapy, can guide milieu practices. Cognitive therapy provides the ideological framework, and its principles can be used consistently in the many staff-patient interactions that take place in a day. The inpatient milieu can become an effective laboratory for the cognitive approach since it resembles many of the social situations and conflicts in a patient's life. The person can test out beliefs with minimal risk and try out alternative methods of coping. Cognitive therapy is essentially a coping model, not a mastery model. In contrast to the psychoanalytic model, it can be effective in short-term inpatient treatment directed toward stabilization [2–4].

Techniques can be educational, cognitive, and behavioral. Daily activities, psychoeducational programs and group therapies are designed to help the patient not only understand but use basic cognitive theories and techniques. The educational techniques help the person adequately process information and set agendas. The cognitive techniques can illuminate and correct illogical thinking. Behavior techniques are often used to increase activity so the patient can begin to feel competent. The final goal of behavioral techniques is an increase in activity to challenge cognitive beliefs about personal inadequacy. Activity scheduling can eliminate indecision as a barrier to action and increase participation. The patient's interactions with the staff can be very effective because of their immediacy. The staff member can identify distorted cognitions almost as soon as they occur and quick and effective interventions can be done while the automatic thoughts and feelings are still fresh in the patient's mind [2–4].

In addition, the patient may be asked to keep a record of dysfunctional thoughts, which can provide data for future interventions. This would include a description of the situation, the emotions around it, the person's automatic response, and what might be a "rational response." For example, when the person wakes up feeling depressed, an automatic thought might be about the inability to do anything. The "rational" response would be to get out of bed and begin to accomplish one small task, then another, and then check out feelings. This can lead to a decrease in depression [5].

Unit community meetings help patients share responsibility for treatment, and the interpersonal issues that emerge can serve as opportunities to apply cognitive therapy principles. Patients experienced with its principles are a helpful source of information and support for newcomers. Schrodt describes a cognitive therapy group for adolescents, with a focus on problems that brought the adolescents to the hospital. The group therapists identify automatic thoughts and use behavioral analysis, cognitive rehearsal, and training in problem solving. The group works to define the problem, generate possible solutions, weigh their advantages and disadvantages, develop a plan and evaluate the outcome. This group format helps to develop skills in problem solving and the response from peers in the group gives different perspectives on the problem and solutions [6–7].

The role of the milieu staff using this model will require careful definition of the cognitive therapy principles that serve as the infrastructure for everything that goes on in the milieu. At a minimum the staff will learn the relationship of dysfunctional beliefs to depressed or maladaptive behavior. Although milieu staff members will not be practicing cognitive psychotherapy, they will be guided by a common philosophy and language that are easily taught and will also make sense. To date, the cognitive milieu has been most effective in the treatment of depression [8].

Cognitive therapy in the milieu employs 3 models: 1) a primary therapist model where the major responsibility for cognitive therapy remains with the primary therapist, with a staff educated in cognitive principles providing the support; 2) an add-on model, whereby cognitive psychotherapy is added to milieu treatment, merely as the psychotherapy component of the model; 3) the staff model, which uses the cognitive milieu as the principal form of therapy. The staff model is the most comprehensive since the cognitive approach guides all therapeutic activities. The entire staff participates fully in cognitive methods and there is a psychoeducational program designed to teach cognitive therapy principles. A comprehensive model would restrict unit admissions to patients who could benefit from cognitive therapy. The clinical staff would be called upon for an accurate reading of each case that can be communicated and understood by all staff members, with cognitive methods designed for each individual patient [9].

References

1. Beck AT, Rush AJ, Shaw BF, Emergy G. Cognitive therapy of depression. New York: Guilford Press, 1979.
2. Davis MH, Casey DA. Utilizing cognitive therapy on the short-term psychiatric inpatient unit. General Hospital Psychiatry 1990 May;2(3):170–6.

3. Perris C. Cognitive psychotherapy and milieutherapeutic processes in psychiatric inpatient units. Journal of Cognitive Psychotherapy 1988;2(1):35–50.
4. Wright JH, Thase ME, Ludgate JW, Beck AT. Cognitive therapy with inpatients. In: Wright JH, Thase ME, Beck AT, Ludgate JW, eds. The Cognitive milieu: Structure and process. New York: Plenum Press, 1993, 61–90.
5. See reference 2.
6. See reference 4.
7. Schrodt GR Jr. Adolescent inpatient treatment. In: Wright JH, Thase ME, Beck AT, Ludgate JW, eds. The Cognitive milieu: Structure and process. New York: Plenum Press, 1993, 273–294.
8. See reference 3.
9. See reference 4.

3. The Medical Model

The medical model is the traditional model of psychiatric hospital practice. It emphasizes psychiatric diagnosis and the placement of the physician at the head of the treatment team, with final clinical responsibility. Challenges to the predominance of this model have resulted in its modification and an incorporation of the tenets of many other disciplines. Consequently, it might be more accurately described as the biopsychosocial model. The remedicalization of psychiatry, based on the discovery of the biochemical and genetic concomitants of psychiatric disorders, helped to reestablish the medical model as appropriate for hospital practice [1].

The medical model usually has a vertical structure with clearly defined lines of authority and unambiguous role definitions. This model is known to bring about predictability and clear rule enforcement [2].

References

1. Engel G. The need for a new medical model: A challenge for biomedicine. Science 1977;196:129–36
2. Alarcon RB, Bancroft AA, Daniels TD. Dynamics of the inpatient psychiatric setting. Psychiatric Annals 1988 Feb;18(2):102–5.

4. The Peer Culture Models

Peer culture models use peers as the primary instrument of influence and change. The model is based on sociological findings that adolescent delinquency is primarily influenced by the peer group, and that peer influences are usually more effective than the treatment efforts of the staff. The values of the peer group can help individual group members to improve. Rose writes of the "gang as therapist," and feels that group identity should be strong enough to support disturbed adolescents through major identity crises. Positive peer culture teaches the basic value of caring for one another. Ideally, participation in such programs usually requires a high level of verbal and intellectual abilities. Such programs have been extremely valuable in residential treatment centers and correctional settings, and are often the treatment of choice in substance abuse programs, since peer pressure strongly influences substance use [1–2].

Since adolescents need to feel important and good about themselves, they will usually respond to helping themselves and each other. The process of caring and helping is based on the belief that one is helped by helping others and that persons consequently grow by participation in this process. The peer culture is made up of cohesive groups which promote prosocial responsible, caring behaviors. These programs empower those in treatment, giving them full participation in the change process. Much of the therapeutic work is done in groups. Residents participate in small groups with an adult leader and are asked to discuss their own personal problems as well as problems involved in living together. Both the staff member and peers identify problems and develop strategies to solve them. The solutions usually bring about changes in attitudes, behavior, values and self-concepts. Problems become an opportunity for teaching rather than behavior to be punished. Members of the groups will approve of positive behavior, disapprove of negative behavior, and help to develop responsibility. The positive peer culture model recognizes the troubled adolescents' potential for decision making and social influence instead of a more conventional view of them as being negative and destructive [3–4].

Principles of Peer Culture Programs

Peer programs are developed in a positive subculture that emphasizes: caring, accountability, peer interventions, and nonpunitiveness.

Caring

The central value of peer culture programs is that people will act in caring ways toward themselves and to others. By their own actions, staff members serve as models for helpful, concerned behavior. They create a climate of concern with high expectations on everyone in the environment [4].

Accountability

Residents hold their peers responsible for their behaviors. Acceptance and approval reinforce positive behaviors. The group challenges negative attitudes. Positive peer cultures need vigilant monitoring to remain positive, and the principle of holding peers accountable is crucial [4].

NONPUNITIVENESS

To hold peers accountable does not mean punishment. The message is to help, not to punish. Residents must never be told that they should do whatever they want to establish discipline. The group teaches the following methods: listening, encouragement, support, feedback, and helpful criticism. In many programs, the staff rather than the group gives or withholds privileges. The group should not be punished for the actions of a member nor decide who should be admitted to the program or remain in it. Their true responsibility is to create a caring environment for members, not to decide who should be excluded from it [4].

LEAST INTRUSIVE MANAGEMENT

Since one of the goals of the program is to develop responsible autonomy, any form of coercion is contraindicated. Residents still respond actively to new peers when they display negative attitudes or behaviors. They do this to help peers learn that their behaviors can't be accepted in the community, or later in society. Despite the principle of least intrusive management, Brendtro and Ness note that the severe emotional crises that may require the most intrusive management are the very ones that can be the most powerful teaching moments in the lives of adolescents and their peers. If peers can assist staff with these situations, they learn to resonate to the needs of others and develop stronger abilities as caregivers. However, the staff has the final responsibility for insuring the therapeutic value of any intervention [4].

NONINTRUSIVE INTERVENTIONS

Nonintrusive interventions include involving peers with staff to decide appropriate rules for the program, supporting peers in crisis by active listening or constructive feedback, calling unacceptable behavior to the peer's attention and encouraging self-monitoring and self-control, discouraging acting-out behavior such as running away or fighting [4].

Techniques of Positive Peer Culture

GROUP COUNSELING SESSIONS

The group sessions build a trusting atmosphere that helps members work to solve each other's problems. Trusting openness should replace confrontation or any attempts to break down defenses. Groups can form a very effective social support system that embraces the total community, affirming the basic value of caring for each other. Both staff and peers point out problems displayed by group members and help to solve them. Residents often find that the best way to solve their own difficulties is to become engaged in helping others with similar problems; the positive peer culture emphasizes giving help to others rather than getting help from the group [4].

The groups usually meet daily. Brendtro and Wasmund outline four typical group stages. The meeting often begins with members reporting on their own problems and others pointing out the problems they might have omitted. The group awards the meeting to the person most in need of help that day. This then leads to problem solving, using methods that arise naturally from the group. The leader can also help the group learn new approaches to helping, such as more effective ways to deal with resistance. During the last ten minutes of the group, the leader evaluates the group's accomplishments, supports the group's successes, and encourages members to continue helping outside the session [5].

Harstad describes peer culture groups that usually begin with each member reporting personal problems that have occurred since the last meeting. Each member has two minutes to describe an incident and the problem. Problems usually include conflicts with authority, lying, stealing, being inconsiderate, misled, easily angered, drug or alcohol problems. Harstad also describes what is called a "fronting problem," when the male adolescent tries to be something that he is not, putting up a front to impress others. After the problems are introduced, group members decide who will own the meeting for the day, based on who needs it most and who will use it best. Asking for help in the meeting is seen as a sign of strength, not weakness. The meeting ends with a summary; the leader gives the group members feedback on how they were able to help each other [5–6].

Relabeling

Negative behaviors are given labels that might reduce their status value for the adolescent, while helping behavior receives attractive labels. Adolescents usually always want to appear "cool," or strong or sophisticated. So instances of hurting behavior are called weak or immature. Care is taken to negatively label the behavior, not the person. The message might be something like: "This is really babyish behavior for someone as 'together' as you are" [5–6].

Reversing Responsibility

One of the most common delinquent defenses is the projection of blame for one's own actions. This technique places responsibility for the action on the person who must do the changing, rather than allowing members to place the blame elsewhere [5–6].

As staff members model helping and caring, relabel behavior and require responsibility, the entire group culture will eventually reflect these values and mold these behaviors. Staff members must be capable of turning the natural peer group into a support group with prosocial values. The acculturation of new members is crucial. When new residents enter a well-functioning positive culture they will notice that group members can share deep feelings without embarrassment, discuss their own problems without fear of punishment, and support all members regardless of their status. Yeager finds that when residents consistently encourage appropriate behaviors, the new residents' idea that "cool" people never think or act positively can certainly change. The residents learn by watching how those around them are acting. The older residents show others that it's okay to admit to problems, show faults and admit to wanting help. Rose describes the young boy's mixed feelings toward the group. It will take him a long time to feel that the group's mature and compassionate views can become a part of him. He may hate the group because of his dependency and vulnerability. When he becomes aware of its power to nourish him, he can begin to lose the fear of his own self-destructiveness and can "love the group gratefully." Rose sees parallels between the group experience and good parenting. Programs based on peer influence have demonstrated that young residents can be effectively involved in almost every challenging situation if the staff trains and supervises them. When a resident is in crisis, staff members most often let group members gather around rather than get away. Successful peer culture programs are usually characterized by a strong sense of staff collaboration. Programs that empower youth should also empower staff [5–10].

Some Potential Areas for Misuse of the Model and Solutions

One of the problems with early peer influence programs was the use of intense and destructive verbal confrontation. Nearly all programs have shifted away from this practice and confrontation with empathy and sensitivity is now the model for group work. The peer groups that began in the 1960s emphasized a highly masculine culture, which became inappropriate as values changed. Confrontations were aggressive, with realistic street language used for emphasis or to express hostility. This emphasis has declined in adolescent peer culture programs. There were also slogans or mechanical verbalizations, some of which are now seen as misleading, simplifying or distorting. There is now a stronger attempt to work for more authentic communication, not automatic slogans. Peer concern replaces peer coercion. Peers learn quickly that the responsibility for helping another person does not establish the right to be punitive. The staff must insure that confrontations about behavior are carried out in ways that will reduce antagonism [11].

A strong peer culture may create a distance between residents and staff and residents and their families. Most programs now maintain family connection with participation as full partners. The ethos of group responsibility may cause staff to avoid leadership and groups can begin to lose direction. Staff members must realize that there are times when adult authority is needed, particularly when group members cannot handle all problems in a responsible and caring manner. Group-oriented work should not preclude individual therapeutic relationships with residents. A strong group orientation threatens individualization and privacy. Individual relationships may not develop when there is a sole focus on the group. Many programs have integrated individual counseling. A "forced togetherness" can also be extreme and residents should be given some privacy as well as the luxury of some unstructured time [11].

Positive Peer Culture Effectiveness

Peer culture programs help change the self-concept of group members. Delinquent adolescents often have a negative self-concept, but Davis and colleagues found that delinquents who had completed Positive Peer Culture (PPC) programs rated themselves as having a more positive self-concept and a higher level of psychological adjustment upon discharge. Changing of attitudes, self-concept and values is fundamental to the PPC philosophy of treatment [12–13].

The ideal group size is from 9 to 11 members. Some populations are especially responsive to this model, particularly persons with conduct disorders and socialized delinquents. It is been used successfully in many correctional settings. Gilliland believes that because of strong Native American cultural values stressing cooperation, that peer intervention groups can help Native American students [13–14].

When adolescents don't respond to peer group influence, it may be because they don't have a feeling of belonging. Those who work with this model believe that programs can be effective if they provide a social climate where members can explore and make a choice between social and antisocial behavior. They need to feel safe in declaring their own beliefs and disbeliefs. They need to be able to test the legitimacy and roles of authority figures. The system must allow peer group decision making which will consider, involve, and recognize others [15–16].

References

1. Lyman RD, Prentice-Dunn S, Wilson DR, Taylor GE. Issues in residential and inpatient treatment. In: Lyman RD, Prentice-Dunn S, Gabel S, eds. Residential and inpatient treatment of children and adolescents. New York: Plenum Press, 1989, 1–22.
2. Rose M. The potential of fantasy and the role of charismatic leadership in the therapeutic community. International Journal of Therapeutic Communities 1982;1(2):79–102.
3. Harstad CD. Guided group interaction: Positive peer culture. Child Care Quarterly 1976 Sum;5(2):109–22.
4. Brendtro LR, Ness AE. Extreme interventions for extreme behavior: peer-asssisted behavior management in group treatment programs. Child & Youth Care Forum 1991 Jun;20(3):171–81.
5. Brendtro LK, Wasmund W. The Peer culture model. In: Lyman RD, Prentice-Dunn S,

Gabel S, eds. Residential and inpatient treatment of children and adolescents. New York: Plenum Press, 1989, 81–96.
6. See reference 3.
7. Eiskovits Z, Guttmann E. Doing competent residential child and youth care work: the normative and experiential dimensions. Children & Youth Services Review 1987;9:271–90.
8. Yeager RJ, DiGiuseppe R, Olsen JT, Lewis L, et al. Rational emotive therapy in the therapeutic community. Journal of Rational Emotive & Cognitive-Behavioral Therapy 1988 Win;6(4):211–35.
9. Rose M. The context for psychological change in a therapeutic community for adolescents. Part II. Residential Treatment for Children & Youth 1987 Fall;5(1):29–46.
10. See reference 4.
11. Brendtro LK, Ness AE. Perspectives on peer group treatment: the use and abuse of guided group interaction/positive peer culture. Children & Youth Services Review 1982;4:307–24.
12. Weber GH. Two studies of positive peer culture: a response. Child & Youth Care Quarterly 1988;17(3):163–4.
13. Davis G, Hoffman R, Quigley JR. Self-concept change and positive peer culture in adjudicated delinquents. Child & Youth Care Quarterly 1988;17(3):137–45.
14. Gilliland H. Discipline and the Indian student. In: Reyner J, ed. Teaching the Indian child: a bilingual multicultural appoach. Eastern Mountain College, 232–41.
15. See reference 5.
16. Wasmund WC. The social climates of peer group and other residential programs. Child & Youth Care Quarterly 1988 Fall;17(3):146–55.

5. The Psychoanalytic/Psychodynamic Model

The psychoanalytic model continues to form the substrate of inpatient psychiatric treatment. Psychoanalytic principles contribute to the understanding of human behavior just as physiology contributes to medicine. While the biomedical model describes a psychiatric disorder through biological mechanisms, the psychoanalytic model describes the mind and personality of the person who has the disorder [1–2].

The fundamental premise of the psychoanalytic model is that behavior has meaning and that the motives and determinants of behavior are often unconscious. Understanding and interpreting the unconscious meaning of symptoms no longer play the predominant role in most inpatient treatment, although psychoanalytically oriented treatment continues in many of the world's most prestigious hospitals. Treatment now usually concentrates on quickly ameliorating the patient's most troublesome symptoms and strengthening coping mechanisms. Psychiatric treatment in hospitals may be now more accurately described as psychoanalytically informed, providing depth and a theoretical basis for most treatment modalities—psychotherapy, psychiatric nursing, and family therapy [3–5].

THE MEANING OF SYMPTOMS AND BEHAVIORS.

Psychoanalytic hospital treatment is organized around at least two basic principles. The first is that symptoms and behaviors have meanings that can be observed and interpreted. The second is that hospitalized patients will repeat their past actions and relationships as well as their characteristic modes of engaging others to meet their needs. The hospital constitutes a social system that allows the patients to essentially live out these interpersonal problems as part of the process of solving them [5–6].

Because behaviors are driven by the unconscious, the psychiatric patient cannot voluntarily control them; nor can reassurance, rules or coercion quickly change them. Instead, in long term treatment, they are initially tolerated and become a major source of significant information. Zee notes that the hospital should tolerate symptomatic behavior within certain limits imposed by time, hygiene, and the law, but should not tolerate others. Hospitalization provides a total picture of the patient's contradictory and conflicting behaviors, information that is not available in outpatient treatment. Behavior is contained so that it can be experienced, observed and understood. Working with patients in a psychoanalytic framework will therefore require a nonjudgmental and nonpunitive attitude [7–8].

THE PATIENT'S ROLE IN THE TREATMENT PROCESS

Patients are not merely acted upon (as their treatment might be described in the traditional medical model) but become active participants in the treatment process. The patient develops self-awareness and self-management by working consistently with a multidisciplinary team and selected peers. If treatment is long term, the patient's behaviors can be observed in a variety of situations, discussed, clarified, and related to earlier life patterns. The process is analogous to the classic psychoanalytic concepts of observation, confrontation, clarification and working through [9].

The patient's psychopathology is not contained within the psyche but rather in relationships with family, small groups, and community. Milieu activities allow the patient's past significant relationships to be as transparent and observable as possible and the patient's relationships provide a rich source of information. The psychoanalytic model brings about change through relationships. Human interactions are planned and integrated; the private relationship with the psychotherapist, group therapy that promotes self-disclosure and provides feedback, peer groups, and community meetings. These group processes and human interactions will help the person to gain a sense of self-acceptance and self-esteem in both social and intimate relationships [10–12].

OBJECT RELATIONS

Object relations theory has revitalized the psychoanalytic/psychodynamic model. This approach views the patient's internal object world as played out in the theater of the hospital milieu. The object relations approach helps to explain the intensity and irrationality of many staff-patient relationships and enables the staff to achieve mastery over countertransference reactions. If staff members come to understand the object relationships played out repeatedly in the milieu, they can control the gratification of the transference, clarify and understand it. Although the patient attempts to reestablish the internal world in the hospital, there is also a yearning for new ways of relating that will lead to interpersonal fulfillment. Gabbard believes that if the staff members resist responding as everyone else has in the patient's internal world, then they can offer the patient new objects and new models [13].

Object relations theory is an extension of earlier work on transference and countertransference, always predominant in psychoanalytic theory. Transference and countertransference were once believed to occur only in the psychoanalytic relationship, but their prevalence in the milieu became increasingly evident, solving many mysteries of staff behaviors. Object relations theory enlarged the dimensions of psychoanalytic treatment and helped to explain the staff's contradictory reactions to the individual patient. The patient re-creates internal object relationships within the hospital. This reenactment is as significant as the individual patient's free association in psychoanalysis. For example, the patient may lack an integrated sense of self and of others, and will vividly demonstrate these contradictions in the relationships made in the milieu. Patients display differing aspects of themselves to staff members and the staff's sharing of observations is a first step in integration. In the hospital the patient is helped to see the distortions that affect relationships with fellow patients, therapist, and staff. Connections can be made between present and past relationships. Object relations theory also helps to illuminate the concept of boundaries. Definition of boundaries, e.g., where the patient ends and others begin, negotiations around boundaries, and the examination of transgressions against them, become part of the psychological work in the hospital [14–15].

Object relations theory seemed to solve many mysteries that had existed in hospital treatment. The theory enabled treatment to focus completely on the "here-and-now," rather than continue the search for all of the reasons behind the patient's behavior. Object relations theory also can explain the final goal of treatment far beyond "the resolution of the transference." As the patient's internal script is played out in the external drama, the staff can study and respond to it in such a way that the patient can internalize stable relationships. Loewald describes this internalization as a transformational process by which the interactions of the person with the environment are changed into inner relationships. While the group processes in the hospital initially transform the intrapsychic into the interpersonal, the interpersonal processes return to the intrapsychic much transformed [16–18].

Transference and countertransference remain significant in the psychoanalytic model of treatment, although object relations provides a more expansive view. Gabbard describes each object relation as a "rewriting of the first attachments of childhood." Transference involves experiencing similar attitudes, impulses, wishes, and conflicts toward the new person as those that occurred with significant persons in the past. Transference and countertransference can be understood as the interpersonal externalization of an internal object relationship. The patient may project a troubled inner world upon the staff [19–21].

Ego psychology also contributed to the psychoanalytic model. The treatment goal in psychoanalytic hospital treatment is often described as strengthening ego functions so that the person can relate effectively and autonomously with the environment. The ego executes the adaptation to the environment, and includes such functions as judgment, perception, attention, recall, imagination, synthesis, impulse delay, reality testing, modulation of emotion, tension control, and anticipation. In the beginning of treatment, staff members must provide auxiliary ego functions for the patients, such as impulse control, reality testing, anticipation of consequences, and the delineation of boundaries between themselves and others [20–22].

Even in the psychoanalytically oriented hospital, the psychoanalytic model is but one of three forces. It combines with the protective and restraining environment contained in the hospital structure and the influence of traditional medicine. The hospital structure protects the patients against excessive stimulation, impulsivity and destructiveness. Although symptoms are tolerated, limit setting and structure help the patient bear anxiety, put actions into words and develop a sense of reflectiveness. Psychoanalytic hospitals must struggle with the need to combine hospital structure with the freedom of expression necessary for an analytic and therapeutic process. While a predominant value of psychoanalysis is that the person must be treated as an individual, the organization of the hospital must often disregard the individual needs of the patients in order to function rationally. There must be clearly stated and consistent treatment principles that will guide the staff's subjectivity. In their absence, the integration of treatment and organizational needs will seriously miscarry. Even when the psychoanalytic/psychodynamic model is not predominant it can provides a strong conceptual basis for much of the treatment that goes on [22–24].

References

1. Ross JL. Principles of psychoanalytic hospital treatment. Bulletin Menninger Clinic 1985;49(5):409–26.
2. Melchoide GA. On teaching today's residents psychoanalytic concepts. Journal American Academy of Psychoanalysis 1991 Win;19(4):548–59.

3. Stamm I. A psychoanalytic model. In: Lyman RD, Prentice-Dunn S, Gabel S, eds. Residential and inpatient treatment of children and adolescents. New York: Plenum Press, 1989, 25–41.
4. Brown LJ. A short-term hospital program preparing borderline and schizophrenic patients for intensive psychotherapy. Psychiatry 1981;44(4):327–36.
5. Gabbard GO. A contemporary perspective on psychoanalytically-informed hospital treatment. Hospital & Community Psychiatry 1988 Dec;39(12):1291–6.
6. Gralnick A. A psychoanalytic hospital becomes a therapeutic community. Hospital & Community Psychiatry 1969 May;20(5):144–6.
7. See reference 1.
8. Zee H. Purpose and structure of a psychoanalytic hospital. Journal National Association of Private Psychiatric Hospitals 1977;8:20–26.
9. Zee HJ. Reflections on the psychoanalytic hospital in the 1980s. Bulletin Menninger Clinic 1985;49(5):417–31.
10. Marmor J. The current status of psychoanalysis in American psychiatry. American Journal of Psychiatry 1968;125:131–2.
11. Rosnick L. Use of a long-term inpatient unit as a site for learning psychotherapy. Psychiatric Clinics of North America 1987;10(2):309–23.
12. See reference 8.
13. See reference 5.
14. Jannsen PL. On integrative analytic-psychotherapeutic hospital treatment. International Journal of Therapeutic Communities 1986;7(3):225–42.
15. Bauer SF. Intrapsychic structure, object relations and interpersonal interaction: treatment process and change in the psychiatric hospital. Journal American Academy of Psychoanalysis 1990;18(4):566–86.
16. Newman CJ. The application of psychodynamic principles to day treatment. In: Zimet SG, Farley GK, eds. Day treatment for children with emotional disorders. Vol. 2. Models across the country. New York: Plenum, 1991, 117–38.
17. See reference 5.
18. Loewald HW. On internalization. International Journal of Psychoanalysis 1973;54(1):9–17.
19. See reference 3.
20. See reference 5.
21. See reference 16.
22. Nammun A. The integrative role of psychoanalysis in the psychiatric hospital. Bulletin Menninger Clinic 1985;49(5):403–8.
23. See reference 1.
24. Novotny PC. The pseudopsychoanalytic hospital. Bulletin Menninger Clinic 1973 May;37(3):193–210.

6. The Re-ED Model

The Re-ED model is a psychoeducational approach that conceives of inpatient treatment as a re-educational process for children and adolescents. It is distinguished by its focus of treatment and by those who provide it. Treatment focuses upon the components of the child's ecology rather than exclusively upon the child and is provided primarily by professional educators as front-line staff: teacher-counselors [1–2].

The Re-ED model and the central role of the teacher-counselor had their origins in the work of Nicholas Hobbs, who was influenced by the role of the educateur in post-World War II Europe. The treatment site is a school, not a hospital, and learning takes the place of therapy. Hobbs attempted to develop a vocabulary that would set no one apart from the normal course of life. The Re-ED program usually provides treatment in centers that are noninstitutional, open, and homelike [3–6].

The Staff

The model usually requires three teacher-counselors who work with a group of eight to ten children. The teacher-counselor who works during the day is concerned primarily with formal teaching in the therapeutic classroom. The night teacher-counselor begins work at the end of the classroom day and engages the children in recreational and leisure activities, field trips, projects, sports, arts and crafts, and fun. The third teacher-counselor, the liaison teacher, who is there to essentially treat the child's environment (3–6).

The Ecological Model

The ecological model defines the child's symptoms, not as individual pathology but as part of a malfunctioning ecosystem. The Re-ED model moves away from the traditional definition of emotional illness as intrapsychic and focuses upon the child's interactions with significant others. Hobbs used the term the "troubled and troubling" child rather than the emotionally disturbed child in order to focus on this interaction. Lewis points out that when others call a child emotionally disturbed, they usually mean disturbing to them. The child so described usually has a long history of behaviors that deviate from the expectations of the adults responsible for socialization. Defining the problem as ecological and directing therapeutic attention to the social consequences of the child's behavior still does not deny biological or psychological determinants [3–7].

The ecosystem comprises a unique combination of persons who frequently interact with the child, an interlocking social system of family, school, neighborhood, and community. These persons have expectations and provide consequences. When the child departs from these expectations and behaves in a way that the system cannot tolerate, this creates discordance in the ecosystem. There is too much or too little of an expected behavior—aggression, temper tantrums, social withdrawal [7].

Each source of discord becomes a target for intervention to increase the ecosystem's effectiveness. The first intervention in the Re-ED model is to develop the child's competence in the valued areas of behavior. Next, the expectations of the child's ecosystem are examined and opportunities are created for the child to meet them and to build confidence. Those assessing the ecosystem may not be able to learn what caused the deviant behavior, but they work both to increase the child's competence as well as the ecological system's effectiveness. This work takes place in the setting where the troubling behaviors occurred in order to achieve a better fit between the child's behavior and the setting. The teacher-counselor and the treatment team work with the child's behavior and the liaison teacher works with the setting [7].

Although many treatment models consider the child's posttreatment environment, the Re-ED model employs a staff member to focus exclusively on working with it. The child must not only develop competence to meet the ecosystem's demands but also learn how to gain its support. The goal is not necessarily to make the child perfect, but to make the ecosystem work. Strengthening the ecosystem's support while also increasing the child's ability to meet its demands will establish the foundation for a successful adjustment after treatment. The ecological assessment and plan are usually worked out in a conference that will usually include the child, the parents, adult friends of the family, teachers, the school psychologist, and caseworker. Before the first conference, the liaison teacher-counselor will have reviewed the child's records, interviewed major participants, and visited the child's home and school. Some examples of possible ecological interventions would include having the school plan special tutoring after discharge, suggesting that a father re-arrange work in order to spend more time with the child, or teaching parents successful behavior interventions to be used at home. While the young child may need help to become integrated successfully into the ecosystem, the older adolescent may learn how to influence the ecosystem in order to achieve some mastery over the external environment [7].

RE-ED PRINCIPLES

Re-ED programs are based on several principles, the primary one being the belief that the disturbance is not contained exclusively within the child but within the ecosystem. It follows from this that children and adolescents can change their behavior without necessarily developing insight. The goal is to establish the child's competence as well as to improve cognitive abilities. Each child and adolescent can develop coping skills and self-control and learn to be good in something. The program does not neglect the child's emotional life. There is a philosophy that feelings should be nurtured and shared and that trust should be built between the child and adult. Treatment objectives are simple and direct, focusing on the teaching and learning of skills within a relatively short period of time, from 6 to 8 months. The staff also formulates objectives for the child's ecosystem.

Each student has daily and weekly objectives, written in behavioral language and in measurable terms [7].

Structured daily activities develop problem-solving skills and remediate social and academic deficits. The Re-ED model actively uses group processes. Group therapy sessions often focus on the children's behavior and performance for the day. Behavioral interventions help to shape behavior and restore social competence. Lewis writes that the use of these interventions does not mean complete adherence to a behavioral program, but rather that the Re-ED model can successfully incorporate such useful techniques as a point or level system or contracts can be without a change in philosophy. The children will set goals at the beginning of the week and discuss their own behaviors at their behavioral group meetings. Children who meet their goals get special rewards or treats. Both problem solving and planning meetings are part of the structure [7–9].

Consultation

Re-ED programs are not set apart from the traditional mental health professions, but are continuously nourished by consultants who bring new and significant findings from medicine, the behavioral and social sciences, and the humanities. Consultants help to design the program, support the teacher-counselors, help to guide the management of problem behaviors, train staff, and provide research and evaluation.

References

1. Gamboa AM, Garrett JE. Re-Education: a mental health service in an educational setting. American Journal of Orthopsychiatry 1974;44(3):450–3.
2. Lochman JE, Bennett Cl, Simmers DA. Residential Re-ED treatment of highly aggressive youth: preliminary indications of effectiveness and the precursors of improvement. Education & Treatment of Children 1988 Feb;11(1):52–62.
3. Hobbs N. The troubled and troubling child. San Franciso: Jossey-Bass, 1982.
4. Hobbs N. Helping disturbed children: psychological and ecological strategies. American Psychologist 1966;21:1105–15.
5. Guindon J. The re-education process. International Journal of Mental Health 1973;2(1):15–26.
6. Kirby TF, Wilson CT, Short MJ. A follow-up study of disturbed children treated in a Re-ED program. Hospital & Community Psychiatry 1977 Sep;28(9):694–7.
7. Lewis WW. Ecological factors in successful residential treatment. Behavioral Disorders 1982;7:149–56.
8. See reference 2.
9. Noshpitz J. History of milieu in residential treatment. In: Szajnberg NM, ed. Educating the Emotions: Bruno Bettelheim and psychoanalytic development. New York: Plenum Press, 1992, 92–102.

7. The Rehabilitation Model

The primary goal of rehabilitation is to alleviate the condition that made inpatient treatment necessary. The rehabilitation model is pragmatic and not concerned with etiology. Treatment based on this model is more supportive than analytical and focuses on restoring or developing the skills that will allow the person to live outside the hospital. The model is adaptable to structured programs with protected living as well as psychoeducational programs or advocacy programs that help clients use community support. A comprehensive rehabilitation program will help the person discover a support system, find housing, and prepare for a job. Although the rehabilitation model is predominantly used for those psychiatric illnesses that have no definitive cure, it has also been adopted as a model for short-term treatment and day treatment for children and adolescents [1–2].

Patient Responsibility

The rehabilitation model encourages the patient's responsibility for self and for others. Patients who take an active role in their own attempts to change can discover their own abilities and raise their self-esteem. Every effort is made to restore autonomous functioning as well as concern for others. Rehabilitation should develop the ability to influence one's environment and manage relationships. Appelbaum and Munich believe that this can be accomplished by psychotherapy combined with experiences that provide successful exercises of power. In the program that they describe, patients had a great deal of power to make decisions and have real control over their daily lives. Interdisciplinary team meetings included patients and met three times a week. The group developed management plans with treatment strategies for each patient and considered such questions as how much freedom, support, and protection each patient needed. The patients made real decisions that affected each other's lives. They lived with these decisions and reevaluated them at each unit group meeting [1–2].

Several years later Munich and Lange wrote about this program, focusing on the work of the administrative unit group, where individual, interpersonal and group problem-solving took precedence over interpretation. The group came to represent a family group in the treatment setting, promoting socialization and the development of bonds with others. Such feelings of belonging promoted the internalization of "adaptive" values. The group supported each person's rehabilitation and respected each private struggle. Working in the group helped patients learn and develop responsibility toward others as well as develop awareness of dysfunctional social processes [3].

Skill Development

In the program that Munich and Lange describe, the schedule of the hospital day resembles a work day. The patients not only learn adaptive skills but know how to apply them in a variety of settings. They could apply what they learned in individual therapy to group therapy and then to family meetings. Adaptive skills cannot be learned unless the inpatient activities approximate real-life problems and situations [3].

The Role of the Staff

In one sense, the rehabilitation model provides higher respect for the contribution of all staff who provide treatment and reflects the increasing professionalization of activity therapies, occupational therapy, and social work. In the program that Munich and Lange describe, the staff relinquishes the parental role, since decision making is given to the patient. In addition, the importance of the staff's feelings toward patients in their work is minimized. Munich and Lange describe this as upsetting a long tradition which focused upon the staff's own emotions as a significant factor in psychiatric hospital treatment [3–4].

The Rehabilitation Model for Schizophrenia

The rehabilitation model is now the treatment of choice for persons with schizophrenic disorders. Its selection comes by default, after other models have failed, and with stronger confirmations of the biological basis of schizophrenia. Psychiatric rehabilitation helps the person with schizophrenia to acquire the social, emotional, and intellectual skills needed to live and work. Rehabilitation will also require social skills training, family education, and enlisting environmental resources and support. Intervention proceeds respectfully at the patient's own level of functioning. Token economy methods may increase social learning to reduce inappropriate behavior. Smith and colleagues describe the rehabilitation model in inpatient work with a woman with paranoid schizophrenia. They contrast it with the medical model and somatic treatment which has little effect on the patient's interpersonal and functional deficits. The rehabilitation model complements the medical model by helping the patient identify personal strengths and self-determined overall rehabilitation goals. This contrasts with the medical model's focus on deficits. They feel that the patient must cling to real functioning strengths to grow away from the world of illness. While most rehabilitation efforts take place in outpatient treatment, the emphasis in inpatient treatment should be to control psychiatric symptoms and establish a treatment alliance so that rehabilitative efforts can continue [5].

The Rehabilitation Model for Children and Adolescents

Blom finds the rehabilitation model particularly appropriate for children and adolescents in day treatment. The model focuses upon skills training and acquisition and building support networks for learning, working and living. Blom believes that this pragmatic, atheoretical approach is appropriate since psychiatric diagnosis does not really specify effective interventions and since skill acquisition rather than symptom reduction has been related to positive outcomes. Skills training involves explaining, demonstrating and practicing specific physical, emotional and intellectual skills. Skills in the physical area would include hygiene, cooking, using leisure time, physical fitness and work [6].

In the emotional domain, residents learn how to achieve satisfaction, socialize, develop self-control and find jobs. They will master such intellectual skills as mathematics. Techniques will include modeling, rehearsal, feedback, reinforcement, homework and practice for skill generalization. The staff must consider the child's social network and help to modify it, since the children will be strongly influenced by their many environmental contexts, including home, school, and community. Children and adolescents particularly will need support networks of caring, guiding, and protective environments. The model that Blom describes derives from the belief that the seriously disturbed child's impairments can be remedied and that interdisciplinary and coordinated services will be the most effective [6].

VOCATIONAL READINESS AND TRAINING

The rehabilitation model has inspired educators to develop innovative programs for chronic patients. Allen and colleagues describe an intensive 8-week vocational readiness program in day treatment which integrated education, support, and case management. Following their placement in jobs or volunteer work, clients were guaranteed an indefinite follow-up and increased rather than decreased support. Brieff describes the use of personal computers for skills training in psychiatric rehabilitation. Patients enrolled in one of two programs: a general education component to improve basic math, spelling, grammar, and vocabulary and a course in advanced computer applications. Brieff believes that computer-assisted instruction can help patients overcome cognitive, attentional, and motivational problems that have interfered with learning. There was a strong link between the mastery of these skills and the person's own self-esteem [7–8].

DISCUSSION

The rehabilitation model is based on the belief that persons are motivated for mastery and competence and that new behaviors can be learned. While the medical model focuses upon the patient's deficits, the rehabilitation model emphasizes the patients strengths, functional capacities and motivation. This model concentrates on the person's healthy functioning and provides a comprehensive approach to vocational, residential, social, educational and recreational services. The model can be used in a variety of settings with a variety of illnesses, including substance abuse and schizophrenia. It stresses self-determination and encourages and affirms the person's ability to make life decisions. Cnaan and colleagues write that even wrong decisions may have rehabilitative value. Self-determination can also include participation in decision-making in the treatment center in planning, policy and evaluation. This is reflected in many rehabilitative settings, where the persons served may be called members or associates, rather than patients. Appelbaum and Munich believe that this model represents a shift from the view of the hospital as a holding environment to one of a community that builds autonomy [9–10].

References

1. Tucker GJ, Maxmen JS. The practice of hospital psychiatry: a formulation. American Journal of Psychiatry 1973 Aug;130(8):887–91.
2. Appelbaum AH, Munich RL. Reinventing moral treatment: the effects upon patients and staff members of a program of psychosocial rehabilitation. Psychiatric Hospital 1986 Win;17(1):11–19.
3. Munich RL, Lange E. The boundaries of psychiatric rehabilitation. Hospital & Community Psychiatry 1993 Jul;44(7):661–5.
4. Stanton AM, Schwartz M. The Mental hospital: study of institutional participation in psychiatric illness and treatment. New York: Basic Books, 1954.
5. Smith TE, Woo-Ming AM, Lang E, DeFelice L, et al. Treatment planning: Rehabilitation psychiatry in the inpatient treatment of a woman with paranoid schizophrenia. Hospital & Community Psychiatry 1994 Dec;45(12):1179–81.
6. Blom G. Developmental rehabilitation perspectives in the day treatment of children with serious emotional disorders. In: Farley GK, Zimet SG, eds. Day treatment for children with emotional disorders. V. 2. Models across the county. New York: Plenum Press, 1991, 65–84.
7. Allen BA, Hodgson WR, Marlow VI, Lindsey JK. A practical model for a vocational readiness program in a day treatment setting. Hospital & Community Psychiatry 1994 Apr;45(4):374–8.
8. Brieff R. Personal computers in psychiatric rehabilitation: A new approach to skills training. Hospital & Community Psychiatry 1994(Mar);45(3):257–60.
9. Cnaan R, Blankertz L, Messinger K, Gardner J. Psychosocial rehabilitation: toward a definition. Psychosocial Rehabilitation Journal 1988;11(4):61–77.
10. See reference 2.

8. Systems Models: Contextual and Cybernetic Model

Systemic therapy results from thinking that is interactional and multicausal, rather than being based on linear causality. The linear paradigm assumes that there is an objective reality, that a person's behavior develops internally and that symptoms may finally be changed by tracing the person's life history, and by gaining insight about the link between cause and effect [1].

A system-circular view regards effect and cause as interacting with each other, as a cybernetic feedback loop: X influences Y and Y then influences X in a circular manner with no point or event highlighted as the cause or effect. Because of this circular influence, persons can become stuck in patterns which they cannot change, since these patterns of interaction are embedded in a complex interlocking system. Since the system operates as a whole, everything in the system influences everything else. So a change in one part of a system can cause other parts to change. Since the person's symptoms may be the least amenable change, systemic treatment focuses on another part of the system that will be more responsive. Systemic thinking considers ways to loosen the symptom's grip [1].

The cybernetic principle in operation in the milieu might involve finding a positive, useful or affirmative aspect of the resident's behavior, highlighting it, and preserving it so that it can become a larger part of the pattern. Any information about a positive difference in the resident's pattern may then alter family, peer, or staff response and then reshape the meaning of behavior. Both verbal and nonverbal behavior function as information in the cybernetic system. The meaning of this information is then defined by the feedback that is returned. All behaviors therefore provide communication, and all feedback affects the meaning of what is communicated [1].

The systemic perspective sees the resident's problem as interactive, so that treatment must focus upon all significant relationships. The treatment of choice then would be family therapy. But in instances when the patient must be removed from the family, systemic solutions must be forged in residential treatment. Pare and colleagues address the redefinitions that must be made to provide a systemic model of residential treatment. These include redefining who will be treated and how the staff will relate [2].

THE IDENTIFIED PATIENT

The identified patient is the person the family identifies as the one with problems requiring treatment. Admission to residential treatment only reinforces this definition. To retain systemic treatment, family members must be made aware that they are valued and that they, too, are responsible for what happens in treatment. They are involved in the treatment plan, and consulted on all issues such as bedtimes, therapeutic leaves of absence, school, and consequences for breaking rules. This kind of consultation keeps the parents constantly engaged in treatment, gives respect to their parenting skills, and empowers them as parents [2].

THE SURROGATE PARENT

The bond between staff and children has usually been a curative factor in residential treatment. The systemic model, with its focus on necessary changes within the family system, would be defeating treatment by merely substituting staff for family relationships. This would block interaction between the family and the resident. The adolescent should not be "triangulated" in such a relationship which often seems to call for a choice between staff and family. Nor should the family be disempowered [2].

Parents often feel so guilty that they abdicate responsibility, and may want to take a vacation from their feelings and investment in the child. In other treatment models, this may have been quite acceptable to staff who wanted to intervene directly in the children's lives without parental interference. Lines of authority must be clearly established so that the child can't play adults off against one another. The most important step is to establish the parental hierarchy as the primary system and to keep all hierarchies secondary to family. Parents must be engaged so they can experience being in charge [2].

In addition to redefining their roles, staff members must be aware of the resident's own reluctance to be treated. The staff is usually asked to provide treatment to the "identified patient" who was admitted more because the family insisted than because of a personal desire to change. The systemic model consistently reframes the treatment context so that the residents know that they are responsible for initiating their own behavior change. Yet change itself may make the child feel disloyal to the family. If residents change, they may be confirming that staff members are better than their own parents. In addition, positive changes can be seen as "losing," backing down under adult pressure. One way to solve this is to have the treatment goals established together by residents and their families. Reluctance to change can be dealt with by using strategic interventions. Essentially this means that the staff members avoid taking on a directive role but use strategic/systemic principles [2].

Pare provides an example of a strategic or reframing intervention with a female resident whose mother believed she was depressed and suicidal. The treatment staff felt that she was overdramatizing her depressed behavior and was too eager to explain to others how sick she was. The staff's goal was to reframe her behavior as an expression of sadness, not depression. She could display this, but the staff did not overload her with empathy when she behaved this way. They avoided a "more of the same" type of response and placed the responsibility on her own shoulders. The hypothesis was that the purpose of the symptom was to communicate a need for nurturance. When the staff accepted the crying and avoided the savior role, this confused the patient and led to new behaviors [2].

The systemic model also requires a change in the staff's discipline, since staff members have traditionally been in charge of managing the residents' behavior. Residential management usually relied upon the staff's "turning up" their power when necessary to gain cooperation, or power struggles or the reenacting of earlier struggles that existed in families. Staff in residential treatment centers are always faced with the basic question of how to provide adequate control without compromising a therapeutic role. The staff must avoid a situation where "more of the same" kind of consequences are applied in an attempt to deal with continued misbehavior. In other words staff must avoid the power struggle which develops when progressively severe consequences are applied. If the resident tries to break a rule, staff should decide upon a novel intervention, based on strategic/systemic principles rather than progressively escalating consequences. By reframing rather than mechanically applying an apparently ineffective sanction staff can avoid situations where the attempted solution becomes the problem [2].

Since the primary goal is to build a more functional relationship within the family, parent-like relationships on the part of the staff will not lead to improved family interactions. Staff members who work within a systemic model therefore retain a "therapeutic maneuverability" which will allow them to assume a position of neutrality when necessary. Although staff members must consistently demonstrate their concern and desire to help, they may need at times to "back off" from intimate intense involvement [3].

Forbes and Maddron describe systems therapy in a day treatment setting for children, defining information management as the essential team task. The team views the child's interactions as providing relational meanings and parallels with family relationships. The team then generates hypotheses about the presenting problem, attempts a family intervention, observes the differences, and reformulates the hypothesis. Interventions are aimed at helping the family begin to begin to rely on its own resources [4].

The systemic model demonstrates how helpful it may be to redefine the focus of inpatient treatment as well as the role of staff members. There is a wealth of literature for systemic and strategic therapy that may eventually be applied to inpatient treatment, much as psychoanalytic principles once enriched the practice of milieu therapy.

Contextual and Cybernetic Models

The contextual and cybernetic models are based on the belief that nothing has any meaning unless it is seen in context. A change in the context of treatment can change not only meanings but also the treatment itself. At the base of this model is the cybernetic/constructivist assumption that reality is contingent on beliefs and validated by consensus. What we perceive is ideological, and perception essentially depends on previous beliefs. Problems develop in the identified patient or family as a result of the activation of cycles of family interaction which occur when a problem situation is mishandled. The family then becomes stuck in its interaction with the problem and one another [5–7].

The cybernetic or contextual model is designed to counteract some of the problematic results of conventional inpatient treatment: the family's feelings of failure, the transfer of responsibility from the hospital to the treatment center, and the family's feelings of helplessness after discharge. The context is the overall framework that provides meaning to placement and against which all experiences and events will be interpreted. The context will determine how the child and family will make sense of themselves and their life situation and the way staff members will make sense of their roles, providing a template against which success or failure will be judged. Admission to inpatient treatment usually indicates to all concerned that the person admitted is at fault, needs fixing, and will only come back when better. When the adolescent improves in treatment, it usually reinforces the family's own feelings of incompetence. The adolescent often returns home to live with a helpless family whose feelings of inadequacy have been validated. Staff members, too, in search for an explanation for the adolescent's difficulties, will consider parental inadequacy as one of the causes. This search for explanation or cause will actually determine how the staff makes sense of the parents' and child's behavior. The staff also sees itself as responsible for the adolescents in treatment and helping to solve their problems. Durrant believes that residential treatment can't be about "fixing" children or adolescents but instead is about helping them to build a conception of themselves as potentially successful and competent and able to build upon their strengths and resources [8–9].

Context

Nothing really has meaning unless it is seen in some context. Context determines the meaning of behavior and relationships. Context refers to the connections that we make between behaviors, how we "punctuate" our experience. We make sense of behavior by reference to our ideas, beliefs, presuppositions. Further, these beliefs are likely to become perpetuated and confirmed since we will make sense of things in the ways that fit [10].

We will then be restrained from noticing things that might provide different information. The family that comes to the mental health system is already stuck in its own version of reality and usually so tied to its own beliefs and behaviors that all members are prevented from discovering any way to replace them. The family's way of making sense of things means that alternative behaviors or chances for solutions aren't possible for them. Contextual therapy can generate a change in the family's description of the problem [11].

Difficulties in residential programs are not necessarily due to program inadequacies, staff competence, or the family's ability to be treated. Difficulties often make sense when the broader context or meaning/frame of the family is considered. No matter how caring the staff the meaning of placement for the family may work against a positive outcome. If the adolescent is admitted in the context of defeat, despair, and failure, everything that happens will be interpreted in those terms. Or if the adolescent is admitted in the context of needing "fixing" that will provide a map which will determine the way the adolescent and family respond [11].

CHANGING THE CONTEXT

Contextual residential care places admission in a different context, providing a frame of meaning that can promote change and responsibility. The aim of contextual therapy is to construct placement in such a way that it can be seen as the first step in a new process or direction rather than as the final step in the old direction of failure. The adolescent's admission is redefined and placed within a context of success and responsibility. It can be framed as a rite of passage which heralds the family's organizing together around the problem. Treatment concepts can be integrated with this definition [11].

Placement begins with a model that tries to give back responsibility. The problem is acknowledged with the recognition that previous solutions did not work and that placement will allow everyone to try a new direction. The adolescent, family, and staff will experiment with this direction intensively and the adolescent can then return home for more practice. Both adolescent and parents are told that coming to the treatment center will give them a new chance to take control over their living together again and to practice fitting together in a new way. In order to place decision making and responsibility in the family's hands, its members are told that they should take some time together to consider whether to take this step. The framing of the meaning of treatment begins immediately. Menses and Durrant indicate that when the adolescent is introduced to other residents, they might be told that the new resident has come to get control over some old habits that have been "pushing him and his family around" [11].

EXTERNALIZATION OF THE PROBLEM

Externalizing the problem takes the blame away from the adolescent and the family and allows for more constructive alternatives. When the problem is seen as external, it is no longer defined as a permanent personality trait. The person is then free to change. Externalizing the problem also allows it to be removed from the symptomatic person. Even the physical layout or equipment in the treatment center may be given a definition which calls attention to the external problem to be solved. An exercise bike, for example, might be called a "monster-fighting" machine. Attempts to resist the temptation to steal might be described as "itch-fighting." An adolescent might be described as "fighting the temper monster when it strikes." Selekman reports helping a family create a new objectified and metaphoric description of substance abuse problems by asking externalizing questions. Cocaine addiction becomes "Coke," and the family is asked such questions as: "Did Coke push Laura around and make her lose her job?" Children will be responsive to a description of the problem as a tyrant or monster with personality characteristics they need to fight. In addition, the family is asked to consider their times of triumph over the external enemies, to speak of times when Coke was "not pushing them around." This helps the family break out of its feelings of failure and examine previous successes. Those who work with substance abuse problems are usually aware of the guilt/blame cycles in families, and externalization helps to break it [12–14].

Externalizing the problem means making a linguistic separation between the problem and the person. This then gives "space" for the resident and family to take steps to escape the problem's effect on their lives. When the problem is clearly distinguished and given a name separate from the child, then blaming either the child or family won't happen. Everyone is now under the influence of the same "troublemaker" and not struggling against each other. Externalization can be a healing process because it takes away negative labeling which defines the person having the problem as the problem itself. When the problem becomes part of the personal identity, it is much more difficult to escape. Once the problem is externalized, everyone can then begin to take action against it. Durrant writes that by framing the problem as an external entity, family members can then see the possibility of doing something to act upon it or to control it [15].

Change in Staff Responsibility

Staff members are told that their role is one of education, not one of primarily caring or control. Their main role is to respond to everything that the residents do, no matter how small, in ways that give new information and allow distinctions to be drawn. They are to respond to any indication of change and highlight it. The introduction of rules must convey that the staff is not responsible for the person. Rules are described, for example, as what will happen if the adolescent stops practice or training. Further, discipline is framed as a way to give information rather than a way to modify behavior. So natural consequences are used whenever possible. If other consequences are imposed they will be designed so that they can be achieved and to provide some information about responsibility [16].

One consequence that is given in the program that Menses and Durrant describe is called "close supervision." The resident is required to stay with a staff member. Residents are told that since their behavior shows that they don't want to supervise their own lives at the moment, they can stay with the staff member for two hours so the staff can supervise it for them. The resident remains with the staff member while normal activity continues and receives information about control and responsibility [16].

Framing Treatment as Information Gathering, Experiment, and Practice

The adolescent's time in residence is defined as one of experiment and practice. An adolescent who had problems with stealing would be provided with chances to steal and then given information about success or failure at resisting temptation. A record of successes would be kept and the adolescent told to call the family after each success. Selekman describes outpatient family sessions which ask parents to expose the adolescent to the frustrating situations which had previously led to substance abuse, and to keep track of both the adolescent's and the Chemical Monster's victories over one another. Special privileges were given to the adolescent for victories over the Chemical Monster [16–17].

Menses and Durrant find that once a problem is given a new description, it is not difficult to design experiments, training, and practice. These might be similar to the homework assignments often given in family therapy. Experiments and tests generate information about success. A resident might be given a certain number of tests about honesty or growing up or temper. These tests allow a new description of treatment. Although the tests are behavioral, their primary purpose is to reframe treatment as providing information. The staff's response to the success or failure is to provide information about control and responsibility [18].

All are told that the adolescent will have a chance to practice growing. Selekman, describing outpatient treatment using a cybernetic model, reports that successes might be responded to with both amazement and celebration. Family members should be asked to distinguish between their past and present ways of interacting so that they can highlight the presence of a difference [19].

PARENTAL INVOLVEMENT

Parental involvement is crucial. Parents should be involved in the planning of the program and the therapy sessions with them involve a review of training. Parental involvement is increased by scheduling regular phone reports from the adolescent into the training or experimenting schedule or regular visits to review the progress chart. The family is also involved in designing further experiments. Family therapy emphasizes the transitional nature of the placement. Family members are given experiments to carry out at home, make preparations for fighting the "monster," and practice doing some things differently. As early as possible, the adolescent goes home on a pass for further experiments, which are framed as practice sessions. The staff tells the family that the real work will start at home, and that the problem will not be resolved at discharge. Placement is regarded as a period of preparation and training with no expectation that the adolescent will be free of problems when coming home [20].

DISCHARGE OR THE END OF TRAINING

Menses and Durrant describe a significant ritual celebration at the end of training that highlights change in a way that allows the family to see itself in a new light. The celebrations are carefully planned as information-giving events. They may include a presentation of temper-taming trophies, monster-fighting certificates, or a ritual enactment of a new path to mark the change in context. These celebrations also act as a marker for other residents, allowing them to measure their own progress. A context of success is enhanced as residents share in each other's achievement [20].

The celebratory rituals place the homecoming in a new context, carefully highlighting what has already been achieved but placed within the context of going home to solve the problem. The family's anxiety is reframed as appropriate nervousness about going on to finally conquer the problem. Family members should leave celebrating the fact that change has occurred and that they are now ready to stand up to the problem as a family. They are taking a triumphant step together [20].

Dealing with Relapse

Since the work is framed as practice, relapses can be normalized or expected, even as "newsworthy" information. Selekman notes that in day treatment for substance abusers, relapses are externalized as interruptions from the "beast" or "monster", and students keep a record of their daily encounters with "relapse monsters" [21].

Durrant and others have essentially reframed residential treatment, placing the experience within an entirely new frame, one that will increase the possibility of the residents' experiencing themselves as competent and successful. This new meaning will give the child or adolescent the opportunity to begin to behave and feel differently. New meaning can make new behavior possible [22].

References

1. Peterson RW. Exploring the application of systemic thinking in child and youth care practice: a shift in paradigm. Journal of Child & Youth Care 1993;8(2):35–54.
2. Pare T, Walter J, Friesen J. A strategic/systemic approach to residential treatment. American Journal of Family Therapy 1992;20(1):52–61.
3. Sachs B. Systemic strategies for dealing with problem children in institutional settings. Contemporary Family Therapy 1986 Fall;8(3):217–23.
4. Forbes E, Maddron T. Systems therapy in a day-treatment setting. International Journal of Partial Hospitalization 1988;5(3):237–50.
5. Menses G, Durrant M. Contextual residential care: Applying the principles of cybernetic therapy to the residential treatment of irresponsible adolescents and their families. Residential Treatment of Children & Youth 1990;7(3):11–32.
6. Sluzki CE. Negative explanation, drawing distinctions, raising dilemmas, collapsing time, externalisation of problems: A note on some powerful conceptual tools. Residential Treatment for Children & Youth 1990;7(3):33–7.
7. Selekman M. Taming the chemical monsters: Cybernetic-systemic therapy with adolescent substance abusers. In: Lawson, GW, Lawson AW, eds. Adolescent substance abuse: etiology, treatment and prevention. Gaithersburg MD: Aspen, 1992,105–119.
8. See reference 5.
9. Durrant M. Residential treatment: a cooperative, competency-based approach to therapy and program design. New York: Norton, 1993.
10. See reference 6.
11. See reference 5.
12. See reference 6.

13. See reference 7.
14. See reference 5.
15. Tomm K. Externalizing problems. Journal of Strategic & Systemic Therapies 1989 Spr;8(1):54–9.
16. See reference 5.
17. See reference 7.
18. See foonote 5.
19. See reference 7.
20. See reference 5.
21. See reference 7.
22. See reference 5.

9. The Teaching Family Model

The Teaching Family model is the most consistently evaluated behavioral treatment for delinquency. It was developed at Achievement Place, a family-type group home for 6 to 8 predelinquents or delinquents, age 12 to 15. The model is designed to help young persons who have been in serious trouble learn the skills necessary to lead self-directed and productive lives. The model was later adopted at Boy's Town in Nebraska, a very large residential treatment center for a similar population. The program includes comprehensive skills training, a token economy, self-government, and a "reciprocally reinforcing relationship" between the young persons and the staff. The model interprets delinquent behaviors as a result of inadequate social learning. Desired behavior is shaped by the use of a token economy. Later, this reward system is replaced by those that occur more naturally and less immediately [1–3].

THE STAFF

The community-based Teaching Family Model is usually administered by two persons, the teaching parents. This title distinguishes them from the more custodial role of a houseparent. The teaching parents have completed one year of professional training that includes classroom and practicum experience. Their role is to form positive, personal teaching relationships with their students that will enable them to teach the skills necessary for productive lives in the community. They will also be the students' advocate in the community and help them to achieve their goals. They establish working relationships on the residents' behalf with the school, juvenile court, social welfare agencies, police, and mental health centers This assures that they will be the first contact with the community agencies if problems arise [4].

Although the Teaching Family model is a behavioral program, much of its effectiveness rests on the strong relationship between the resident and the teaching parents. The strength and satisfaction of these relationships become the strongest motivating influence on learning and behavior. Teaching parents must learn to balance their interventions with recognition of the residents' need for independent functioning [4–5].

The Teaching Interactions

The teaching parents spend time with the residents alone and in a variety of environments, developing the ability to observe and describe their behavior. These observations permit them to identify situations that the residents have difficulties handling. They then have a background for suggesting behaviors that would be more effective, and use the new outcome as a reason for change. Essentially, every interaction can become an occasion for teaching. One specialized interaction that is used to change a maladaptive behavior includes initial praise, a description of the inappropriate behavior, a negative consequence, description of an alternative behavior, practice, a positive consequence, and final praise. Teaching is essentially the treatment. Yet learning itself is a complex skill and some of the residents need to be helped to learn. Blase and colleagues give an example of how a complex skill, such as how to follow instructions, is broken down into simple steps: looking at the person, listening to what is said, completing the task, checking back when done, then calmly discussing the instruction and accepting criticism. The way to accept criticism is also taught: e.g., look at the person, don't argue or pout, calmly discuss issues or concerns [4–5].

The Behavioral Program

The skills training program is based on the belief that delinquencies arise from a deficit in essential skills. These deficiencies are not the result of individual psychopathology but due to inadequate motivation, examples, or training. The behavioral program attempts to develop competence in social, academic, vocational and family living skills. The program uses instruction, modeling, feedback, and support [4–5].

Self-Government

The residents can make and change the rules, evaluate the motivation systems, and constructively examine each other's behaviors. The family conference in the evening makes them aware of how their own behavior affects others and how they can help others to change [4–5].

The Model in Operation

The token economy is essential in the beginning phases of the program and helps to motivate the learning of behaviors. In the beginning, the residents exchange points for privileges each day. After the resident has learned some skills and self-control, a weekly exchange system replaces the daily exchange. The program is individualized, with goals established to improve competencies and remediate deficiencies of each resident. Residents progress from the point system to a merit system, at which time no points are taken away and all privileges are free. There can be a demotion from the merit system if the resident does not maintain the newly acquired skills and behaviors. All privilege systems are carefully monitored to be respectful of residents and their rights [4–5].

Residents have daily report cards, which they take to school for teachers to complete. Students can gain or lose points and privileges on the basis of their school performance. Some of the evening is spent in a family conference, the self-government part of the program. The residents and teaching family discuss the happenings of the day, talk about rules that are needed, and make decisions on consequences for violating the rules. They are specifically trained in group decision-making, how to make constructive criticism, negotiation, and compromise. The family conference helps residents learn fairness as well as concern for others. Many residents also have individual counseling with the teaching parents. The teaching parents will help them seek alternative solutions for problems and may also focus on specific skills [4–5].

EVALUATION

The effectiveness of each component of the models has been tested: the token economy system, the self-government system, the elected manager system, and the daily report card system. The evaluations examine not only the effects of these components on the residents but also which they prefer. Even their preferences in helpful teaching-parent interactions are evaluated and are used to improve the teaching parent training program. The model has been continuously refined following each evaluation [6–8].

THE INFLUENCE OF THE MODEL

The development and careful evaluation of each component of the Teaching Family model has led to its successful replication in many group homes, both in the United States and Europe. Forst and colleagues describe the psychoeducational treatment model at Boy's Town, which was influenced by the Teaching Family model and adapted some of the techniques for a much larger residential treatment center. They report on a training program to guide the staff in both planned and spontaneous interactions with residents. With a foundation in the token economy, residents are taught social skills and how to solve problems. Adaptive skills are continuously reinforced, and corrective teaching is used to respond to problem behaviors. The community meeting, which includes staff and residents, provides opportunities for teaching and practicing adaptive skills [8–9].

The training sessions help the direct care staff to teach social skills. They learn the principles of learning and behavior theory, systems for motivating residents and the levels of tolerance for distinguishing between acceptable and non-acceptable behavior. In addition, the staff is taught problem solving and techniques for patient government. The teaching methods that they master embrace techniques for preventive, corrective, and intensive teaching. Preventive teaching is used for residents who show no problematic behavior, while corrective teaching identifies and responds to problematic behaviors, linking adaptive behavior to the treatment plan. Intensive teaching helps residents regain control of their behavior and develops skills to maintain it. Staff members learn the technique of effective praise as a way to reward positive behaviors. The behavior is identified, described, and praised, its rationale discussed, and a positive consequence provided [9].

The Teaching Family model has also made a practical application of the ecological approach, with a recognition that not only the resident, but also the resident's interactions with all significant others in the environment require therapeutic attention. The model provides a family style of treatment that works intensively with the child's community, which must continue to provide support.

Although the model has been extremely effective in promoting change while the resident is in treatment, even this widely acclaimed and widely-replicated model cannot guarantee a permanent successful adjustment after a return to the community [10].

References

1. Werry JS, Wollersheim JP. Behavior therapy with children and adolescents: a twenty-year overview. Journal American Academy of Child & Adolescent Psychiatry 1989;28:1–18
2. Wolf MM, Phillips EL, Fixsen DL, Braukmann CJ, et al. Achievement Place: the Teaching Family model. Child Care Quarterly 1976 Sum;5:92–103.
3. Baron L. Skill-based management training for child care program administrators: the Teaching-Family Model revisited. Child Care Quarterly 1984 Win;13(4):262–77.
4. See reference 2.
5. Blase KA, Fixsen DL, Freeborn K, Jaeger D. The Behavioral Model. In: Lyman, RD, Prentice-Dunn S, Gabel S, eds. Residential and inpatient treatment of children and adolescents. New York: Plenum Press, 1989,43–59.
6. Fixsen DL, Phillips EL, Wolf MM. Achievement Place: Experiments in self-government with predelinquents. Journal of Applied Behavior Analysis 1973;6:31–47.
7. Phillips EL, Phillips EA, Wolf MM, Fixsen DL. Achievement Place: Development of the elected manager system. Journal of Applied Behavior Analysis 1973 Win;6(4):541–61.
8. Bailey JS, Wolf MM, Phillips EL. Home-based reinforcement and the modification of predelinquents' classroom behavior. Journal of Applied Behavioral Analysis 1970;3:223–33.
9. Furst DW, Boever W, Cohen J, Dowd T, et al. Implementation of the Boys Town psychoeducational treatment model in a children's psychiatric hospital. Hospital & Community Psychiatry 1993 Sep;44(9):83–8.
10. Kirigin KA, Braukmann CJ, Atwater JD, Wolf MM. An evaluation of teaching-family (Achievement Place) group homes for juvenile offenders. Journal of Applied Behavior Analysis 1982;15:1–15.

10. The Therapeutic Community

Although many therapeutic community practices are no longer used, the principles of the therapeutic community model have been incorporated into hospital psychiatry. There is a distinction between the therapeutic community model and the therapeutic community approach which adopts only some of the ideology and practices of the therapeutic community and blends them with traditional hospital psychiatry [1–2].

The therapeutic community had its roots in social psychiatry—the study of social and psychological factors in the origin, maintenance and treatment of mental disorder. Since personality theory indicates that personality traits are not determined solely by internal factors but also by the environment, then treatment that combines psychotherapy and sociotherapy should be more effective. If it is social forces that produce harmful effects, then correcting social forces can also be mobilized for the patient's treatment. The ideal was to transform social processes into a therapeutic force. The therapeutic community can be conceived as a social field. Since personal problems often have to do with relationships with others, living in a community with a therapeutic emphasis allows behavior to be observed, understood and corrected [3–6].

In England in the 1940s, Thomas Main conceived of the hospital's reorganization as a community where the primary therapy would be done, not by physicians, but by the community itself. The social unit of patients and staff became the primary therapeutic agent. Maxwell Jones expanded the work of the therapeutic community, believing that it would be possible to design an understanding and permissive environment where patients could become aware of their interpersonal patterns and get help in changing both their behavior and ways of relating to each other. Jones believed that changes were possible because the members of the therapeutic community would not provide the response to behaviors that the patient had come to expect. For example, if the group responds to the aggressive male's provocations, not with rejection, but with an interest in the meaning of his behavior and a desire to discuss it, they can create an opportunity for change [7–9].

Principles of the Therapeutic Community

The treatment philosophy of a therapeutic community is based on the belief that character traits and intrapsychic conflicts are displayed as interpersonal problems. They can then be better understood and support and feedback from others can test new behaviors. The fundamental principles of the early therapeutic communities were: democratization, permissiveness, communalism, and reality confrontation [10–11].

Democracy

The ideal of democracy extends the responsibility of treatment to both patients and staff, so that each patient can responsibly participate in the treatment of others. The resident is no longer a passive recipient of treatment but a person with increased autonomy, who helps to provide it. Full participation in the unit distributes power. Jones and Rapoport note that when patients who have been powerless or destructive have a share in running the unit, they can see for themselves the problems that antisocial behavior creates. This sharing of power also changes their beliefs about authority [12–13].

However, the ideal of democracy in the therapeutic community deserves scrutiny. Democracy should not mean that there is no leadership; nor is it really true that everyone is equal. When an authority structure disappears, informal relationships or subgroups will often reestablish one. Morrice finds it potentially harmful to insist that there is no distinction between trained and untrained persons. Most treatment centers have abandoned a total democratic approach since it usually led to role blurring and role confusion. Clinicians now realize that when boundaries between patients and staff become confused, it can lead to intense involvements and acting out for both patients and staff. Sacks and Carpenter note that although the therapeutic community supports patient responsibility, the staff members covertly function as though patients are irresponsible. Still, the long term influence of the therapeutic community approach has allowed patients to make many more decisions in their care, either individually or as a group [14–16].

Despite the ideal of democracy, the staff's authority to set limits on residents is usually stronger than the residents' authority to set limits on staff. While it is usually acceptable for the staff to challenge the residents' maladaptive behavior, the residents' ability to impose limits on staff is more restricted. The ultimate power of the community to set limits on members depends on each member's wish to belong and to build good interpersonal relationships [17].

Permissiveness

Active resocialization can take place only within a background of permissiveness. The ideology of permissiveness in inpatient treatment usually interprets deviant behaviors as a symptom of an illness rather than a reason for punishment. The patient's acting out behaviors should not be so much controlled as brought to light. Main referred to the therapeutic community as a culture of inquiry. Behaviors provide data about the person's needs and motivations. As the person becomes more aware of these patterns, a willingness to try out new behaviors can develop. Permissiveness in the therapeutic community gives members the necessary latitude for rehearsing new behaviors which not only meet their needs but are socially acceptable [18–20].

REALITY CONFRONTATION

Since all interactions in the therapeutic community become public knowledge, members cannot split the staff by displaying various parts of their personality. They quickly become aware of the bad effects of their behavior on others and can develop an improved ability to empathize through identification with the community. Jones calls this development of empathy the most significant change brought about in a therapeutic community. Whereas the person alienated from society once acted out conflicts, relationships with others and knowledge of how this behavior affects them can bring about changes. The response from the group provides a variety of checks and balances for reality testing. The feedback of information from the multiple social situations in the community serves as a check on individual perceptions. Personal views of reality can always be checked with the group. In addition, this feedback helps to provide correction and control in the therapeutic community. The signals are usually clear as to what sort of behavior will lead toward recovery [21–23].

Other Characteristics of the Therapeutic Community.

OPEN COMMUNICATION

Therapeutic community members must have the freedom to express feelings which they have previously hidden. Privileged communication is discouraged. It is the free flow of information which allows therapeutic work to continue, and any restrictions upon it will make it less effective. Open communication assures that the behavior of everyone will be open to examination [24–25].

THE PATIENT CULTURE

The therapeutic community requires a strong patient culture. Informal social situations provide the setting for members to display as well as observe their own maladaptive social relationships. They soon become aware of their effect on others and are motivated to improve their social learning because it brings approval. They can provide each other with support to overcome difficulties and help absorb the stress of the treatment process. They can actually keep each other in treatment. Peer relationships provide powerful incentives for therapeutic effort. The culture of the therapy groups is continued in daily life and members can continue group work beyond the group and with other persons in their life.

RELEVANCE

Therapeutic communities can be described as a form of milieu therapy in which everything that occurs can take on relevance. Yet how does the regular life of a therapeutic community become "therapeutic?" McKeganey and Bloor explain that in a therapeutic community, even an everyday event can be redefined as therapeutically relevant. They describe a community member's cleaning a toilet as a simple event that can be given meaning and interpreted as a sign of recovery. Almost any event in the community can be redefined, set apart or transformed, much as an everyday object becomes sacred when used in a ceremony. This redefinition can transform the everyday social life of the unit as an agency of therapy in its own right. McKeganey and Bloor note, however, that this occurs only if the community maintains a free flow of information and does not confine work to formal meetings [25].

The therapeutic community becomes the concrete living out of the treatment center's primary values. Stern and colleagues describe the therapeutic community as a "play" space which is temporarily set apart from the world outside. Within this space, the members are able to play out the problematic and rehearse the more mature aspects of their personality for the group's responses. They can experiment with and learn about new ways of being. The group becomes a playground for corrective learning, both cognitive and emotional, facilitated by mutual caring and by mixing reality with play and fantasy [26–27].

Forms of Motivation

Many therapeutic communities provide a system of status changes, which are often based on staff and patient discussion and majority votes. This arrangement makes a concrete connection between privileges and responsibilities to the community. Status changes provide a mechanism for reviewing the individual member's relationships with the community. The status system internally motivates the person to become responsible and is based on observable behaviors. It is a system of social reward which provides group approval of positive behavior, greater responsibility and upward mobility [28].

Some Goals and Results of the Therapeutic Community

Social Learning

Social learning is acquired in many ways in the therapeutic community. The sense of belonging to the community makes both peer influence and behavior change possible. Inappropriate behaviors can be dealt with by the group as they occur. Group discussion replaces punishment and any enforced isolation occur only when safety is threatened. The community must also focus on the patient's assets as the foundation for growth [29].

The resolution of personal problems and conflicts within the group also leads to social learning. The members will need support when they express private feelings and will require freedom to try on new ways of relating. They are encouraged to take an interest in fellow patients and to help each other. This learning to care also helps members develop feelings of responsibility toward each other. Identification with fellow patients and responsibility for the community eventually develop. At the same time, Morrice challenges the myth that only the group can help, and warns against what can happen if the resident in the therapeutic community gets "lost in the crowd." Although the group is the most vital therapeutic instrument, it must not be used exclusively [30].

Social change can occur in the therapeutic community as members develop bonds with each other. As they experience the rewards of being accepted and cared for by others, they will also need assurance that their own individuality will not be lost. However, respect for individuality does not really mean that the treatment program adapts to the patient. Rather, the goal is for the patient to adapt to a sane environment, by both learning and conflict resolution. The therapeutic community becomes an entity with which the patient must eventually negotiate, assimilate, and accommodate. At the same time, the sanity of the community and the member's own motivation must provide a protection against coercion and the potential tyranny of the group [31].

Responsibility

Social learning also occurs as community members develop responsibility. The staff usually will stress to residents the value of regulating their own behavior and being considerate of others, rather than being externally controlled by rules or sanctions. Since a great deal of responsibility is turned over to the residents, staff members must tolerate disruption and disorganization. Their own role in increasing responsibility may be to influence residents to confront irresponsible behavior when it happens. Norman believes that patients will constantly struggle to reject the personal responsibility that the therapeutic community demands. Their strong wish is to be cured by the doctor, cared for by the nurse and to generally retreat from worldly cares. They would prefer that their illness be seen as someone else's fault. The patient community often does its best to maintain dependence and thrust power back to the staff [32].

Increase in Self-Esteem

The patient's self-esteem can be increased by a sense of belonging to a community and receiving help from others with similar problems. The patient's own ability to help others by sharing experiences also builds self-esteem [33].

Current Status of the Therapeutic Community

The medicalization of psychiatry and the shorter length of stay contributed to the decline of the therapeutic community. The model is not used in treatment today because it takes time for meaningful relationships and an assimilation of therapeutic community values to develop. Rapoport found that it takes at least 100 days for a person to be affected or accepting of the unit's values. Caine and Small found that it took at least 6 weeks before a patient became an active therapeutic community participant [33–35].

The therapeutic community's success has often been dependent upon strong, even charismatic leadership. Morrice challenged the belief that the therapeutic community can be leaderless, even though decision making is usually described as shared. He states that in no other situation is the exercise of authority more necessary, yet so difficult. The most successful therapeutic communities usually had a dedicated leader who infused the community with hope, the expectation of improvement and a sense of how it could happen. This brings up a question whether the therapeutic culture has absorbed the ability to carry on following the loss of a leader. Another interesting question is whether patients or staff will regress when they leave such a community. The leader must be skilled at both interpretation and confrontation and be able to maintain an authority which is not undermined by the ideal of the community's democracy. The leader truly stands at the boundary between the group and the external society, aware of the group's life, but also outside of it and thus preserving a therapeutic influence. The leader embodies the leading ideas of the therapeutic community and brings influence, authority, and stability to it [36–38].

The therapeutic community is helpful for only a few of the mental disorders that lead to inpatient treatment. There are always problems in designing treatment that will be equally helpful to persons with varying degrees of ego impairment. There can also be destructive interactions among different types of patients. Even finding a staff equally skillful in treating all kinds of patients is difficult. In addition, there has never been solid research to define the therapeutic value of the specific methods of treatment, or of comparative outcomes. Although in the United States the therapeutic community is more prominent in chemical dependency treatment, hospital psychiatry and residential treatment programs have incorporated many of its principles. The idea of honesty and open communication so central to the therapeutic community has become a guiding principle in most treatment. The therapeutic community's experiment with patients' full participation in treatment has influenced all inpatient treatment so that most patients learn to help, support, and take responsibility for each other. The patient's own information and opinions are taken seriously in the design of treatment. At the same time, therapeutic community principles cannot always be grafted on to programs with stronger philosophical commitments. Bell and Ryan found that in a biologically oriented milieu, the emphasis on providing support clashed with the attempt to achieve practical goals such as helping the patient restore functioning. They found that the philosophy of the therapeutic community could be better integrated into psychosocial rehabilitation programs than psychoanalytic or biologically oriented milieus. Stern believes that the ideals of the therapeutic community can function to limit the therapist's need to manage the patient's environment. Interpersonal difficulties are more apparent and can be brought more quickly into therapy sessions to be clarified and interpreted. The therapeutic community provides psychotherapy with a "firm but negotiable reality" which will help the patient gain self-knowledge. When the daily life with other residents becomes a therapeutic agent, the therapist can preserve neutrality. Stern even extends the psychoanalytic concept of the holding environment to the community, believing that it draws in its members rather than holding them apart [39–41].

Although the therapeutic community helps to change the person's own sense of responsibility and self-esteem, it is not clear how well it can prepare for post-community living. Rapoport's four-year study of Jones' Belmont experiment found that the therapeutic community members had developed skills that were inappropriate outside the hospital and that patients were not able to generalize their new behaviors to the community environment. Karterud, in discussing the modern therapeutic community, believes that it should refer only to specialized treatment which can establish a culture of inquiry and not simply be a term to describe milieu therapy or wards which treat their patients as fellow human beings. Karterud agrees with most others that therapeutic community treatment is best suited for those with personality disorders and severe neuroses. Papiasvill believes a therapeutic community model can be helpful for neurotic persons since they can often become passive and dependent and blocked in their capacity to solve problems. The therapeutic community is particularly helpful for those with personality disorders, in that it can counteract a passive or helpless role or identity. Peer authority is also much more welcome than hierarchical authority for this group. Their self-esteem can be protected when they accept help from others with similar problems and it can be enhanced as they help others with similar problems [42–44].

Therapeutic communities are quite varied, but most have a structured daily program with multiple therapeutic activities. Social interactions become significant learning experiences and communication problems between staff and patients create therapeutic interventions. Community meetings, group therapy and staff conferences build a unit culture. Community members are regarded as responsible persons who can share decision making. The failure to establish satisfying relationships with others decreases self-esteem and may lead to isolation and alienation from reality. The therapeutic community provides not only psychotherapy but sociotherapy, treating those who are both psychologically and socially disabled. The goal of the therapeutic community model is not only to teach more effective social skills through active resocialization but also to help residents work through their personal problems and develop caring and responsible relationships with others [45]. For information on its application to a specific population, see the section on Substance Abuse for the Therapeutic Community in Chapter VI.

References

1. Stauble WJ. Therapeutic community: a Canadian update. Canadian Journal of Psychiatry 1988;33:213–7.
2. Oldham JM, Russakoff LM. Dynamic therapy in brief hospitalization. Northvale, NJ: Aronson, 1987.
3. Millard DW. Generative rules and the therapeutic community. British Journal of Medical Psychology 1981;54(2):157–65.
4. Trauer T. Current status of the therapeutic community. British Journal of Medical Psychology 1984;57(1):71–9.
5. Sivadon PD. Techniques of sociotherapy. Psychiatry 1957;20(3):205–10.
6. Clark DC. The therapeutic community—concept, practice and future. British Journal of Psychiatry 1965;111:947–58.
7. Main TF. The hospital as a therapeutic community. Bulletin Menninger Clinic 1946; 10:66–70.
8. Jones M. The treatment of personality disorders in a therapeutic community. Psychiatry 1957;20:211–20.
9. Mandelbrote B. The therapeutic community. British Journal of Psychiatry 1979;136:369–71.
10. Karterud S. What are the prerequisites and indications of the therapeutic community proper? A comparative study. Acta Psychiatrica Scandinavia 1988;77:658–69.
11. Rapoport R. Community as doctor. London: Tavistock, 1960.
12. Erickson RC. Viewing the therapeutic community through Adlerian spectacles. International Journal of Group Psychotherapy 1981;32(2):201–16.
13. Jones M, Rapoport R. The absorption of new doctors into a therapeutic community. In: Greenblatt M, Levinson DJ, Williams RH. The patient and the mental hospital. Glencoe, IL: Free Press, 1957, 248–62.
14. Morrice JKW. Myth and the democratic process. British Journal of Medical Psychology 1972;45:327–31.
15. Norman A. Double messages in a therapeutic community. Psychotherapy & Psychosomatics 1972;20:143–7.
16. Sacks MH, Carpenter WT. The pseudotherapeutic community: an examination of anti-therapeutic forces on psychiatric units. Hospital & Community Psychiatry 1974;25:315–8.
17. Stern DA, Fromm MG, Sacksteder JL. From coercion and collaboration: two weeks in the life of a therapeutic community. Psychiatry 1987;49(1):18–32.
18. Rees TP, Glatt MM. The organization of a mental hospital on the basis of group participation. International Journal of Group Psychotherapy 1955;5:157–61.
19. See reference 6.
20. See reference 7.
21. See reference 8.
22. See reference 13.

23. Killiam LM, Bloomberg S. Rebirth in a therapeutic community: A case study. Psychiatry 1975;38:39–54.
24. Page RC. Social change in a therapeutic community. International Journal of the Addictions 1983;18(6):769–76.
25. McKeganey NP, Bloor MJ. Teamwork, information control and therapeutic effectiveness: A tale of two therapeutic communities. Sociology of Health & Illness 1987;9(2):154–78.
26. See reference 17.
27. Knobloch F. Knobloch J. Letter. American Journal of Psychiatry 1989 Dec; 146(12):1643–4.
28. See reference 12.
29. Skinner K. The therapeutic milieu: Making it work. Journal of Psychiatric Nursing & Mental Health Services 1979;17(8):38–44.
30. See reference 14.
31. See reference 17.
32. See reference 15.
33. McGlashan TH. Residential Treatment. In: American Psychiatric Association Task Force on Treatments of Psychiatric Disorders. Treatments of Mental Disorders. v. 2. Washington, DC: American Psychiatric Press, 1989, 2689–2706.
34. Caine TM, Small DJ. Attitudes to treatment of medical staff in therapeutic communities. British Journal of Medical Psychology 1966;39:329-34.
35. See reference 11.
36. See reference 14.
37. Cohen MB. Editorial notes: the therapeutic community and therapy. Psychiatry 1957;20:173–5.
38. Whiteley JS. Dilemma of leadership in a therapeutic community. Group Analysis 1978;(2):40–7.
39. Edelson M M. Ego psychology, group dynamics and the therapeutic community. New York: Grune & Stratton, 1964.
40. Bell MD, Ryan ER. Where can therapeutic community ideals be realized? An examination of three treatment environments. Hospital & Community Psychiatry 1985 Dec;36(12):1286–96.
41. See reference 17.
42. See reference 11.
43. See reference 10.
44. Papiasvill E, Papiasvill A. A residential therapeutic community for neurotics. International Journal of Group Psychotherapy 1983;33(3):387–95.
45. Lehman A, Ritzler R. The therapeutic community inpatient ward: Does it really work? Comprehensive Psychiatry 1976;17(6):755–61.

11. The Wilderness Challenge Model

The wilderness therapy or wilderness challenge model has its roots in the Outward Bound Program, which demonstrated that certain challenging experiences shared in a group context could produce prosocial values. The model has a resemblance to systemic therapy, in that it does not focus on a pathological behavior, but rather attempts to challenge some other aspect of the personality that will unlock a habitual way of acting to produce new results. The focus is upon the healthy and functioning part of those who participate. It helps to dislodge old behavior patterns and gives a renewed sense of personal worth and confidence [1–2].

The wilderness program includes a series of progressively difficult challenges. It will involve such activities as hiking, climbing, canoeing, or specially designed challenges that will provide experiences in solving problems and working together. Such experiences can serve as metaphors for other daily living situations to be carried over into peer group discussions. A crucial aspect of the challenge is that members learn to cooperate and to rely upon each other. Mastery of the challenges requires persistence, creativity, and the application of skills. The challenges appear more difficult and dangerous than they really are, so that the sense of mastery is enhanced. The challenges at first will seem overwhelming, but the group members learn that they can be mastered if approached systematically. They can leave their previous experiences of failure or weakness behind them when they take part in this transforming experience. The person can attain mastery by a strong ability to focus in the novel environment, support of the leader and the group, and the quality of the problems themselves that are arranged in such a way as to develop mastery [2–3].

Although the challenges are significant, group process and the establishment of a community are the core of wilderness therapy. The group, isolated from all other influences, becomes a way of life. The group forms a powerful bond with strong feelings of trust in each other. Just as earlier social processes shaped behaviors, the group process can reshape them. The group confronts the tasks at hand and organizes to accomplish them. The group evaluates performance, gives feedback, helps to solve problems. The adolescents learn a lot about themselves in the group process. Bacon and Kimball report that many self-centered and maladaptive behaviors can be corrected when the adolescent receives and respects feedback from peers. The leaders manage the group process in such a way that group members can distill appropriate social values from the wilderness experience. Wilderness therapy can strengthen the sense of competence, improve the self-image and significantly decrease antisocial behavior. The experience does not solve all of the participants' problems, but it is a breakaway experience from old behaviors, and provides a new sense of strength, self-respect and social skills. Insights from this experience develop emotional controls and interpersonal experiences that translate into behavioral control and an increased ability to plan actions rather than simply acting on impulse [2–4].

References

1. Berman DS, Davis-Berman J. Wilderness therapy and adolescent mental health. Administration & Policy in Mental Health 1991 May;18(3):373–9.
2. Reid WH, Matthews WM. A wilderness experience treatment program for antisocial offenders. International Journal of Offender Therapy & Comparative Criminology 1980;24:171–8.
3. Stich TF, Senior N. Adventure therapy: An innovative treatment for psychiatric patients. New Directions for Mental Health Services 1984;21:103–8.
4. Bacon SB, Kimball R. The Wilderness Challenge model. In: Lyman RD, Prentice-Dunn S, Gabel S, eds. Residential and inpatient treatment of children and adolescents. New York: Plenum Press, 1989;115–44.

CHAPTER

IV

The Organization of Treatment

The manner in which the human milieu organizes itself around the patient has powerful effects, not only upon the patient's treatment, but also on the staff's satisfaction with its work. Can a psychotherapist concentrate on therapy if burdened with day-to-day concerns about the patient's behavior? Does the amount of time spent in team meetings each week bring equivalent results in treatment? Is there a way to respect and reward clinical administration (managing the details of the patient's life) so that it has equal status with psychotherapy?

Staff members may feel most effective organized into departments in order to bring the full force of their own professional training to patient care. Are these professionals effective when they operate as a team? Can they can function effectively being supervised by both department and team? Team-centered treatment has become the preferred arrangement. There still remains a need to determine the individual therapist's role in relation to the team. Should the therapist be the team leader? Does the therapist continue to make immediate decisions for the patient or is this left to the nurse or milieu manager? Or is it always a team decision?

1. The Treatment Team

The social worker who overlooks the findings of biology, the behavioral psychologist who scoffs at unconscious motivation, the psychiatrist who does not believe in treating the family—each would ignore powerful therapeutic forces if solely responsible for the patient's treatment. The team concept arose from the recognition that a single profession or person cannot fully understand the patient's difficulties. In a medical setting, the psychiatrist usually leads the team and carries primary responsibility for the quality of treatment, overseeing the biological asessment and coordination of treatment. The team includes the milieu staff and nurses, all adjunctive therapists, the psychotherapist, and the social worker. Team members with varying professional backgrounds can stimulate, support, and complement each other with great effectiveness. The team's interaction can be synergistic in generating new solutions. Although a therapist manager or therapist/administrator combination can still be a part of the organization of treatment, when the therapist helps to direct the team and the team helps direct the therapist, integration of interdisciplinary treatment is achieved. Gralnick believes that the team structure can protect both therapist and patient from countertransference complications. If the team members are to do their work, the confidentiality between therapist and patient must be expanded to include them. Kerlinsky warns that if any staff person conspires with the patient or family to keep secrets from the team there is a risk of recreating old pathological family situations. The basic function of the team is to structure coherent, integrated transactions with and around the patient. The way a therapeutic team interacts around a patient crisis is an indication of its organizational structure [1–5].

THE INTEGRATION OF PROFESSIONALS INTO A TREATMENT TEAM

The professionals who work as a team expect to reach final agreements in their approach to each patient. Yet each profession has different values and models of intervention. Members of one profession often dominate. Moreover, there is always the question of who is competent to make decisions in areas that are not within the traditional domain of any of the professions. Bernard and Ishiyama believe that the team allows its members to contribute to the extent that they prove capable of doing so. Team members should finally have latitude to define their own roles. Krueger notes, however, that not all decisions can be team decisions, since some must be made by particular team members with specific expertise or administrative accountability. For example, the team does not prescribe medication, the psychiatrist does. At the same time, the psychiatrist will turn to team members for their observations about the need for medication or its effects. Since the interdisciplinary team evolved to coordinate professional services for the patient with a minimum of duplication, roles should be clearly defined and each profession understood and respected. Membership on the team is justified only by having something to contribute that cannot be done as well by other members [6–9].

In addition to seeing the patient from the vantage point of varying professions, team members will also have derived an image of the patient that may have evolved from their own countertransference responses. When the team comes together, it may seem as if several people have come to discuss a book, each having read only one chapter [10].

The professions that make up the team represent a storehouse of knowledge, which no individual member will have. When team members share their knowledge, professional identities combine to create a new professional, a composite of the professionals who compose the team. Pruyser describes each team member as having a unique agenda that finally contributes to a superordinate agenda of a holistic kind. Keliher uses the word transdiciplinary to describe the team that can move beyond interdisciplinary boundaries and fuse as a new entity. At times, the team becomes an educational seminar with emphasis on the conscious synthesis of information. The task of every team member is to contribute knowledge not available to other members, a willingness to recognize the contribution of others and an ability to carry out decisions. Pruyser believes there is a need for balance between the sharpening and leveling of the differences between disciplines. If there is too much sharpening the team becomes a Tower of Babel. With too much leveling, everyone thinks and acts nearly the same way, ignoring the patient's complexity. In addition, this leveling will most likely be in the direction of adopting the concepts of the profession that is culturally, if not politically, dominant in the treatment center [11–13].

Merkel points to the work organization in Saab automobile factories as a model for clinical teams in a behavioral treatment unit. The clinical teams derived two important principles from these Swedish experiments. The Swedish teams were free to design their own methods to accomplish their task and they were also protected from any external interference from the administrative hierarchy. The second principle had to do with accountability. If the team's production or success was not adequate, it was up to team members to design ways to solve it. (Measuring effectiveness, of course, is easier in a behavioral unit than in a psychodynamic milieu.) The clinical teams had a true sense of ownership, both for their work and its results. The preservation of this team arrangement is not always easy. Merkel writes that the behavioral unit's boundaries and the boundaries around each clinical team were robust enough to resist the continued efforts to invade them for organizational or personal needs. There was also a constant pull to consolidate power once again into the familiar vertical structure that every worker knows so well. Pruyser reports that the team's multidisciplinary work can be counteracted by an administration that continues to see the team as part of an organizational chart rather than the living organism it can become [12–14].

Team Communication

The interdisciplinary team makes decisions after hearing from all members. When communication is not clear and accurate, information is incomplete and treatment suffers. Communication problems may reflect dysfunctional group processes that can result in the distortion or withholding of information. Butterhill and colleagues write about team members who appoint themselves gatekeepers of information, deciding what to share and what to withhold, causing a breakdown in communication. They believe that knowledge of team dynamics is as crucial as those of the patient and that the team must often pull back in order to examine itself [15].

TEAM LEADERSHIP

It seems wise to select the professional who carries primary responsibility for the patient as the team leader. Abramson writes that physicians usually become the team leaders and that their higher status will influence definition of the patients' problems, types of intervention and decision making as well as team interaction. Crawshaw and Key believe that if the psychiatrist is the team leader members may have to work through their own resentment with authority, although the team can usually withstand anger and resentment if it can still respect the leader [16–18].

The leader builds the team culture. Abramson stresses the need for an optimistic culture with a belief in change and the team members' abilities to bring it about. Even though members have commitments to their own professions, the leader forges an identification with the team. Whereas early in the formation of the team the representatives of each profession will struggle to identify their own contribution, they later identify themselves as members of the group as a whole. As Modlin and Faris write, the team member's problems become the group's problems, and the team's success, their success. Group cohesiveness can grow from internalizing the value system of the team; the beliefs of the team should be congruent with that of the treatment center, and reference to its treatment philosophy will be helpful. Krueger recommends that the leader express the congruence between individual and team goals for the patient and for the team. Whereas status factors may have once played a role on the team, the leader tries to create a culture where status and the hierarchy can finally disappear. The leader can change status differences by giving full support and attention to team members who may wish to disagree with "higher status" members. The leader must also assure that all members have equal time and are asked for their opinions. Krueger notes that since team members often don't remember participating in a decision, one way to change this is to ask each member to comment before consensus is reached. The leader also makes the hierarchy fade and team identity develop by taking full part in all team functions, even physical interventions, and joins all team activities with patients. The leader must show confidence in the team and instill that confidence by implicit expectations that all members of the team will operate on the highest therapeutic level [16–20].

It should be clear how decisions are made. If the administration will also have a voice in some of the team's decision, this should be clear. There will always be external pressures on the team and the team leader should define the pressures that are external so that they will not affect team cohesiveness. All team members should expect disagreements. Peters believes that a team culture should view conflict as signaling improved functioning rather than regression. Osborne suggests that there be a belief in collaboration based on creative conflict. The leader must pull back sufficiently to maintain an overview of the team process. It will be the leader who makes or catalyzes decisions that seem too difficult for the team. If the treatment plan simply isn't working, it is often the leader who should acknowledge that it needs to be changed [20–23].

The leader's very effectiveness, however, can cause the team to be dependent and see the leader as the only person qualified to carry the overwhelming responsibility of treating the patient. This helps the team members to control their own overwhelming anxiety at the magnitude of the task. To keep this in check, the leader must value and empower the team members to help them internalize their own sense of confidence. The team leader must be able to tune into team concerns that have the potential to intensify feelings. The leader needs to understand what it is like to be the target of the patient's devaluation in order to empathize with the staff members' struggle to control their anger or restore their own confidence. When the leader validates the team members' efforts and instills them with value, it will strengthen their self-esteem and sense of belonging. At the same time, the function of the team is not to treat its members, but to increase effectiveness with patients. The leader's knowledge of psychodynamics, transference and countertransference will be of help. A frank acknowledgment of feelings about certain patients will help others to discuss their own hopelessness or anger. The team can then be in touch with its own reactions sufficiently to begin to understand the patient's emotional predicament. All team members have become members of the patient's interpersonal world and will be projected upon, devalued or idealized, and each should be open to share this experience with other team members. Psychotherapeutic teams can recognize and understand countertransference much better than the single worker in the milieu [23–24].

Some Disadvantages of Teams

Teams may simply carry on a circular "buckpassing" without end and create a situation where no one person accepts responsibility and accountability. Individual members may use collaborative decision making to escape their own responsibility for team decisions. Rae-Grant and Marcuse write that teams may be a good place to hide, since the individual member's own clinical effectiveness escapes evaluation. Patients and their families simply have no way of knowing who on the staff takes responsibility for what. When decisions are announced as being made by the team, no one person can be singled out as responsible. Appelbaum and Munich report that patients often directed their frustration about decisions on whomever they could find—even cooks who served them food—while the team members remained protected by the anonymity of decision-making. Team members may also take greater risks as group members. Seeking a consensus and democratic decision-making take up a great deal of time and this process may be too cumbersome to provide quick responses when they are necessary. Rae-Grant and Marcuse believe that meeting schedules, team coordination and the emotional interaction in teams drain the staff members' energy—an energy that would be better directed toward patients. Finally, they believe that to praise the treatment team is to underestimate the psychotherapist and the therapeutic potential of confidential clinical work. Seeking to equalize all members of the team may finally have nontherapeutic effects on patients [25–28].

TWO MODELS OF ORGANIZATION: DEPARTMENT AND TEAM

The departmental model organizes separate responsibilities such as psychotherapy, teaching, social work, and recreation into separate departments with the work directed by a professional in each field. Bettelheim feels that this division into departments dilutes the worker's commitment to the patient who will be pulled in as many directions as there are departments, all of which have a professional bias as to what the patient needs and exaggerate their own contributions. Butterhill and colleagues describe some of the difficulties presented when both a team and department model are expected to co-exist. Most team members are directly accountable to department heads, not to the team leader, despite the fact that the team leader is usually medically and legally responsible for the patient's care. The team leader must work very closely with department heads to insure that all team members are functioning effectively and develop alliances based on mutual trust, respect and open communication [29–30].

Garner argues that this departmental organization causes each group to develop its own treatment philosophy, values and perceptions of other departments. Their theories target the symptoms that only their expertise can treat. Group cohesiveness develops with an associated resistance to the philosophies and values of other departments. Each department comes to expect misguided behaviors of other staff members and makes plans to counter their moves. Garner outlines several disadvantages of the departmental model: 1) Staff members who spend the most time with clients are rarely consulted and have the least power to make vital decisions; 2) Staff sharing responsibilities of patients can avoid developing relationships with each other; 3) Staff members have no reason to share a treatment philosophy and often make conflicting rather than compatible responses to children; 4) There are few arenas for combined problems solving and treatment planning for individual residents, and 5) All significant decisions are left to top administrators. Garner believes that the departmental model simply fails to mobilize staff together around the residents that the institution is "organized" to serve [31].

Garner recommends that the supervisory function, which often remains with the department even when there is a team structure, should revert to the team. Team members have direct experiences with staff performance and the team is the most comfortable place to receive feedback—essential for growth for the team and its members. Garner witnessed many positive benefits with the change from a departmental to a team structure. All staff members came to feel more central to the treatment and more confident that good things were happening to patients as a result of team effort. Teams were able to respond quickly to new information that emerged from sharing, and address behavioral problems quickly while they were still minor. Because the staff was confident that team members were best equipped to handle crisis behaviors, there was less need for back-up staff. Elopement decreased, and children were no longer caught between staff members with conflicting opinions. The staff felt much more significant in the children's lives, a satisfaction that had previously been difficult when so many different professionals seemed to have a somewhat exclusive segment. As a result, staff turnover decreased. In the team model, as opposed to the departmental model, the administrator's role also changes. The administrator attends team meetings from time to time, and writes policies in the form of proposals to the teams. Staff members find these easier to follow since they have been asked to evaluate them beforehand. This also helps those closer to the action to help formulate policies [31].

The Total Team Approach, Team Primacy, and the Generic Team Approach

Some believe that the staff members' responsibility to both department and team keeps the team from operating in full capacity and often generates stress. In what has been called the Total Team or Team Primacy approach in residential treatment, teachers, social and child care workers form a team that becomes a department unto itself. The team's leader becomes the department head. Teams administer and supervise all members. Team members become accountable to each other, constituting a self-supervising and decision-making group [32].

The Generic Team approach in residential treatment goes even further in abolishing professional divisions. Departments are abolished completely. This approach stresses direct interaction in the milieu by all members; team members divide indirect responsibilities such as writing reports and evaluations. Persons with varying backgrounds (education, social work, and child care) are hired with one job title, receive equal pay and spend equal time with residents. Although they contribute their own expertise, such as family therapy, they work in other aspects of the program as well. The approach is based on the need to eliminate unnecessary professional boundaries by challenging team members to work together in assuming all responsibilities. It is based on strong beliefs that teams will work most effectively when all members have equal authority in the organization and equal opportunity to advance to team leadership positions. Krueger and colleagues conclude that although making such a change causes staff members to sacrifice their status, a hierarchy, and central control, it liberates their great human gifts to the children [32]

References

1. Kerlinsky D. Integrating interdisciplinary team-centered treatment. In: Hendren RL, Berlin IN, eds. Psychiatric inpatient care of children and adolescents: A multicultural approach. New York: John Wiley, 1991, 94–111.
2. Hulse WC, Schiffer M. The psychotherapeutic training of the team members and its influence on the team. American Journal of Orthopsychiatry 1960;30:63–70.
3. Toseland RW, Palmer-Ganeles J, Chapman D. Teamwork in psychiatric settings. Social Work 1986;31(1):46–52.
4. Gralnick A. The socially-oriented psychiatric hospital. International Journal of Social Psychiatry 1987;33(3):218–55.
5. Lewis JM. The organizational structure of the therapeutic team. Hospital & Community Psychiatry 1969;20:206–8.
6. Abramson JS. Making teams work. Social Work with Groups 1990;12:45–63.
7. Bernard SE, Ishiyama T. Authority conflicts in the structure of psychiatric teams. Social Work 1960 Jul;5(3): 77–83.
8. Krueger MA, Fox, RG, Sampson J. The generic team approach. Child & Youth Care Quarterly 1987;16(2):131–45.
9. Keliher MN. In defense of the interdisciplinary team and the role of the child and youth care worker. Journal of Child & Youth Care 1992;7(1):25–33.
10. Harty MK. Countertransference patterns in the psychiatric treatment team. Bulletin Menninger Clinic 1979;43(2):105–22.
11. Bowen WT, Marler DC, Androes L. Psychiatric teams: myth and mystique. American Journal of Psychiatry 1965 Dec;122(12):687–90.
12. Pruyser P. Religion in the psychiatric hospital: a reassessment. Journal of Pastoral Care 1984;3 8:5–17.
13. See reference 9.
14. Merkel WT, Pollard CA. Applying modern management principles to clinical administration of a behaviorally oriented inpatient unit. Hospital & Community Psychiatry 1987 Feb;38(2):152–9.
15. Butterhill D, O'Hanlon J, Book H. When the system is the problem, don't blame the patient: Problems inherent in the multidisciplinary inpatient treatment. Canadian Journal of Psychiatry 1992 Apr;37:168–73.
16. See reference 6.
17. Crawshaw R, Key W. Psychiatric teams: A selective review of the literature. Archives of General Psychiatry 1961;5:397–405.
18. Yank GR, Barber JW, Hargrove DS, Whitt PD. Mental health treatment team as a work group: Team dynamics and the role of the leader. Psychiatry 1992;55:250–64.
19. Modlin H, Faris M. Group adaptation and integration in psychiatric team practice. Psychiatry 1956 Feb;19:97–103.
20. See reference 8.

21. Peters CP. The inpatient treatment of severe personality disorders: the borderline spectrum. New Directions for Mental Health Services 1990;47:65–85.
22. Osborne OH. Issues in achieving effective professional alliances. Hospital & Community Psychiatry 1973 Apr;26(1):207–13.
23. See reference 18.
24. See reference 21.
25. See reference 3.
26. Rae-Grant QAF, Marcuse D. The hazards of teamwork. American Journal of Orthopsychiatry 1968;38:4–8.
27. Appelbaum AH, Munich RL. Reinventing moral treatment: the effects upon patients and staff members of a program of psychosocial rehabilitation. Psychiatric Hospitals 1985;17(1):11–19.
28. Green DO. Anti-therapeutic group processes: Potential dangers to the hospitalized patient. Journal for the National Association of Private Psychiatric Hospitals 1973;5(1):19–21.
29. Bettelheim B. Home for the heart. New York: Knopf, 1974.
30. See reference 15.
31. Garner HG. A trip through bedlam and beyond. Child Care Quarterly 1977;6:167–79.
32. See reference 8.

2. The Therapist/Administrator Split

This approach is variously called the therapist/manager split, the therapist/administrator approach, as well as the manager/therapist approach. Many early psychoanalytic institutions organized treatment so that the psychotherapist did not work with the patient's behavior. Goodrich believes that this therapist/administrator split serves many psychodynamic and sociodynamic functions. Problems from the patient's daily behaviors do not contaminate the psychotherapy session. The therapist can concentrate on what the patient says and not be distracted. The patient is freer to talk and to select the topics for discussion, and cannot distract from the therapeutic process by concentrating on behavior. The therapist can avoid numerous difficult and time-consuming relationships. When both the therapeutic and administrative responsibilities are taken care of, the staff can focus on creating a holding environment for the patient that will enable new social learning [1–2].

The manager usually meets daily with the patient to deal specifically with problems in living and behavior on the unit. In some settings, the manager will offer supportive psychotherapy. The manager also meets with the team to discuss problems, provide instructions, and directs specific adjunctive therapies. The manager also meets frequently with the therapist and uses this information to continue the ongoing reality-oriented, here-and-now therapy with the patient and supervision for the staff. In some settings, the manager will also have regular phone contact and conferences with the family. Cowan describes the manager's psychoanalytic function as a "constant object" for the patient, the person who sets limits, meets with staff and family, and orders privileges. The manager also becomes a constant object for the patient's distortions and can assist the patient in understanding these primitive mechanisms. Free of the burden of management and negotiations with staff, the therapist becomes more able to contain, decode and interpret in the psychotherapy session itself. Cowan warns that there are large groups of less severely disturbed patients for whom management might be countertherapeutic, infantilizing and undermining of self-esteem [3].

Indeed, the effectiveness of the therapist/manager organization may often depend upon the population it serves. Cohen and Grinspoon write about the manager/therapist split in the treatment of three antisocial female adolescents and ascribe their improvement to the firm, consistent stance of the administrator. Johansen describes the therapist/administrator split as helpful for the patient with borderline personality disorder. Patients transfer feelings from the parental relationship to the administrator, and the therapist is free to analyze this transference while remaining more neutral and reflective with the patient. Conrad and colleagues find the division of therapy and administration helpful for patients with eating disorders. While the nurse retains responsibility for handling issues of weight, bingeing, and dieting, the therapist is in charge of psychological factors. The nurse promotes new behaviors, helps the patient delay acting out behaviors, and teaches proper nutrition. This approach made it possible to use behavioral methods to deal with problematic eating behaviors and yet correct the underlying psychological disturbance. The plan came about after many turf battles between the nurses and the attending psychiatrist [4–6].

Levine and Wilson compare the organization of the psychiatric unit to the nuclear family. As with parents, there will be conflicts over privileges. The parental task of absorbing frustration and aggression inevitably rests with the person who makes decisions about privileges, and in the hospital program they describe, the unit administrator performs that function. Levine and Wilson see the nursing staff as "a nonfamily peer group" in that they help the patient develop more socially acceptable ways to interact [7].

Beck and colleagues describe several disadvantages to the manager/therapist split. The inevitable disagreements between the therapist and administrator weakened the consistency of the staff's attitude toward the patient. Nurses found it took much more time having to deal with both the therapist and the administrator. There was some evidence that patients were slow to learn what was therapy and what was administration. Many believe that the therapist-administrator split will produce serious consequences, and that excluding the psychotherapist from the decision-making process deprives the administrator of vital information. Greben writes that psychotherapy should not operate artificially in a vacuum. Separating therapy and management can lead to a natural resentment in administrators, who may see psychotherapists as unwilling to get their hands dirty, while the therapists in the ivory tower may come to believe they are the only ones who truly understand the patient and blame lack of progress to management errors [8–10].

References

1. Goodrich, W. Symbiosis and individuation: The integrative process for residential treatment of adolescents. Current Issues in Psychoanalytic Practice 1984;1(4): 23–44.
2. Harrison SI, McDermott JF, Chethik M. Residential treatment of children: the psychotherapist-administrator. Journal American Academy of Child Psychiatry 1969;8(3):384–410.
3. Cowan NN. The manager-therapist team approach. Journal National Association of Private Psychiatric Hospitals 1981 Spr;12(2):69–74.
4. Cohen RE, Grinspoon L. Limit setting as a corrective ego experience. Archives of General Psychiatry 1963;8:74–9.
5. Johansen KH. Separation of therapist and administrator in hospital treatment of borderline patients. Hospital & Community Psychiatry 1980;31(4):259–62.
6. Conrad N, Sloan S, Jedwabny B. Resolving the control issue on an eating disorders unit. Perspectives in Psychiatric Care 1992 Mar;28(3):13–18.
7. Levine I, Wilson A. Dynamic interpersonal processes and the holding environment. Psychiatry 1985;48:341–5.
8. Beck JC, Macht LB, Levinson DJ, Strauss M. A controlled experimental study of the therapist-administrator split. American Journal of Psychiatry 1967 Oct;124(4):467–74.
9. Greben SE. The multi-dimensional inpatient treatment of severe character disorders. Canadian Journal of Psychiatry 1983;28:97–101.
10. Silver D, Cardish RJ, Glassman EJ. Intensive treatment of characterologically difficult patients: a general hospital perspective. Psychiatric Clinics of North America 1987;10(2):219–45.

3. The Therapist-Manager

Bettelheim has always given the strongest human reasons for the therapist-manager, for one person to be involved in every aspect of the patient's life: he believed that the unity of treatment came from the person who took care of the patient and that the staff members struggle toward their own self-understanding by working through this process. This self-understanding became a motivation and the source of meaning. Jules Henry, an anthropologist, analyzed various organizational structures and related them to the psychiatric hospital. He described the structure of the Orthogenic School as a model of simple undifferentiated subordination. It was undifferentiated in that there were no departments. Subordination refers to the model of one director who is responsible for and directs the counselors' work. The counselors are therapists who are also responsible to attending to all of the child's needs. The worker's motivation comes from the potential for self-realization derived from the satisfaction of working so intensely with the children and at the same time satisfying an inner need to achieve autonomy. Henry contrasts this with the structure in other hospitals. While the way for advancement is often to become a supervisor (and thus to become more distant from patient care), workers achieve status at the Orthogenic School by becoming involved with patients. He describes the counselor as "internalizing the children," which is the school's ideal. Bettelheim believed that for very young regressed patients it was impossible to separate administrative and psychotherapeutic roles from caretaking. Treatment had to be based on satisfying their needs and then continuing from there [1–2].

The therapist-manager system was extremely successful at the Orthogenic School. In another treatment setting, which is not so simply constructed, it may present more problems. Staff resistance often occurs when the therapist takes complete responsibility for the child. Staff members always feel "on the line," as if the therapist is testing their competence. They can be confused about the therapist's theoretical stance and their own role in the treatment. They may suppress such doubts with their own feelings that they know much more than the therapist about what the child needs. Staff members who feel left out of participation and decision making can unconsciously collude against everything the treatment is trying to do [3–4].

The child's therapist is often a consultant for the staff, the person responsible for creating the environmental conditions that can energize and facilitate, the pivot around which treatment turns, with a stake in every aspect of the child's life. Noshpitz describes a structure where the therapist has the real authority to make all decisions about the child's life, but can do this only by participating fully in the child's environment. The therapist comes whenever the child is in need and works directly with the staff around all problems it has in relationships with the child. Cohen describes the ego weakness of the adolescent patient population and advises that the therapist function as a strong reality-oriented limit-setter during early treatment. Although this system may prove successful with children, it may not be as successful with other groups [5–7].

Gutheil believes that administrative transactions with the patient are as significant as psychotherapeutic ones and that successful clinical administration usually comes before successful psychotherapy. He argues that clinical administration and psychotherapy should be united within the same person. Indeed, administrative interventions may be the predominant factor in the patient's psychological growth. Administrative considerations should come before psychotherapeutic issues in treatment because psychotherapy cannot succeed without administrative stability. Administrative decisions may be constructively discussed in psychotherapy sessions. A mutual focus on these decisions are valid materials for the patient and therapist's investigation and an opportunity for the therapist to model problem-solving. This also means giving proper attention to behavior change as a sign of improvement. Gutheil and Grunebaum indicate that for severely ill patients, the clinical administration may be the only therapy. The decompensated patient may be helped only through verbal interventions that are part of clinical administration: milieu, medication, changes in status and physical space. Gutheil finds that the therapist can achieve both a therapeutic and an administrative alliance with the patient [8–9].

Peters, in describing the treatment of severe personality disorders, recommends that the inpatient therapist also serve as an administrator for the patients. This therapist needs to assess the patient's behaviors in the unit, process information from the team, and make administrative decisions. Ploye′ advises that when the therapist is also the patient's manager it is vital that the patient be shared with other staff members and that the therapist be willing to take opposition. The therapist-manager must adjust to the team's consensus even when it is difficult, respect staff judgments and feelings as much as the patient's feelings, and simply not expect other staff members to be an extension of the therapist. Ploye′ describes this consensus as important in the treatment center as it is for two parents at home when they make significant decisions about their child. Ploye′ finds, however, that the therapist-manager may end up being primarily managed by the team [10–11].

Organizing Treatment by the Integration of Theoretical Orientations

Treatment must also be organized so that the therapist's theoretical orientation is congruent with the treatment philosophy of the milieu. When individual psychotherapy is the primary form of treatment there are possibilities for disagreements between therapist and milieu staff. They may mistrust each other or fail to support each other in work with the patient. Blotcky and colleagues describe the staff members' insecurity when they wonder if the therapist disagrees with the unit's philosophy. They can perceive the therapist as threatening their competence as well as the quality of their relationships with children [12].

Frank and Gunderson studied two milieus. The first, which they describe as control-oriented, was based on the medical model and was designed for containment of disturbed behavior, the removal of symptoms, and short-term treatment. The unit discouraged regression and firmly set limits. The second, the insight-oriented milieu, helped patients toward self understanding and improved ego functioning. It encouraged open expression of feelings. They then examined certain characteristics of the therapists. They characterized the therapist's theoretical beliefs as reality-oriented or insight-oriented. They were either administratively involved or administratively uninvolved. They found that patients in the study were more likely to engage in therapy and remain in it longer if the therapist and milieu theoretical orientations were the same. However, even when the therapist and milieu staff's orientation did not match, if the therapist did not become administratively involved with the patient's care, harmful effects were not evident. Therapists who shared the treatment orientation with the milieu staff who also conformed to the staff's conception of a therapist's proper administrative role had the most success in engaging and maintaining patients in therapy. Milieu staff are most successful with therapists who share both theoretical and role expectations [13].

The staff of control-oriented milieus works best with therapists who share its beliefs, take an authoritative role in treatment, and will make decisions and support and implement administrative decisions. The staff of insight-oriented milieus works best with therapists who share beliefs, are willing to help the staff understand the psychodynamics of patients, and restrict their administrative decision-making to merely providing an overview of the patient. Although the authors caution that while the study indicated that there had been some benefit from having the therapist administratively uninvolved with the milieu, they don't believe that inpatient therapists can be uninvolved in administrative decisions [13].

ORGANIZING THE RELATIONSHIPS OF NURSES AND CHILD CARE WORKERS

Rindner discusses two models of organizing milieu management in a children's psychiatric unit. In the first model, nurses take responsibility for milieu management and supervise the child care workers. In the second model, child care workers manage the milieu and report to a milieu director. Nurses also work in the milieu but report to the director of nursing [14].

Placing both nurses and child care workers in the same department, as described in the first model, assures that they have the same treatment philosophy and policies. The nurse's actual direct experiences with patients are curtailed, however. In the second model, where both groups work side by side, nurses' time with patients is increased. Child care workers who demonstrate management abilities can advance in responsibility and may eventually be able to direct the milieu. The disadvantage of this model comes in supervision, since when persons are supervised by different department heads there can be confusion and splitting and a blurring of roles when two groups are performing similar tasks. For this model to work, there should be good lines of communication between nursing and milieu program directors [14].

THE PRIMARY CARETAKER

Selecting one person as the primary caretaker for each patient is not only helpful for the patient, but provides great satisfaction for the staff member. Although the needs of the patient come first, experiments can teach how staff members can best be organized in order to fully use their interpersonal abilities and maintain dedication. Primary caretakers are particularly important in child and adolescent inpatient treatment, both for the patient who needs that primary attachment and for the staff who experience fulfillment in providing it [15].

Habel and Biggs describe a child-ally system in residential treatment. The child care worker who becomes the child ally guides the child in relationship to all aspects of treatment and is the person who insures continuity across shifts and treatment modalities. The child-ally coordinates the treatment and records the child's progress. The child ally system carefully matches the staff members' skills with the children they are most likely to be able to help. Beyond coordination and recording, the most crucial function is to establish an attachment with the child, a relationship that can be used later as a form of influence and role modeling [15].

Population as a Determinant of Organization.

Some organizational models have evolved from the treatment of children and adolescents. The generic team approach and the team primacy models were developed in children's residential treatment. However, the therapeutic necessity of the primary relationships with children and adolescents should not be sacrificed in the name of a well-functioning team. Other models, such as the therapist/manager split, arose in psychoanalytic settings and may not be effective in short-term treatment. However, when a conventional plan does not work with special populations, such as with the borderline patient, or the patient with eating disorders, the organization of treatment should be scrutinized for a new arrangement of human resources that will be more effective.

References

1. Bettelheim B. Home for the heart. New York: Knopf, 1974.
2. Henry J. Types of institutional structure. Psychiatry 1975;20:47–60.
3. Blotcky MJ, Wiggins KM, Sheinbein M, Forgotson JH. The development of a therapist-staff alliance on a children's inpatient unit. Acta Paedopsychiatrica 1978;43:233–41.
4. VanderVen KD. Towards maximum effectiveness of the unit approach in residential care. Hospital & Community Care Administration 1979;1(3):287–98.
5. Cohen RL. The influence of child guidance practices on children's inpatient units. Journal American Academy of Child Psychiatry 1964;3:151–60.
6. Noshpitz JD. Notes on the theory of residential treatment. Journal American Academy of Child Psychiatry 1962;1:284–96.
7. Cohen RE, Grinspoon L. Limit setting as a corrective ego experience. Archives of General Psychiatry 1963;8:74–9.
8. Gutheil TG. On the therapy in clinical administration: Part I: Introduction and history: Administration and its relation to psychotherapy. Psychiatric Quarterly 1982;54:3–10.
9. Gutheil TG, Grunebaum HU. The teaching of clinical administration. Psychiatric Quarterly 1977;49(4):259–72.
10. Peters CP. The inpatient treatment of severe personality disorders: The borderline spectrum. New Directions for Mental Health Services 1990;47:65–85.

11. Ploye' PM. On some difficulties of inpatient individual psychoanalytically oriented therapy. Psychiatry 1977;40:133–45.
12. See reference 3.
13. Frank AF, Gunderson JG. Matching therapists and milieus: Effects on engagement and continuance in psychotherapy. Psychiatry 1984;47:201–10.
14. Rindner EC. Recruiting, developing and training staff for work in a multicultural setting of a children's psychiatric hospital. In: Hendren RL, Berlin IN, eds. Psychiatric inpatient care of children and adolescents: A multicultural approach. New York: John Wiley, 1991, 235–49.
15. Habel JC, Biggs TE. Child allies: A staffing technique in children's residential programs. Child Care Quarterly 1983–84;12(4): 272–7.

CHAPTER V

The Creation of the Treatment Environment

This chapter is about the challenges of creating a therapeutic culture. There is an implicit hope that the environment the milieu provides will be different from the world outside and that these differences will prove to be curative. The creation of this culture involves the translation of beliefs about mental illness into a viable treatment philosophy and an examination of the values that will be transmitted to both patients and staff. The therapeutic culture develops in a physical environment that conveys both clear and hidden meanings that will affect the residents' well being. Bettelheim emphasizes the significance of both the physical and symbolic messages of the environment. Melvyn Rose carries it further, attempting to create a magical experience, a "space apart" that will compensate for earlier emotional deprivation. These writers recapture the magnificence of the enterprise and inspire those who are usually grounded in everyday reality.

The writers discussed in this section are treated as if their work is still current, as if all of them worked at the same time in continuous dialogue. The dialogue is merely in print. The study of milieu management and therapy is not more than 50 years old and those who studied the hospital staff and organization in the 1950s built a solid foundation for future work. These early works, such as Greenblatt's edited volume, *The Patient and the Mental Hospital*, and Stanton and Schwartz's *The Mental Hospital* still make good sense today.

The therapeutic culture, philosophy and values influence the human environment, both staff and patients. The therapeutic results of the milieu should be measured by their effect on staff as well as patients. Regardless of the treatment model or philosophy, human relationships will continue to be the primary therapeutic force. The patients, the most important part of the treatment environment, are not discussed in a special section. No one can presume to speak for them. The best writing comes from the patients themselves, particularly the first-person accounts in *Schizophrenia Bulletin. Psychiatric Services* (formerly *Hospital and Community Psychiatry*) now also includes this valuable writing. Plum's review of 20 autobiographies of mental patients provides the kind of material that will be helpful for scrutinizing treatment [1].

There are two other sections covered in this chapter on the treatment environment. One reviews the attempts to study the therapeutic characteristics of treatment centers or ward atmosphere. The final section is an examination of the literature on partial hospitalization. Although partial hospitalization may not strictly be defined as inpatient treatment, it simply cannot be overlooked in any discussion of treatment environments.

1. The Hospital and Treatment Center Culture

The psychiatric hospital or treatment center create a culture which molds and shapes both patients and staff. Smirchich describes the culture as the "social glue" that holds the treatment center together and makes life there both predictable and stable. It determines what is important and what is not and creates a grammar of behavior. The treatment center's history, leaders, values and beliefs combine to create a culture. Values and beliefs are expressed in a special language and in legends, rituals, ceremonies and myths. The treatment center develops a personality, which transcends the people who make it up. At times it seems to function as a person [2–4].

Guiding metaphors often shape the culture's identity. Metaphors are not always consciously chosen, but evolve from the life, the leaders, and the residents of the treatment center. Redl consciously chose the identity and the name "Pioneers" for the children in a residential treatment center, an identity that seemed to inspire them. Dederich at Synanon created a kind of a family that resembled a preliterate tribe with a strong father figure dispensing justice and concern. The father figure was a role model with the old-fashioned virtues of honesty, sobriety, and a belief in hard work [5–6].

A family metaphor is comfortable for those who work in centers for children and adolescents. Boje and colleagues point out that a culture using a family metaphor will establish behaviors and rewards quite contrary to a setting where the metaphor is one of "empire builders." The family metaphor was helpful when psychiatric centers assumed the socializing functions of the family. Staff members often define their role as that of good parents. Symbolic roles can be unconsciously assigned to duplicate those of the family. Treatment centers often have avuncular psychiatrists, sibling relationships among patients, and symbolic father and mother figures. Meaningful life experiences bind this group together, as well as such daily family rituals as putting the "children" to bed at night. Patients and staff celebrate birthdays and holidays together. The living out of the family metaphor creates cohesion and a sense of belonging [6–7].

When both patients and staff enter the treatment center, their acculturation begins. They slowly take in its values and beliefs, find role models, discover individual identities, and become immersed in a therapeutic culture. As long as there are new patients or new staff, acculturation never ends. A group of new patients or staff too large be absorbed by the culture may form a counter-culture instead. "Antitherapy" leaders may arise, either staff or patients, who present alternatives to the unit's treatment approach [6–8].

The treatment center's culture has evolved to nurture sanity, but there may be times when it seems not too sane itself. The hospital culture is integrated around unconscious defenses and myths. Reality is often tenuous in its world of projection and counterprojection, transference, and countertransference. The treatment center can continue to be a self-validating closed system. Brent believes that systems often come to resemble their clients and describes how professionals can so identify with clients that they "blur the interpersonal boundaries" between them. Interpersonal tensions are probably higher in hospitals than in other settings. The input of psychiatric treatment centers—serious human conflicts—affects its culture. Caudill and Stainbrook describe the psychiatric hospital as subject to "mood swings of undetermined origin." The emotion of events in the hospital culture travels much faster than the cognitive knowledge about them. Hinshelwood describes the hospital's social milieu as a relationship network, with emotions as a "psychic substance" that flows from one person to another. The transfer of emotions may occur through projection by one person and introjection by another [9–13].

If the hospital culture can be said to develop a personality, it can also develop a personality disorder. When turmoil occurs, the personality can acquire paranoid or narcissistic characteristics. The staff may distrust people outside the group. In earlier days, this distrust often centered on patients' families. There may be counterattacks on outside systems that seem threatening. (In the last decade, managed care has become a natural scapegoat.) To escape potential criticism the institution may react defensively and thus be deprived of helpful information. In addition, there are often strong taboos against internal criticism with the fear that it will affect patient care. Harris, describing narcissistic features of hospital cultures, reports how a hospital can begin to create a "false self," with its staff spending as much time recording the treatment (in order to look good) than in treating patients [14].

The hospital culture must continually defend against the anxiety that comes from working with mental disturbance. Mohelsky describes the front-line staff as straddling two worlds, the world of mental illness and the world of health, with a need for boundaries to separate them. Rosenberg describes the hospital's social structure as primarily designed to meet unconscious needs of the patients and secondarily to maintain the defenses of the staff. Sacks and Carpenter believe that staff members often operate in a "pseudotherapeutic" mode to avoid anxiety-producing feelings, impulses and insights [15–17].

One way the staff defends against anxiety is to conceive of the treatment center as a dynamic entity that is powerful and superior to the persons who comprise it. Fenichel states that social institutions arise through the efforts of human beings to satisfy their needs but that these institutions then become external realities. This demonstrates what Berger and Luckmann write about the concept of reification—the paradox that humans create a world that society then experiences as something other than a human product. What Jeffers and Britton call the Myth of the Clinic refers to this reification. The Myth of the Clinic provides a barrier against the chaos that is just below the surface, a condition dramatically true in psychiatric hospitals. The staff feels overwhelmed by the magnitude of the task of curing the patient, but it takes comfort in knowing that it shares the responsibility with a great number of people. The great number provides security, becomes externalized or abstracted, somewhat superhuman, and the Myth of the Clinic evolves. The Myth of the Clinic serves as a defense against the burden of responsibility. The Clinic becomes greater than the sum of its parts. It diminishes anxiety and provides a sense of security. The Clinic will continue even if people change, so there is a feeling of stability. Having one's ultimate faith placed in the Clinic neutralizes conflicts and antipathies of individual staff members. Although one may dislike certain staff members, one can still have faith in the Clinic. The staff will often accept decisions that may be disagreeable because they are important to the "Clinic." The myth helps generate the staff member's commitment to something larger than the self and provides identity for members. This commitment helps staff members to perform everyday organizational tasks on the way to some grand scheme of things. The person attached to the Myth of the Clinic is carrying out the dictates of a higher order, which gives meaning to work [18–20].

The myth can be dysfunctional when responsibility seems to always be directed upward and becomes abstract. Menzies describes how anxiety causes nurses to project their burdensome responsibility to senior nurses and attribute or project their irresponsible impulses to junior nurses. They then tended to feel very dependent toward their superiors upon whom they had projected the best parts of themselves. The Myth of the Clinic, with its projection of responsibility upward can prevent staff members from having a sense of confidence in carrying out responsibility [21].

Myths, Rituals, and History

Myths, rituals, and history help to form and preserve the treatment center culture. The events that happen in the milieu become a part of the cultural history and will determine the meanings that the staff gives to later events as well as their emotional reactions to them. The center's history may come into prominence during periods of turmoil, giving order and meaning to conflicting events. The body of cultural beliefs established over time can organize and give meaning to the ongoing difficulties in the milieu. At the same time, this cultural transmission may produce what Levine calls the "fantasy residue"—enduring nontherapeutic ways of dealing with patients that have become habitual. Although the staff's irrational response to stress brought about these methods, they tend to remain active long after the specific conditions that prompted them have ceased to exist. As one example, Levine mentions the misuse of limit-setting to protect a professional image [22–23].

Experienced staff pass on their memories to newcomers, who will become the keepers of the center's history for the next generation. This process allows the center to use its history for understanding and controlling myths and traditions so that treatment can integrate the wisdom of the past. Rituals strengthen the values of a culture and their use helps the patients and staff know that the healing process continues. Ceremonies, for example, can bring attention to success in the culture [22–23].

One cultural myth prevalent in many treatment centers is the myth of uniqueness and superiority. The institution needs to defend its distinctive competence and ability to do its work in a special way. This myth establishes the confidence of new patients and the commitment of all. The myth states that the staff and patients are among the chosen few. This feeling of uniqueness, if successful, can establish what Almond calls "healing charisma," a sense of specialness that makes people believe that they can become what they would like to be. It is also the sense of specialness that lets the leader act dramatically and therapeutically, in the confident belief in an ability to heal others. In many rituals of the psychiatric center, the most frequently voiced word is "special." One article about treatment says it all: "A special being, doing a special job, in a special place" [24–25].

This feeling of specialness enhances everyone in the institution. Stotland and Kobler's writings on "Crest Hospital" describe this myth. In the beginning the staff believed that Crest had a pioneering approach to treatment, whereas in reality its treatment methods were probably similar to that in most other private psychiatric hospitals. When one feels among the special few, nothing should let the vision die. Staff enthusiasm can contribute to healing the patient. This sense of uniqueness also creates a belief that the "outside world" cannot truly understand the treatment center. This perception of an outside threat increases the group's attachment to an ideology. The staff can come to feel that they are special people doing important work against some opposition. Other rituals reinforce the feeling of specialness. The more rigorous and lengthy the selection process for staff, the more the new employee will feel a part of a selected few. Ceremonies for those who leave can highlight the "specialness" of each person. The feelings of uniqueness and superiority can become dysfunctional if they close off learning from other institutions, since an organization with too much investment in its own superiority will find it difficult to integrate new ideas into the system [26].

Without history or myths, values cannot be transmitted to the next generation. A rich mythology lies behind a transformative culture. The cultural mythology can be illuminated by listening to what staff members believe, reading materials published by the treatment center, and learning about the center's heroes and heroines, both patients and staff.

BELIEFS ABOUT PATIENTS

The cultural mythology will also affect the staff's attitudes toward patients and the patients' attitudes toward each other. For example, in most treatment centers, there is an inviolable belief that the patient comes first. There are varying professional attitudes about the patients' abilities to function. Kahne writes that nurses sometimes use great ingenuity to maintain illusions of normalcy about their patients with the hope that this will maximize their potential and become a self-fulfilling prophecy. Sacks and Carpenter write about the "pseudo-therapeutic" community whose staff subscribes to the belief that patients are capable of assuming responsibility and developing self-understanding while covertly functioning as if they were not. Although the unit may see itself as a group of adults, it operates on the unconscious assumption that responsible adults (the staff) and irresponsible children (patients) constitute the population [27–28].

Some professions and treatment centers have a stake in viewing the patients as seriously incapacitated. Novotny describes the countertransferential wish to see patients even sicker than they are. Exaggerating the patients' pathology gives full recognition to the difficulties of the work. Levine writes that certain psychiatric hospitals condone "crazy" behavior because this allows the staff members to view patients as so ill that they feel less personally responsible for their cure [29–30].

Treatment centers will differ in the division or boundaries between patients and staff. The division is wider in treatment centers that tolerate dependency and acting out and much narrower where peer pressure and individual responsibility are part of the treatment. Magnifying the differences between patients and staff will minimize the healing process that is available through identification. Perlman believes that this division prevents patients from developing a sense of self that will enable them to grow and puts an artificial space between patients and healers. Identification can be a therapeutic ingredient for both patients and staff. Both learn by choosing role models and hearing stories about exemplary staff or patients. Patients and staff with some experience are the culture bearers and role models for those new to the treatment center. Each institution has its share of what Perrucci has called "culture heroes" who become a potential source of aspiration for group members. The staff tells stories that emphasize the pathology of former patients when they were first admitted and the dramatic changes they made before leaving: "Horatio Alger myths." These stories not only help staff members and patients believe in the treatment center, but give patients hope that they too will join the ranks of the "cured." [31–33].

Leadership in the culture

The most powerful role model in the culture is often the treatment center's leader. The dramatic histories of treatment centers often tell of an inspirational leader with dedicated followers bringing a new ideology and treatment approach. After some success, the new approach may be reexamined and then replaced by a new ideology. Charismatic leadership can lead to treatment success. The leader's interactions influences the sense of identity and self-worth that patients and staff experience. The hope a charismatic leader instills protects the staff from the depression that often comes with the care of difficult patients. Gutheil and Grunebaum describe the leader as a kind of tribal elder, a repository of information, folklore, precept, and myth. The need for leadership springs from many conscious and unconscious sources and a desire to know that someone is in control in a chaotic world. Kernberg describes the leader as a "pseudopaternal merchant of illusions" who brings the group an ideology. Group members may want to merge with the leader and absorb the leader's power. Kets DeVries and Miller describe this need for oneness and security that comes from the protection of a good leader. The leader operates on the boundary between the unit and its social environment and becomes a transference object for the staff. The leader must understand how this social environment and all the elements of the treatment center interact and work toward integrating them. This integration can come about by developing cohesion. The treatment center's cohesiveness is critical in developing the positive impact the culture will have on the care of the group. However, if the staff sees the unit director as omnipotent, the success of treatment will become the director's sole responsibility and not a collaborative effort between patients and staff. If the staff perceives the leader as omnipotent and omniscient, it may in turn see itself as inadequate, immature and incompetent. Kernberg writes that this idealization may be combined with desperate efforts to extract knowledge, power and goodness from the leader in a "greedy and forever-dissatisfied" way. The leader's failure to live up to this idealization may finally result in devaluation or a search for another leader. There may be a shared fantasy of the leader as arrogant or not understanding or as ready to take revenge. When leadership is in decline in the treatment culture, Colyar writes that patients may fill the void by trying to dominate the group processes in a "bizarre" way [34–38].

CHANGES IN LEADERSHIP

Although a center with a strong treatment philosophy and orientation may function effectively with the change or loss of a leader, mourning, regression and instability often follow. Kaplan describes the death of such a leader, finding that an institution can mourn in the same way as a family. The institution can't easily replace a lost leader and yet replacement is essential to its survival. When morale seems centered in a single person, the leader, the staff seems unable to maintain its therapeutic aspirations. The staff group Kaplan describes had never been open to ideas and influences beyond those developed by the leader. It had strong feelings of loyalty and had built a coherent group identity in the image of its maker. All goodness and meaning had come from this leader, and with his death came the loss of meaning and a feeling of worthlessness. The treatment center Kaplan writes about was not able to work through this loss. A change in leadership may result in a crisis that is even more complex. If the transition is not handled carefully, regression may occur, complete with defenses such as projection and splitting by the staff work group. The person in the new leadership role is likely to become a transference object and become part of the regressive process [39].

Even temporary losses may be difficult. Persaud describes the results of a consulting psychiatrist's four-week absence from a unit. Eight of the 11 patients under his care developed disturbed behavior, although they had all had been stable for many months before. Of the other 11 patients on the same ward who were under the care of another consulting psychiatrist, only one developed similar problems over this time. Persaud speculates that the consultant psychiatrist, who was really rather distant from these 11 patients, somehow embodied authority. When he left, it seemed to have disappeared. His absence apparently symbolized this lifting of authority. The absent consulting psychiatrist had not left many definite patient management guidelines and instead had encouraged staff members to use their own initiative [40].

CHANGES IN THE TREATMENT CENTER

Although a change in leadership is always difficult, changes made in the treatment center's program often contribute toward its health. The culture of the treatment center produces growth and change, and in so doing must change itself. The treatment culture seems to need continual revitalization. New programs can generate excitement. Crabtree and Cox find that the most creative and meaningful periods of community life occurred when the program was developing, before there were few clearly defined routines. It was not merely the patient's experience in the program but the process of being a part of its creation that was meaningful. Patients who came along later felt that the program was imposed on them. They then changed the program again, with full patient participation and reestablished a feeling of excitement. Nathan and Slovak write that if a unit is designated as a "special" unit, and a program is new, different, or innovative, the unit will produce better results than other units in the same treatment center. Such units can develop extremely high spirit, although these superior results will also probably not last forever[41–42].

Greenblatt is one of the first to discuss the importance of change, describing it as challenging old, stagnant practices, mobilizing patients and staff and releasing energy. He finds that the culture develops strength through these successive trials to produce change. There is always a question of how to introduce change, since almost everyone in the beginning will resist it. He notes, however, that many who resist programs requiring new adjustments later show pride at having met the challenge. Greenblatt feels that to remain the same is to decline and that the search for something better is a never-ending process. Hirschowitz describes the homeostasis that often develops in the treatment center culture, comparing it to the homeostasis in family patterns. He describes the entry of a resident psychiatrist that disrupted the center's equilibrium by forcing a discussion of the center's ideology, making differences of opinion and tensions much less covert. This disrupted the "security operations" of the treatment center that had previously exercised control and managed to avoid conflicts [43–44].

Treatment Philosophy and the Hospital Culture

Love is not Enough, the title that Bettelheim chose for his early book on work at the Orthogenic School, refers to the need for a theory, careful planning, and a consistent treatment philosophy to support the loving care that will rehabilitate the patient. The treatment philosophy is a set of values and principles that will guide the staff in its work. It is composed of written policy statements or in procedures and traditions of the staff. A coherent philosophy will support the staff members and guide their perception and management of the problems they confront [45].

The treatment philosophy is built on beliefs about the causes of mental illness and how it should be treated. It will consider how staff members should help patients, how permissive they should be, and whether they should accept deviant or symptomatic behavior. Beliefs about the causes and cures of mental illness influence the staff's feelings about patients and ability to work with them. If staff members feel that a patient is bad rather than ill, they may feel punitive rather than understanding. This will only strengthen the patient's need to stay ill. Staff members may neglect treatment when they feel a patient's condition is hopeless. Their need to believe in what the treatment center is doing will always affect the treatment they provide. When they truly share a common philosophy, they will be able to create the stable environment that patients so desperately need [46].

Novotny writes that if the psychoanalytic hospital does not provide a firm philosophical commitment, physicians may simply have the illusion that they are carrying out psychodynamically oriented treatment when they are not. Then, when inconsistencies arise, work may simply continue in the name of eclectic treatment. This can result in what Novotny calls the "pseudopsychoanalytic" hospital. Even when there is an integrated treatment philosophy, how to implement it concretely is not always sufficiently clear. There may be no way to distinguish arbitrary interpretations from sound clinical judgment. Novotny believes, however, that psychoanalytic principles can translate into a hospital approach. There is a fundamental belief that if patients are not psychotic, their emotional illness can be modified by changing their interactions with others. Although patients at first recreate their earlier pathological life situations, their behaviors and relationships can be altered by special ego support and the development of insight that they receive from both formal and informal psychotherapy. Perry and Shea describe how psychiatric theory used in case conferences can serve an intellectual and social function for the staff. When the problems created by the patients' behavior are explained in terms of psychiatric theory and a treatment ideology, this reduces the staff's own stress and patients can become easier to manage [47–48].

The treatment philosophy in therapeutic communities for drug abusers is often comprehensive and explicit, embracing not only a philosophy of life but a prescription for personality change. In many treatment centers, members refer to it as the Concept, a belief system complete with sayings, mottoes, and jargon. Rachmann finds that such a belief system is helpful for confused adolescents and can give them a sense of meaning. When everyone in the program seems definite about what is right and wrong, the adolescent can gain a strong feeling of direction and purpose. A rigid or dogmatic treatment philosophy, however, can be harmful in that the expectations for conformity disrespect individual differences. In addition, Rachmann believes in encouraging adolescents in treatment programs to explore their own philosophical beliefs [49].

Colyar describes two dimensions of staff behavior influenced by the treatment philosophy. Empathetic staff behavior is characterized by emotional support and a caring response to the residents' feelings and behavior. Expectation behavior is task-oriented and focused on what the resident must accomplish. There is attention to structure, limits, rules and treatment objectives with reminders of consequences. The treatment philosophy will usually take both dimensions into account. A philosophy emphasizing the empathetic dimension may stress permissiveness and tolerance for symptomatic behavior, with the belief that this behavior will change once the resident develops self-awareness and self-acceptance. A philosophy stressing expectations will require adaptation to routine and compliance with expectations and the staff will be expected to establish behavioral goals [50].

The philosophy will influence not only staff but resident behavior. There will be more limit testing against a philosophy of expectations. A program stressing the empathic dimension will often face noncompliance from residents who refuse to become involved. Colyar finds that whether there is a clearly established treatment or whether it simply evolves (often in contradiction to the official philosophy) the residents will establish their own patterns of behavior. When the administration and clinical staff develop a treatment philosophy they are creating a group climate or tone for the resident population as well as the staff. The staff will need support, training and resources in order to manage behavior consistent with the philosophy [50].

There will always be a gap between a stated belief and actual practice. If the treatment philosophy is grandiose and unrealistic, it will breed staff cynicism. Ideology in the abstract can be rejected personally. To test these discrepancies, Rappaport and Zieger asked 336 staff members to rate hospital practices. One half of the group was asked to rate the program theoretically, as staff members, and the other half as if they were patients. More negative responses came from the group who rated as patients, regardless of their seniority, position or age. Bettelheim writes that the "soul" of the institution is not always in its philosophy and describes institutions with inspirational philosophies that were by no means therapeutic. He believes that the institution's soul is its philosophy only when it is carried out by staff [51–52].

Staff members will more willingly invest time and energy when their work is supported by a treatment ideology. Their involvement with such a belief system will allow them to make choices consistent with it and examine these choices for consistency. In this sense, it will ultimately increase the staff's autonomy. A treatment ideology helps staff members to invest in the goals of the treatment center, can create greater autonomy, mutual involvement in their work and greater work satisfaction [52].

Values

One function of the hospital culture is the formation of a consistent value system. Values are ways of thinking, feeling, and acting that are preferred in the treatment culture and communicated to new members. Redl speaks of the value system that "oozes out of our pores." The value system may include a basic philosophy of life, some beliefs about the origin of mental illness, how people get well, and what constitutes mental health. Part of the value system may be resemble that of the larger society, while part is unique to the treatment center. Some values supported by the treatment community will be explicitly stated and others will remain implicit. Implicit values may be inferred from pronouncements by staff members, the institution, procedures, and everyday decisions. Values are not just for the staff, but usually have meaning for patients, particularly in long term treatment. One simple shared value is the value of inquiry into the meaning of behavior. A shared set of values and beliefs will help patients face many of their problems. Some of these values will be translated into action. Many can be simply stated. Being open is good. Being responsible is good. Taking responsibility for others is good. Dependency is bad. Learn from the consequences of behavior. Adoption of the treatment center's values can lead to growth and change [53–54].

Almond and colleagues describe the assimilation of values in milieu therapy. In the beginning, the patients learned to talk about problems and share them with the staff and others. Later changes in values and behavior included confronting problems, learning self-soothing, and developing a sense of responsibility for other patients. Almond and colleagues believe that the patient's value change occurred because of the influence of a powerful ward culture and social structure rather than because of psychotherapy. Role-playing, too, may facilitate change by the process of identification and internalization. Patients begin to take up behaviors and values that are modeled by staff members they like. Perrucci describes patients as able to leave the hospital when they "speak the language" of the staff group. In other words, they have adopted the staff values and norms that have been transmitted through personal relationships [55–56].

Astrachan and colleagues studied behaviors in inpatient group therapy in order to learn whether patients were influenced by the staff's value system. They found that the treatment community's value system had permeated the patient culture. The group members had learned to give feedback, and be critical toward each other. There was stress on being open and being responsible. Patient-led groups reflected even the subtleties of the staff's emotional tone [57].

THE PATIENT VALUE SYSTEM

The most effective value system will be one that is not the staff's system but one that has been absorbed and has meaning for all levels of staff and patients. A shared patient-staff value system is not easily accomplished. Even when the patient's value system is congruent with the treatment community, it operates with considerable autonomy and its norms are not necessarily shared by the staff. Dimsdale used a goal profile questionnaire to study the goals of therapy on psychiatric units and found no significant correlation between patient and staff goals. Astrachan writes that some patients can become so deeply involved in the unit value system that a special patient value system simply does not develop. However, if a patient value system develops that opposes the treatment community values, patients are caught between systems, have divided loyalties and function less effectively [57–58].

LEADERSHIP AND THE VALUE SYSTEM

A charismatic and forceful leader can have a strong effect on the value system of the treatment community. In addition to custom and traditions, the leader's own values and way of operating will influence the values of the treatment center. Although new staff members will usually share many of the attitudes in the treatment community, they should quickly become aware of how they are applied in everyday situations.

STUDYING THE VALUE SYSTEM

Astrachan and colleagues studied values in the psychiatric setting and found that the assimilation of values depended on the kind of value given, the frequency and length of time of value induction, the directness or indirectness of the introduced values, the relationship of the staff to patients, and the extent to which competing values exist in the community. Research on value change must consider how central values are to the setting, how specific they are to the treatment center and how easily they can be generalized [60].

References

1. Plum K. How patients view recovery: What helps, what hinders. Archives of Psychiatric Nursing 1987;1:285–93.
2. Smirchich L. Concepts of culture and organizational analysis. Administrative Science Quarterly 1983 Sep;28(3):339–58.
3. Miyake S, Trostler RJ. Introducing the concept of corporate culture in the hospital setting. American Journal of Occupational Therapy 1987;41(5):310–4.
4. Dean JC. The treatment facility as a co-alcoholic. International Journal of the Addictions 1982;17(6):1091–8.
5. Redl F, Wineman D. Children who hate. Glencoe, IL: Free Press, 1951.
6. Bassin A. Proverbs, slogans and folk sayings in the therapeutic community: a neglected therapeutic tool. Journal of Psychoactive Drugs 1984 Jan-Mar;16(1):51–6.
7. Boje DM, Fedor DB, Rowland KM. Myth-making: a qualitative step in OD interventions. Journal of Applied Behavioral Science 1982;18:17–28.
8. Bloor MJ. Therapeutic paradox—the patient culture and the formal treatment programme in a therapeutic community. British Journal of Medical Psychology 1981;54:359–69.
9. Kahne MJ. Some implications of the concept of position for the study of mental hospital organization. Psychiatry 1962;25:227–43.
10. Brent DA. Systems which resemble their clients: the metatherapeutic role of the administrator. Administration in Mental Health 1983;11(1):57–63.
11. Kernberg O. Leadership and organizational functioning: Organizational regression. International Journal of Group Psychotherapy 1978;28:3–25.
12. Caudill W, Stainbrook E. Some covert effects of communication difficulties in a psychiatric hospital. Psychiatry 1954;15:27–43.
13. Hinshelwood RD. Social dynamics and individual symptoms. International Journal of Therapeutic Communities 1987;8(4):265–72.
14. Harris M, Bergmann HC. The narcissistically vulnerable system: A case study of the public mental hospital. Psychiatric Quarterly 1986–7;58(3):202–12.
15. Mohelsky H. Mental hospital and its environment. Canadian Journal of Psychiatry 1982;27:478–81.
16. Rosenberg SD. Hospital culture as collective defense. Psychiatry 1970;33:21–35.
17. Sacks MH, Carpenter WT. The pseudotherapeutic community: An examination of anti-therapeutic forces on psychiatric units. Hospital & Community Psychiatry 1974;25:315–8.

18. Berger PT, Luckmann T. Social construction of reality. Garden City, NY: Doubleday, 1966.
19. Fenichel O. Psychoanalytic theory of neurosis. New York: Norton, 1976.
20. Jeffers J, Britton N. Some necessary assumptions in private psychiatric treatment centers: the functions and dysfunctions of myths. Psychiatric Quarterly 1985 Spr;57(1):59–71.
21. Menzies IEP. A Case-study in the functioning of social systems as a defence against anxiety. Human Relations 1960;13:95–121.
22. Binder JL, Urist J, Looney J. The use of a ward's history in training psychiatric child care workers. Child Care Quarterly 1978 Spr;7(1):21–34.
23. Levine HB. The fantasy residue: an antitherapeutic force on the psychiatric inpatient service. Psychiatry 1982;45:262–70.
24. Almond RA. The Healing community: Dynamics of a therapeutic milieu. New York: Jason Aronson, 1974.
25. Traber J. A special being, doing a special job, in a special place: A fresh look at the institutional taking into care of children and adolescents. International Child Welfare Review 1987;61:22–36.
26. Stotland E, Kobler AL. Life and death of a mental hospital. Seattle: University of Washington Press, 1965.
27. See reference 9.
28. See reference 17.
29. Novotny PC. The pseudopsychoanalytic hospital. Bulletin Menninger Clinic 1973;37(3):193–210.
30. See reference 23.
31. Edelson M. The Practice of Sociotherapy. New Haven, CT: Yale University Press, 1970.
32. Perlman G. Some problems with the medical model. Journal of Urban Psychiatry 1982;2:31–7.
33. Perrucci R. Circle of madness: On being insane and institutionalized in America. New York: Prentice-Hall, 1972,117.
34. Guthiel TG, Grunebaum HU. The teaching of clinical administration: opportunities and problems of role ambiguity. Psychiatric Quarterly 1977;39(4):259–71.
35. See reference 11.
36. Kets de Vries M, Miller D. Group fantasies and organizational functioning. Human Relations 1984 Feb;37(2):111–31.
37. Oskarrson H, Klein RH. Leadership change and organizational regression. International Journal of Group Psychotherapy 1982;32(2):145–62.
38. Colyar DE. A model for conceptualizing variation in staff-resident behavior. Child & Youth Care Forum 1992 Jun;21(3):165–76.
39. Kaplan T. Death of an institution. British Journal of Medical Psychology 1991;64:97–102.
40. Persaud RD. The psychopathology of authority and its loss: the effect on a ward of losing a consultant psychiatrist. British Journal of Medical Psychology 1994;67:1–11.
41. Crabtree LH, Cox JD. Overthrow of a therapeutic community. International Journal of Group Psychotherapy 1972;22:31–40.
42. Nathan RJ, Slovak JP. The effect of change of director in a psychiatric inpatient unit. Journal of Nervous & Mental Disease 1976;162(2):113–8.

43. Greenblatt M. The psychiatrist as social system clinician. In: Greenblatt M, Levinson DJ, Williams RH, eds. In: The patient and the mental hospital. Glencoe, IL: Free Press, 1957, 317–23.
44. Hirschowitz RG. The maintenance of institutional homeostasis: a case study. International Journal of Social Psychiatry 1973 Fal;19(3–4):277–83.
45. Bettelheim B. Love is not enough: the treatment of emotionally disturbed children. Glencoe, IL: Free Press, 1950.
46. Mathai J, Taylor B. Staff perceptions of adolescent behaviour problems. Journal of Adolescence 1985;8:243–54.
47. See reference 29.
48. Perry SE, Shea GN. Social controls and psychiatric theory in a ward setting. Psychiatry 1957;20:221–47.
49. Rachmann AW, Heller ME. Peer group psychotherapy with adolescent drug abusers. International Journal of Group Psychotherapy 1976;26(3):373–84.
50. See reference 38.
51. Rappaport H, Zieger C. An assessment of staff complicity in attitudes toward the therapeutic milieu. International Journal of Social Psychiatry 1974;20(3–4):251–7.
52. Bettelheim B. Home for the heart. New York: Knopf, 1974.
53. Redl F. The concept of a "therapeutic milieu." American Journal of Orthopsychiatry 1959;29:721–36.
54. Tuck I, Keels MC. Milieu therapy: a review of development of this concept and its implications for psychiatric nursing. Issues in Mental Health Nursing 1992;13:52–8.
55. Almond R, Keniston K, Boltax S. Patient value change in milieu therapy. Archives of General Psychiatry 1969;30:339–41.
56. See reference 33.
57. Astrachan BM, Harrow M, Flynn HR. Experimental introduction of values into a psychiatric setting. Comprehensive Psychiatry 1969;10:161–9.
58. Dimsdale JE, Shershow JC, Klerman GL, Kennedy AM. Social press and its influence on psychiatric treatment goals. Social Psychiatry; 13(3):153–7.
59. See reference 12.
60. See reference 57.

2. The Physical Environment

Bettelheim warns that the treatment center should be designed primarily to serve the needs of patients, not to protect the staff or ease its anxiety. It must offer patients a comfortable, safe, nonthreatening and intelligible environment. When a psychiatric hospital is built or remodeled, the architect becomes a part of a therapeutic endeavor, attempting to understand its messages and interpreting them architecturally. Remen advises the architect to assume nothing and question everything. He describes the goal as simple one—to create a caring setting that will inherently feel good, be understandable and work easily for both patients and staff. The architecture of the hospital has always been guided by the medical theory and practice in effect at the hour of construction. Later modifications may be the product of changes in medical discourse. Prior notes that now that the patient has become the "client," and illness a "behavioral disorder," architects should no longer think about the psychiatric hospital in terms of beds. There is now a continuing emphasis on home-like settings with a stress on domesticity. An analogy to canopied birthing rooms in the hospital comes to mind [1–5].

The Conception and Messages of the Treatment Center

A guiding image of the treatment center can integrate the sensory messages that the patient will receive. Craig describes an image of the new hospital as a small town. The room represents the patient's house, the nearby alcove, the neighborhood, while the lounge at the end of the hall becomes the town square. Some writers use the metaphor of the body. Bettelheim believes the treatment center should be an attractive and secure shell giving protection while the patient discovers the boundaries of the self or should be a chrysalis for the emergence as a full person [6–7].

The center should have a unity, which is more than a sum of its parts. It must be compact enough to be understood and not so large that the patient feels insignificant. Kirkbride's 19th century psychiatric hospital, the model that served as a prototype for many U.S. mental hospitals, had grand halls and 17-foot ceilings. Although these buildings were designed to uplift patients, they also must have overwhelmed them. All who live and work in the building should be able to grasp its intelligible organization. Patients should understand how all the parts will work together to serve them. Bettelheim notes that this is important because different areas have special messages for patients. For one, a pantry near the kitchen will symbolize security. For another, security will be a window seat on top of a radiator. However, intelligible organization should not rule out architectural delight. Remen writes that any number of captivating "events" such as a fountain or a greenhouse where corridors intersect can offer gentle stimulation and comforting surprises [7–9].

Planning the Physical Environment

The architect must understand how psychiatric hospitals work, the types of mental illness and therapies, and the varying needs of different patient groups. There are many ways to learn this. The architect can form new ideas and change incorrect ones by visiting other facilities. Some architects spend days and nights in psychiatric hospitals, visiting staff and patients, assessing space needs, and thinking about features that will make the new hospital more comfortable. Both present and former patients provide valuable information. Remen advises architect and planners to meet with neighborhood groups to help to improve the hospital's inclusion into the community. Crosbie writes about the removal of a hospital's brick wall that faced the community after the neighborhood residents complained that it made them feel excluded. The wall was replaced by a metal fence that allowed viewing from both sides. This response to the community's wishes may have preserved the exterior from graffiti. The hospital can also be integrated into its context by echoing traditional and regional forms that are pleasing and noninstitutional, and by using indigenous building materials and familiar decorative touches [9–10].

Even though patient stays are shorter, the architects of the modern hospital still work toward making the building more like a home, thinking always about privacy and human dignity. This new home must be noninstitutional. St. Clair writes about window coverings as an example of this thinking. Although shades or blinds are the most efficient way to regulate light in buildings, patients usually prefer drapes because they feel more home-like and secure. The feeling of home and respect for the resident's individuality and privacy should be primary. Sanders writes about trying to give each Orthogenic School classroom its own character, although school rooms are usually very much alike. Each class was given a different flooring, wall covering, and color, and each conveyed a different feeling [11–12].

All parts of the building provide a message to those who live there, beginning with the front door and the reception area of the building. Well-scaled clearly defined entrances are welcoming. Entrances should not be monumental, obscure, or confusing. Remen finds that reception areas work best when they are not dramatic and when they provide a simple but understated message of reassurance. Reception and interviews of the newly admitted patient and family should be conducted in a living-room setting, large enough for the patient to establish a comfortable interpersonal distance from the interviewer. There should be many opportunities for privacy. These first experiences can help diminish some of the patients' fears [13–14].

The Arrangement of Space

The most basic decision in the arrangement of space in a new treatment center is whether the building should be a series of small living spaces or a unified whole: centripetal or centrifugal. Bettelheim found that the arrangement of the Orthogenic School, which unifies the residents' activities with the living space facilitates all interactions between staff and patients and adds comprehensibility to treatment. The cottage system, a centripetal system that provides small, family-like living spaces, has become an attractive alternative to a single institutional building. Bleeker and Frohn-de Winter describe a treatment center with independent units housed in home-like structures connected by corridors, patios and gardens [14–16].

Space is an active ingredient in social life. It can construct or constrain it. The treatment center's design must respect the significance of human spatial relationships. The architectural plan integrates territory, space, closeness, and comfortable distances. Patients who need to improve their reality testing, personal relationships and daily functioning will need spaces that will help them accomplish this task. They will need spaces to be alone as well as to be with other patients and staff. There should be intelligent plans about where the patient will spend private waking time or where time can be used most productively. Space should always be on a human scale. Rooms that are too close will not allow a natural flow of social interaction or transition form one social moment to another. Rooms that are too open will speak against the intimacy of social groupings [14–17].

Patients will suffer if they feel crowded or claustrophobic. Bettelheim notes that even in the most luxurious psychiatric hospitals, patients have a much smaller living area than the average family member, although most psychiatric hospital units are designed to be larger than medical surgical units. The same area that accommodates 30 to 35 surgical beds is only adequate for a 20-bed psychiatric unit. There must be good planning for areas where the patients will spend waking hours. If there is insufficient space and lack of intelligent planning they will want to spend more time in bed or wander aimlessly. Crowding can lead to elopement, runaways, self-mutilation, or suicidal behaviors by patients and to punitive measures by staff. The perception of crowding varies with the activity. People may be content to have a large number of people in a given space during social activities than during nonsocial ones. Light colors generally make the space look larger and dark colors smaller. Architectural design can focus interaction to specified areas on the unit and therefore use staff resources more effectively. At the same time, the patients' needs should remain primary. Bettelheim writes that if it is not clear for whose benefit architectural arrangements are made, decisions may be made exclusively for the staff's convenience [18–20].

The space that should not be forgotten is the space of the great outdoors. Psychiatric services have often been located on the top floors of high-rise hospital buildings, which enforces separation from other people and from everyday life, which cannot even be seen from the hospital windows. Comfortable visual and physical access to the outdoors should always be a priority. The design philosophy should incorporate the outdoors with outside views selected and framed for interest and variety. The residents will need generous access to a wide variety of enclosed and outdoor activities space. Indoor activity space is crucial in parts of the country with severe weather. It is often preferable for a therapist to take a disruptive child to a small gymnasium or activities space to release energy rather than using a quiet room. If younger patients are not kept involved in various therapies and activities, the physical environment is vulnerable to destruction [20–22].

Hospital corridors have long conveyed some feelings of threat and alienation, distorting space and time, producing strange shadows, and isolating patients in their rooms. There are ways to make these corridors seem shorter or wider. Each room entrance can be made interesting and individual by graphic designs. Paintings or murals can creative visual stopping places. Textured walls and floors can also make corridors more comfortable and inviting. In new buildings, rooms can be arranged so that hallways are interrupted by alcoves with seating areas where patients or staff and sit and talk [20–22].

Rooms

The traditional hospital was often laid out with a progression of patient bedrooms or double-loaded corridors, hallways with rooms on each side. Modern design allows grouping rooms in clusters, interspersed with connecting kitchens, lounges and space for physical activities. There is also the question of how many should be in a room, particularly for children. Bettelheim found that children in double or single rooms did not relate to others as quickly or seem to take advantage of what the school had to offer. Privacy could still be maintained when several children shared a room and they felt less isolated. Bettelheim writes that eight is the maximum number for a group room. Double rooms for adults can still allow privacy. They can be designed with built-in desk units separating beds and individual seating units. Sharing bathroom facilities is more comfortable if the shower is separated from the toilet and wash basin. Although in well-staffed psychiatric settings with good programming, patients will spend little time in bedrooms, individual areas are important personal territory and a source of refuge [20–23].

Giving the person as much control as possible over the physical environment will help to take away the sense of helplessness that comes from being a patient. Patients should be able to rearrange furniture, hang things on walls, and participate fully in any renovation projects. Lacy reports that patient groups developed color schemes and graphics for their units, and did much of the painting under the supervision of the maintenance department. This helped to insure their own care and protection of the unit. In another facility, where writing on the walls was a problem, a large white bulletin board in the community room now invites graffiti. It is simply painted white again at regular intervals. Bettelheim feels that the children can sense the feelings of the staff by the way their rooms are decorated and their freedom to make it and keep it the way they want it [20–23].

Color and Visual Stimuli

The environment becomes boring if all surfaces are alike. In psychiatric facilities there may be too many shiny, smooth, and cold surfaces made of metal, plastic, tile or vinyl. These materials may always be necessary for some purposes, but when they are used too much the effect is sterile and alienating. A varying sensory environment is vital for all human beings. Of all messages from the five senses, vision accounts for 85%. Color and texture create variety in the environment and texture also appeals to the sense of touch. Instead of plastic and vinyl, designers should consider fabric and carpeting. Although carpeting has a shorter life than tile, if chosen for durability and stain-resistance, it can last for as long as five years and has many acoustic, visual and tactile advantages. Variations in materials have communicative value. All materials evoke tactile and thermal images—smooth, silky, cool or rouge, abrasive and warm. Carpeting increases tactile and visual warmth. Color seems to be the simplest way to provide variety in the environment. Studies indicate that a room with differently-colored walls is visually more interesting. Color variation can be accomplished not only by the color of the paint but also by its value and strength—not just yellow and blue but light yellow and deep blue. The psychiatric setting should never be monochromatic, nor are fashionable colors necessarily appropriate. Distinctive colors can be used to enhance activities and spaces. Warm colors work well for areas associated with more active pursuits and cool colors for less activity. Juxtaposing warm and cool colors shortens and widens long narrow halls. Color may also be used to help patient and staff know where they are on the unit. Craig describes a treatment center that gives each unit an identifying color that is used on entrance walls and as an accent band for the nurses' station. This color also marks offices that serve the unit. An identifying color can also be used for departments. Medium to light colors reduce glare but it should be not be assumed that bright or deep colors should be avoided since they accent a color scheme. Window coverings should be chosen for contrast. Research on colors cannot guarantee a positive response from residents since everyone responds to color in an extremely personal way. Studies have made it clear, however, that most young children and older adults prefer bright colors. Because color preferences are so subjective, the use of color in bedrooms might be used neutrally, in ways to create an airy home-like feeling. Residents can then choose bedspreads and upholstered colored accents [20–24].

LIGHTING

The need for natural light cannot be overestimated. Natural light preserves the body's response to night and day. Clerestories, skylights, and internal courtyards can bring natural light to external areas. Sunshine should be let in wherever possible, although this will require design innovations to reduce the glare at certain times of the day and at various seasons. Artificial light should be used with sensitivity and color corrected so that it will not be too stimulating or confusing. Diversity is a keynote of an effective lighting pattern. There should be strong efforts to illuminate shadows that distort perception, and sources of light should be easily identified. People naturally walk toward light so it can be used to direct the flow of movement. Maximum brightness is recommended for dining rooms and pantries since patients seem to respond favorably to more illumination and bright colors in these settings. Fluorescent lighting, however, will not enhance the appearance of food or the dining area. Brightness is not always the only consideration, since a lower level of illumination with light fixtures and portable lamps are more appropriate than overhead lighting [23–24].

Sound and Smell

Sound and smell must also be considered in the psychiatric environment. Sound readings can be taken to learn which activities produce excessive noise so that soundproofing can be installed. The effect of pleasant sound must also be thought about. Courtwright and colleagues studied the effect of dinner music on 109 older chronic psychiatric patients and found that it reduced disruptive behavior at meals. An earlier study investigated the effect of recorded music played three times a day on a ward for disturbed patients. There were fewer violent episodes during the times the music was played. Several patients reported more pleasant moods which lasted throughout the day [25–26].

Bettelheim, who gives excessive attention to all environmental details, describes the smell of a place. He writes that if an institution smells "clean," it may be a cold smell, rather than a refreshing clean one. Bettelheim felt that patients would find the use of fragrant sprays to cover up odors as yet another deceit. He found the antiseptic clean smell of institutions even worse and less human, an "ominous" odor. It took time for the Orthogenic School to achieve its warm and friendly odor—an effort that required continuous washing, cleaning and redecorating so that the good smell would not be overpowered by one of dustiness. He described it as a combination of whiffs from the kitchen, air from outdoors, and from the those who lived there [27].

Bathrooms

Both Bettelheim and Rose have written about the care that should be involved in planning bathroom facilities for children. Bathrooms need to provide a message that the child is loved and respected. Bettelheim writes that bathrooms should make clear to the child that elimination should be enjoyable and free from shame. Rose feels that bathrooms should somehow establish a "therapeutic dialogue" with adolescents to help restore their injured psychological self. Teenagers need to be able to see themselves naked and feel secure in their nakedness. Their baths, a soothing light, and soft towels can help restore love for the body. They must enjoy and feel deserving of the pleasure that they receive from caring for their bodies in order to dissolve this physical self-doubt. Cotton and Geraty advise that bathrooms for children need to be considered high security areas with alarm switches since children are often alone there [27–29].

The Nursing Station

Practical factors such as sight lines influence the design of the nursing station but patients need reassurance that they are not constantly being watched. While it was once believed that patients should be observed at all times, it is now realized that many features designed to ease staff anxiety violate the patients' privacy and dignity. For example, the glass-enclosed nurse's station made casual and enjoyable interaction with patients virtually impossible. St. Clair's design solution was to install a softly curved wall of counter height without glass or barriers above the counter. Remen describes L-type configurations with nursing support tucked away at the vertices, still maintaining good slight lines. Architect Frank Gehry envisioned the nurse's station as a "soda fountain counter" where staff and patients could sit and pleasantly interact. However, none of the staff members agreed with the concept since they were desperate for a private glassed-in space where they could relax and not be heard. Had they had a private staff lounge, this might not have been necessary [30–33].

Other Physical Amenities

The patient lounge should be designed for varying activity, with moveable furniture, areas for games and places available for TV and conversation. Recreational spaces might also be combined with the occupational therapy area with electronic games and ping pong. Equipping the stereo with headphones for individual listening will expand the music room's use. An exercise room on the unit will be very helpful for those patients who are confined and will provide a message that physical health is also an important part of the total person. Small dining areas might also be provided for patients, with small kitchenettes and enough facilities to allow patients to cook and bake. Electrical power in these areas can be key-operated to insure staff supervision. There are many advantages in encouraging patients to make food and dine in a noninstitutional fashion [34–35].

Furniture

Furniture in psychiatric environments is best provided by a combination of built-in furniture and modular units. Built-in furniture can shape each person's private space in a shared bedroom. A standard size for the units, drawers, and doors can make replacements easy and inexpensive. Patient rooms with built-in beds, desks and seating provide safety and make cleaning easier, and there can be many ways to individualize each room. Loose cushions can be arranged for a couch, stacked on a built-in bench, or used as floor pillows on other occasions. At the Orthogenic School, patients were given a selection of colors, materials and pieces of furniture. The finite number of selections eliminated distress and confusion over having too many choices [36–37].

Modular units are recommended for furnishing the lounge. Since couches seem to encourage lying down, modular pieces that usually form a couch can be divided into sections or grouped in various formations appropriate for all activities. The choice of furniture will also depend on the age of patients, since younger patients prefer lower seating and soft cushioning while older patients need stronger back support, arms on chairs, and higher seating. Furniture creates social spaces, liveliness and animation. Even small changes in furnishings and furniture arrangement can have a therapeutic effect. Many studies have shown that the arrangement of furniture can increase social interaction. Conversational clusters, with chairs around small tables make interaction easier [36–39].

The environment is made as home-like as possible. This often means a choice of wood over plastic; soft upholstered furniture and cushions can provide a feeling of comfort and domesticity. Wood furniture that is sturdy and difficult to break, such as butcher-block furniture, can often be used. Another alternative for children and adolescents in many living areas is carpeted platform seating with pillows, since they don't always use seating in a conventional fashion. Wood remains a good choice for tables. It can be repaired when chipped or scratched. Plastic laminate seems acceptable for shelves and storage pieces in bedrooms. Maintenance must be considered in planning the floor covering, but esthetic factors such as color, texture and pattern are also important. Hard-surface flooring is suitable for areas of heavy circulation and carpeting for bedrooms and residential living areas. A large part of the wall in each room can be specially designed as a bulletin board, where posters, photos, schedules, and pictures can be hung, protecting the remainder of the wall from nail holes and tape. Plants will benefit every setting. Research has documented nature's great contribution to human well being, and a profusion of plants is an inexpensive way to begin [36–39].

Varied Populations

Research may finally indicate what environments might be most beneficial for solving different problem behaviors, such as apathy or violence. There is available information on the varying residential needs of adults, children, and adolescents. Geriatric patients will benefit from optimistic settings and great care must be taken in designing for diminishing physiological states and reduced mobility. Patients who have lost vision and hearing will need a maximum of environmental reinforcement. Lighting for geriatric patients should be at higher levels and strong colors should mark where floor and walls meet. Glare should be eliminated from large surfaces [40–41].

Treatment Centers for Children

The treatment environment for children should provide a welcoming, encouraging, and secure haven. Cotton and Geraty describe environmental planning for a 12-bed children's unit that included six bedrooms, a living room/activity room, kitchen and dining room, two quiet rooms, nursing station, and administrative offices. As each space was planned, clinicians described the kinds of behavior that would take place there, the kinds of behavior the treatment approach would prescribe for the space, and, significantly, the kinds of behaviors that should be discouraged in that space. These discussions enabled the architects to fully understand the behavioral and psychological requirements of each space. They then converted these requirements into design ideas, which the unit staff, the patients and their families then reviewed. Cotton and Geraty describe this process as similar to the medical model, progressing from observation, to diagnosis to prescription, and then to treatment [42].

They documented their combined thinking in a design log that translated theoretical treatment principles and patient needs into architectural concepts. The log documents the clinical reasons, behavioral and design requirements for each decision. With this format, everyone could review decisions and the reasons for them at each stage of the process. Maintenance representatives also participated in the design process, helping to advise on the choice of materials. This participation often brought about agreement on the selection of "warmer" materials, such as carpeting or cloth rather than vinyl, which might have been easier to maintain [42].

Cotton and Geraty describe the treatment messages for a new unit. It should provide a setting that can accept psychological difficulties without avoidance and despair. It should give a sense of firm external controls that could be adapted to the needs of patients as their capacity to use internal controls vacillated and redirect disturbed behavior into more adaptive behavior. It should support all levels of development and provide opportunities for both peer interaction as well as private moments [42].

Many of the walls of the unit were bulletin boards displaying the children's artwork. Spontaneous, timely art creations seemed the perfect substitute for permanent murals. Happy images were not used as room decorations, given the contrast between them and the way children often felt. The paint schemes, however, did communicate positive messages, with strikingly different color schemes far from any institutional connotation. Quiet rooms were painted in warm tones, to encourage a change of mood. The quiet rooms themselves were designed to be very safe with tamper-proof screws, carpeting glued under nailed wooden baseboards, an absence of pipes or throwable objects. They were small and cozy, with a carpeted window bench, and a window looking out on a pleasant scene [42].

The selection of durable furniture and materials anticipated destructiveness. There were short and interrupted corridors. Loose objects in the living or play rooms were soft or too heavy to throw. Children could make "swearing boards" to write on in their room, and were also given the option to use the quiet room whenever they needed it [42].

SAFETY

Designing a safe environment requires knowledge of the severity of mental illness and the levels of risk from various patient groups. In order to prevent harm to self and to others a treatment center may require locked units, seclusion rooms, or short-term intensive care environments. Windows are a primary hazard, particularly in multistory hospitals. Remen writes that security screens with their message of incarceration are not recommended and that Lexan plastics should not be used because of their high smoke production during fire. Polycarbonate glass laminates provide exceptional strength and a normal appearance. The kind of mirrors used in bathrooms and the best light bulbs that can be safely installed must also be considered [43].

Seclusion Rooms

Seclusion room design must insure easy observation and safety. The walls should be made of durable material that will not splinter or fragment, without moldings or free edges. They should be a clear, definitive color, not white or gray. Softer surfaces should be considered for all parts of the room, although there should be no suggestion of a "padded cell" kind of environment. There are damage-resistant materials available that can still be comfortable. The room can be lined with heavy duty industrial carpeting, tight-weave low-pile carpeting or washable synthetics such as nylon with jute backing. Even the wall panels can be wrapped in carpeting before they are installed or carpeting can be applied over a raised platform to make a bed [44].

Ceilings should be too high to reach, with lighting, heating and cooling openings safely located. If a high ceiling is not possible, a lower ceiling should be solid, not tiled. The room will usually need individual controls for heating and cooling. Lights should be inaccessible and out of reach and not excessively bright. The door should have an unbreakable window for observation of the whole interior. A window to the outdoors provides a view, regulates day and night rhythms and supplements artificial lighting. Although it may be updated by later writing, Gutheil's 1980 article provides detailed information about seclusion room design [44].

Cotton and Geraty write that quiet rooms in the children's unit should be used for multiple purposes so that they will not just signify "bad behavior." Staff can use the room for interviews and paperwork. Children can be free to use it for quiet games, play, reading or napping. One of the two quiet rooms was placed next to the director's office, separated by a transparent wall. This allowed the child to curl up on a bench and watch the director at work [45].

The design of quiet rooms affects behavior in them. Glod and colleagues report on the redesign of a quiet room for hospitalized children. The following changes were made: changing the white walls to a pastel color, carpeting the vinyl floor, and painting a picturesque mural on the wall. Total aggression rates for children placed in the renovated quiet room were 45% lower, and initial aggression scores fell by 50% during the first 5 minutes in the renovated quiet room compared with 20 minutes of placement in the standard room. This preliminary report demonstrates that changes made in quiet rooms can help to calm aggressive and agitated children [46].

PREVENTING DAMAGE AND DESTRUCTION

Bettelheim believes that the attractive surroundings created for children will safeguard against deliberate or careless destruction. Patients begin to take pride in their surroundings and want to take care of things entirely on their own. Remen writes that poorly conceived buildings invite destruction and will be abused. When damage occurs, repairs should be carried out immediately. Rivlin and Wolfe warn of a self-perpetuating quality about destruction. Children prone to aggression will feel stimulated when they see damage that goes unrepaired. When the children know that repairs are being made, they can develop self-control and more responsibility, and may even join in the effort [47–49].

Planning for Changes

Even when the treatment center is old, small changes can be made to benefit the environment. Gutkowski and colleagues describe making a change in hospital entrances to signify a closer connection between the hospital and its neighborhood. The hospital, which had two patient entrances, was remodeled to have five additional doorways. Four were to the main hospital grounds and three connected the surrounding street with other parts of the hospital. One new entrance led to the garden. The new entrances and the opening of the doors had great importance for staff and patients. It helped the patients to know that treatment did not mean the loss of freedom. The entrances also clarified the individual identity and therapeutic values of each unit [50].

A cardinal rule in contemporary planning for treatment centers is that the building will probably have many futures. Change will be needed in the course of time, to adjust to new methods and changing length of treatment, expanding or diminishing populations. Change can not always be anticipated. Crosbie's article on Frank Gehry's design for an adolescent psychiatric center vividly demonstrates how impossible it may be to design a psychiatric hospital for future years. This center is a case study in how changing psychiatric theories and health insurance affect architecture. Gehry designed the center in the middle 1980s for the long term care (6–9 months) of emotionally disturbed adolescents. He conceived it as a "therapeutic village, a miniature community built as a progression of spaces that patients would occupy as they continued to improve." By the time the building opened, however, the length of stay allowed was so restricted that there was no opportunity for progression. The vision of the architecture of the building as an integral part of the therapeutic process was not realized [51].

The well-designed physical environment provides visual stimulation and pleasure and helps the resident make sense of the living space. The good environment is one that requires little attention to understand. The environment must be created on a human scale that does not intimidate but relates its physical whole to the parts and makes the person the clear measures of all things. Although large rooms may have high ceilings, they will also need signs and symbols of intimacy and protection so that residents feel comfortable. The physical environment of the treatment center will have both clear and hidden meanings that will influence the residents' life. The psychiatric center is an emotionally charged environment and every object can carry a symbolic action that could be uniquely meaningful to the patient [52].

References

1. Bettelheim B. Home for the heart. New York: Knopf, 1974.
2. Sanders J. Culture and residential treatment. Residential Treatment of Children & Youth 1993;10(3):37–48.
3. Remen S. Signs, symbols, and the psychiatric environment. Psychiatric Hospital 1991;9(2):113–8.
4. Remen S. Planning psychiatric hospitals—human design considerations. Psychiatric Hospital 1987;18(1):11–6.
5. Prior L. The architecture of the hospital: A study of spatial organization and medical knowledge. British Journal of Sociology 1988 Mar;39(1):86–113.
6. Craig JL. Goal of West Campus planners: Achieve comfort, human dignity. Menninger Perspective 1980; 27–31.
7. See reference 1.
8. Fort JP. Editorial: Buildings. Psychiatric Hospital 1987;18(1):7.
9. See reference 4.
10. Crosbie MJ. Critique: Village Not: The unfulfilled promise of Yale's Psychiatric Institute. Progressive Architecture 1993 Jun;100–3.
11. St. Clair R. Psychiatric hospital design. Psychiatric Hospital 1987;18(1):17–26.
12. See reference 2.
13. See reference 4.
14. See reference 3.
15. See reference 1.
16. Bleeker JAC, Frohn-de Winter ML. The principle of separate responsibility in clinical psychiatric practice. Psychiatrica Clinica 1981;14:189–95.
17. See reference 5.
18. Wax D. E. Humane ecological perspectives. Child Care Quarterly 1977;6(1):51–60.
19. Whitehead CC, Polsky HH, Crookshank C, Fik E. Objective and subjective evaluation of psychiatric ward design. American Journal of Psychiatry 1994 May;141(5):639–44.
20. See reference 1
21. Lacy M. Creating a safe and supportive treatment environment. Hospital & Community Psychiatry 1981 Jan;32(1):44–7.
22. See reference 6.
23. See reference 4.
24. See reference 11.
25. Courtwright P, Johnson S, Baumgartner MA, Jordan M, et al. Dinner music: Does it

affect the behavior of psychiatric inpatients? Journal of Psychosocial Nursing 1990 Mar;28(3):37–40.
26. Michel DE. A study of the sedative effects of music for acutely disturbed patients in a mental hospital. Unpublished masters thesis, University of Kansas, Lawrence, 1950.
27. See reference 1.
28. Rose M. Treasure Island: the metamorphosis of deprivation and injury in the residential setting. Residential Treatment for Children & Youth 1992;10(2):75–87.
29. Cotton NS, Geraty RG. Environmental planning for a 12 bed psychiatric unit for latency age children. American Journal of Orthopsychiatry 1984;54(4):624–36.
30. See reference 11.
31. See reference 19.
32. See reference 4.
33. See reference 10.
34. Gershon HJ, Voorheis H. Planning and design considerations for general hospital psychiatric units. Administration in Mental Health 1984 Spr;11(3):205–12.
35. See reference 6.
36. See reference 1.
37. See reference 11.
38. See reference 21.
39. Devlin AS. Psychiatric ward renovation. Environment & Behavior 1992 Jan;24(1): 66–84.
40. See reference 19.
41. See reference 4.
42. See reference 29.
43. See reference 4.
44. Gutheil TG, Daly M. Clinical considerations in seclusion room design. Hospital & Community Psychiatry 1980 Apr;31(4):268–70.
45. See reference 29.
46. Glod CA, Teicher MH, Butler M, Savino M, et al. Modifying quiet room design enhances calming of children and adolescents. Journal American Academy of Child & Adolescent Psychiatry 1994 May;33(4):558–66.
47. See reference 1.
48. See reference 4.
49. Rivlin LG, Wolfe M. The early history of a psychiatric hospital for children. Environment and Behavior 1972;4:33–72.
50. Gutkowski SI, Ginath Y, Guttmann F. Improving psychiatric environments through minimal architectural changes. Hospital & Community Psychiatry 1992 Sep;43(9):920–3.
51. See reference 10.
52. See reference 3.

3. The Symbolic Environment

The treatment center is alive with meaning and there are times when the meaning of the great enterprise becomes explicit. Lives depleted must find meaning again. Melvyn Rose of Peper Harow is a writer who seems most aware of the need to create meaning and is the most successful in doing it. Rose writes that the symbolic environment can provide the means for residents to become absorbed in the community. Those who create the symbolic environment usually have an appreciation of the unconscious, as both Rose and Bruno Bettelheim do. They both believe that the treatment center environment must compensate for earlier deprivation. Rose describes this as providing maternal care, or as giving the emotional security of a primitive tribe. Rose describes the treatment center as restoring a golden childhood to those who never had one and giving the resident powerful messages about self-worth. Edgar refers to this as the myth of symbolic compensation. Bettelheim believes that children can finally develop mastery over the forces in their lives because unconditional gratification of their basic needs is available to them at all times [1–3].

Although adults may design the surroundings for treatment, it is the children who bring them to life. The residents create their own symbolic meanings for the physical environment—such as secret, cozy places for intimate talks. Bettelheim describes how children found symbolic meaning in the circular sunken pool and sandbox at the Orthogenic School, treating the circles as nourishing breasts. Those who live in the physical surroundings will find much more meaning than conscious planning allows. The ordinary experiences of life, such as eating or taking a bath, become symbolic forces in the treatment of the child. Bettelheim, for example, describes the child's bath as a way to change the image of the body and develop pleasure in the sense of touch. Such corrective sensations originate in being able to take a bath undisturbed [4–5].

The New Resident and the Creation of a New Experience

Rose believes that those who come to the treatment center should receive the promise of a new experience, more intense and meaningful than ordinary life. He describes the new resident as emotionally depleted, with little energy to invest for future rewards. The experience must be so dramatic that it jolts the newcomer out of habitual expectations and negative experiences. Moreover, this first perception needs to be recalled over and over again, so that it remains alive, as a contrast to those earlier negative expectations. It can continually provide the message that this new experience heralds the beginning of a new life [6].

What are some of the differences that the new resident may find at a place like Peper Harow, what Rose calls a "space apart." The new resident must know that the center is there to serve the child, not the family or those who arranged placement. At Peper Harow, each resident's framed photograph is hung in the hall with great care. The newcomer can sense affection among members of the group or notice that unpleasant behaviors are not immediately condemned. Bettelheim warns against giving the new resident a hearty welcome. The newcomer is not ready for such a greeting and may find it insincere. The newcomer does appreciate being taken around and shown where everything is, being helped to feel at home and to understand how everything works together. The resident must also feel free to explore every nook and cranny at leisure. Menses and Durrant show how the introduction of the new resident can begin to frame everything that will happen in treatment. Adolescent residents in the treatment program they describe are introduced as having come to get rid of some "bad habits" that have been "pushing them around." At Peper Harow, the present residents will show potential residents, parents and social workers around. This gesture alone begins to create the feeling that the place belongs to children, not to adults. It is also the child or adolescent who will make the final decision to come. When offered a place after the initial interview, the adolescent is asked to write a letter, to provide a written commitment to the community's task. This is a new idea for the adolescent, being given a choice about what to do. Since the adolescent's life is taken seriously at Peper Harow, the expectation is that all who live there will take it seriously, by choosing to engage in the mutual task of changing lives [6–8].

FOOD

Food is an excellent example of how the ordinary can be invested with great symbolic meaning. Eating and being fed are synonymous with feelings of love and security. Bettelheim writes that at the Orthogenic School there was hardly a time when one child or another was not eating. Children can experience an abundance of food as an abundance of all good things and begin to feel secure. Deprived children will experience food as a symbol of all pleasures, not just nourishment. Food can be a symbol of having all basic needs fulfilled, even if they were not in the past. Rose describes the dining room as providing an atmosphere that gives the residents the pleasurable feeding experience they might have missed in infancy. This sense of abundance is so vital that Rose indicates that the children may even need to waste food to be sure there will always be enough [9–12].

Food not only nourishes but also stimulates the visual and auditory senses while providing oral and gastronomic pleasures. Rose finds similarities to the pleasures of feeding in babyhood, and says that nose, fingertips, eyes, and ears are busy reading the messages that pass between mother and child. Bettelheim feels that meals can give the children the infantile pleasures they so desperately need but can't really request. Food can restore security in times of stress, and demonstrate that satisfaction is available. Both Bettelheim and Rose write about having snacks and food continuously available for the children, providing much more than nourishment, a symbol of all pleasures. However, some children have had negative experiences with food. Many have had food allergies; others may fear that food will poison them. Bettelheim writes that seeing staff members eat the same food reassures the children. The school prints weekly menus so the children will know there will be enough to eat and food that they like [9–12].

Food brings people together when nothing else can and serves as a great socializer. The preparation and serving of food in the treatment center can add to the therapeutic atmosphere for children, families, and staff. Rose describes the dining room as creating the experience of good mothering and writes about special Sunday breakfasts at Peper Harow that last all morning. Religious and ethnic rituals involve the preparation and eating of special foods, a well as the denial of others, to demonstrate beliefs. Rose writes of the many great feasts at Peper Harow, astounding occasions that transform the dining room into various fairy tale settings [9–12].

History, Stories, Naming, and Slogans

The new resident has neither a sense of belonging nor a proud history. The treatment center can often fill this void. Edgar describes Rose's ability to create myth at Peper Harow. Names, for example, can be extremely significant. Names can be chosen to symbolize growth, hope, the change in identity. Bassin writes about the naming of and the philosophy of Phoenix House, a successful therapeutic community for drug abusers. The name was derived from the Egyptian myth of the great bird that destroyed itself by fire and rose again from its own ashes. It symbolizes the belief that those who destroyed their lives by drug addiction can also rise from the ashes of their own defeat and take their place in society. Rose changed what was once called the "Approved School" to Peper Harow, an Anglo-Saxon place name. The new name provided the community with ancient and historical roots, and created a psychological place where roots could be found. This link with a historic past gave adolescents without roots a sense of secure belonging. There may be legends that are passed on through the years—stories of early struggles, legendary staff members, stories about residents, their mischievous tricks, and their successes. Such stories give a sense of unity to all who live there. The name of the treatment center, the stories of all who have lived and work there can write a sacred story that creates an intensity of community and makes everyone in it feel special [13–14].

Rose describes how Peper Harow was personified, how residents seemed to relate to the place as if it were an actual person. For some deprived adolescents it may initially feel safer to relate to a symbolic community rather than to a single adult. The community becomes a group ego and the feeling of belonging creates an emotional participation. Names given to the staff members at Peper Harow are also carriers of meaning. A resident's primary staff member might be called "the personal member of the staff," or was also called the adolescent's "guru" throughout the program. Both terms foretell how special the relationship will be [14–15].

Statements of belief, proverbs, folk sayings, and songs can help to create identity and cohesion. Bassin writes about entering a treatment center with a large life preserver on the wall emblazoned with the words "hang tough." He soon realized that it was an important slogan in this therapeutic community for drug abusers. Such slogans, if they speak directly to the residents' experiences, become symbolic mechanisms for strengthening social ties and building cohesion in the group. Intense group identity has been described as one of the forces that can help a person break the drug habit. Bassin mentions the serenity prayer, as well as some of the slogans and proverbs written on the wall in places where Alcoholics Anonymous (AA) meets, such as "One Day at a Time, "Let Go and Let God, "Call Your Sponsor before, not after You Take the First Drink." Zeitlyn cautions, however, that the use of slogans increases the power of words to distort reality. The members of the therapeutic community must constantly scrutinize what they are really doing [14–16].

RITUALS AND CELEBRATIONS

Rituals and celebrations intensify the meaning of life at the treatment center. There are special times when the residents' lives are celebrated and when the values of the treatment center are stated most clearly. Edgar refers to the rituals and celebrations at Peper Harow as a "calendrical structuring of events" that provides anticipation and excitement as well as predictability and stability. Parsons and Imhof write about the celebration of the Field Day in day treatment. It eventually became a Festival Day, complete with displays of the children's schoolwork, yearbooks highlighting each child's years complete with autographs, favorite drawings, reports about favorite foods and activities. The ritual created a transition for the children, a nostalgic review of the past and a therapeutic focus for a new beginning. The staff soon discovered, however, that the preparation for festival day had become an obsession that overshadowed the other work of the center. This high-pressure celebration was then changed into a low-key recognition ceremony and lunch. Each child receives a memory book with written messages from other children and staff and photographs recording the time spent there. Menses and Durrant describe the graduation ceremony for residents, which not only recognizes the adolescents' achievement but continues the framing of problems as external. At the Orthogenic School, the anniversary day of each student's coming to school is celebrated, with a gift for each year. The gifts are chosen as a symbol of the student's achievement over the year. Residents and staff can spontaneously create rituals. Redl mentions, for example, that all groups have certain rituals by which a member can return to the good graces of the group after having done something wrong. There are many natural opportunities to create rituals: birthdays, farewells to both staff members and residents, graduations, reunions, and holidays [17–21].

Sanders writes that the celebration of holidays at the Orthogenic School develops a sense of time because holidays are significant and obvious time markers in the revolving course of years. It also helps the children feel part of a larger community. Sanders believes that holidays satisfy some basic human needs, and the holidays at the Orthogenic School are organized to consider them. As school director, Bettelheim began the tradition of talking with all of the young people together about the significance of the holiday. The holiday message was not always the conventional one. On Thanksgiving, the theme of the Pilgrims' successful survival was made significant for children who also came to a new world and have to survive what to them seem to be very great hardships. Since the Orthogenic School students are of varying backgrounds, a religious celebration of Christmas is optional, but everyone celebrates the holiday. The Christmas message is that the child is of great value. There is a theme of hope in the midst of darkness. Easter and Passover, the holidays of spring, provide symbols of hope and new beginnings. The children receive the message that they are not alone in winters of despair and that such winters can end with springtimes of birth and hope [21].

It is not only the celebration of the holidays but also the celebration of the person that invests the treatment center with meaning. For that is what the essential work is about. Rose describes the young person as being sent away from the everyday world to a special place that looks like something from a storybook, led into a "pied piper" community with relationships, values, behaviors, and activities that are different from anything ever experienced before. There are great feasts, fireside music-making in the winter, stories at bedtime, rowdy games in the snow, adventures in the mountains and journeys by water. These opportunities are given to young persons who have learned few good lessons about their own worth and potency. Later, when they struggle with life's ordinary difficulties, they will be able to call upon that absorbed security that was their gift from the symbolic environment of Peper Harow [22].

References

1. Rose M. The design of atmosphere: Ego-nurture and psychic change in residential treatment. Journal of Adolescence 1986;9:49–62.
2. Edgar I. Myth at Peper Harow. International Journal of Therapeutic Communities 1985;6(3):239–51.
3. Bettelheim B, Sylvester E. A therapeutic milieu. American Journal of Orthopsychiatry 1948 Apr;18(2):191–206.
4. Bettelheim, B. Home for the heart. New York: Knopf, 1974.
5. Bettelheim B. Love is not enough: the treatment of emotionally disturbed children. Glencoe IL: Free Press, 1950.
6. Rose M. The context for psychological change in a therapeutic community for adolescents. Part II. Residential Treatment for Children & Youth 1987 Fall;5(1):29–46.
7. See reference 4.
8. Menses G, Durrant M. Contextual residential care: applying the principles of cybernetic therapy to the residential treatment of irresponsible adolescents and their families. Residential Treatment of Children & Youth 1990;7(3):11–32.
9. Zimet SG, Schultz GF. The cook, the kitchen, the cafeteria and beyond: Food in the day treatment program. In: Zimet SG, Farley GK, eds. Day treatment for children with emotional disorders. v. 1. A model in action. New York: Plenum, 1991, 113–28.

10. See reference 4.
11. See reference 2.
12. Rose M. Treasure Island: the metamorphosis of deprivation and injury in the residential setting. Residential Treatment for Children & Youth 1992;10(2):75–87.
13. See reference 2.
14. Bassin A. Proverbs, slogans and folk sayings in the therapeutic community: A neglected therapeutic tool. Journal of Psychoactive Drugs 1984 Jan-Mar;16(1):51–6.
15. Rose M. The function of food in a residential treatment process. Residential Treatment for Children & Youth 1988;6(1):43–60.
16. Zeitlyn BB. The therapeutic community: fact or fantasy? British Journal of Psychiatry 1967;113:1083–6.
17. See reference 2.
18. Parsons PC, Imhof R. Special projects in the treatment program: their birth, development, and emotional demise. In: Zimet SG, Farley GK, eds. Day treatment for children with emotional disorders. v.1. A model in action. New York: Plenum Press, 1991, 143–61.
19. See reference 8.
20. Sanders J. Culture and residential treatment. Residential Treatment for Children & Youth 1993;10(3): 37–48.
21. Redl F. When we deal with children. New York: Free Press, 1966.
22. See reference 1.

4. The Human Treatment Environment: The Staff

The therapeutic milieu represents the creation of a human and social environment to restore mental health. The therapeutic work is about entering into the lives of others with caring, respect, and appreciation to form a relationship committed to their personal growth. No psychiatric treatment modality will replace the help that comes through interpersonal experiences and the staff works to make daily experiences with patients constructive steps in their recovery. The staff provides consistent adult relationships that will allow residents to try out their own interpersonal skills with a feeling of safety [1–3].

There is a comprehensive body of literature providing both guidance and comfort for all who work in inpatient treatment. The nursing literature is not only extremely helpful but is also relevant for all who work in inpatient settings. The residential treatment and child care literature is an impressive testament to the development of the child care professional. The literature of psychology and psychiatry now deals less frequently with staff questions; when it does, it is of high quality. The earlier sociological literature is still of interest today. This section examines what has been written about the treatment staff that has relevance to all who work in the interpersonal environment. It is about all staff members and "generic" staff issues, rather than exclusively about psychiatric residents, psychiatric technicians, child care workers, or nurses.

An organization that is serious about healing needs the services of very special people. Bettelheim writes that the staff needs to internalize the teaching of the institution and develop a truly positive attitude about its task. The primary task may not only be the healing of patients but also the re-creation of all who are part of the interpersonal environment. Staff and patients constitute a single social system. The institution needs to recruit and socialize both staff and patients in order to perpetuate itself [4–5].

The Staff: Power, Authority, Responsibility

The staff must be organized rationally in order to work and the system of authority and decision making is significant in determining the milieu's therapeutic effectiveness. The delegation of responsibility and the lines of authority must be clear, understood and accepted in practice. If not clear and accepted, if there are unresolved contradictions and ambiguities, the staff may be confused and anxious. Since mental health professionals usually have strong beliefs in equality, it is usually more difficult for them to enter a hierarchical system. Many may choose to deny its existence. Wells writes about persons in high administrative positions who somehow try to pretend that they and the custodial staff are doing the same work—a type of condescension with no place in the reality of hospital practice. Leeman warns against the pretense of complete equality in decision making but recommends equal consultation before making decisions, since it is helpful if all can be heard [6–8].

Administrative leaders can hold an egalitarian philosophy regarding the potential of each staff member to exert a therapeutic influence upon patients. They should deemphasize status when it can limit relationships that could be beneficial to patients. Bettelheim writes that we can never develop a therapeutic community if it is divided between those who create it and the others who do what they're told. Although there is a hierarchy of persons who make decisions and take responsibility, Greben writes that there cannot be a hierarchy based on helpfulness to patients. It is a myth that the most significant person is the doctor and that other staff members' contributions are inferior to that. The reversal of that myth is that there is no hierarchy and that staff members are interchangeable. A hierarchy produces some natural feelings against authority. Staff members working in direct care often feel that they know much more about the patients than the administrative or medical staff. If staff members challenge authority, the result is often tighter policies and procedures. This then puts the staff in a position of having to defend policies they don't really like. Colyar describes how adolescent patients can find and push the buttons of staff members' own dissatisfaction with authority. When both patients and staff members challenge authority it may indicate that staff members have received little affirmation from administrators about their own performance or about the running of the program [9–12].

ROLE AMBIGUITY AND PROFESSIONAL ALLIANCES

Indeed, there is an overlap among professionals, particularly in that all of them must be experts in listening and talking to patients. Yet each discipline has its own role to play. Role ambiguity exists if staff members don't know the expectations of each position, if there are no clear performance guidelines and if responsibilities overlap. Overlapping roles can result in competition over patients [11–13].

Boyd and Paisley found role ambiguity to be the strongest predictor of emotional exhaustion and depersonalization on the job. Role ambiguity can occur in a treatment setting when objectives are not clear and not communicated. It can be reduced by clarifying treatment objectives and procedures and monitoring them for consistency. Role ambiguity also affects patients. Clarity for the patient can come from knowledge of what to expect from each professional group. Most patients need order in their environment with clear role models who do the same things day in and day out. The therapeutic community concept allowed a blurring of roles, but this structure was successful only for selected patients [14–15].

The leaders of the treatment center should have strong interdisciplinary commitments in order to build sound professional alliances. Carefully written job descriptions are an essential first step in achieving good role relationships and reducing ambiguity. Yet if it becomes a situation of limiting some of the roles of one profession so as not to overlap with another, the result might also be a limiting of a person's professional potential. The nursing profession often presents a good example of the underutilization of knowledge and skill [16].

The Organization of the Staff's Responsibility

STAFF CONFLICTS

Eliminating role ambiguity will not automatically eliminate staff conflicts. Martin believes that hospital environments are characteristically in a chronic state of strained staff relations, and that psychiatric residents training in the hospital are often prime targets for criticism. The psychiatric resident who must serve two divisions, training and clinical, may become vulnerable by neglecting one role for the other. Despite having sufficient authority, residents have many reasons to feel insecure. They may have particular problems with their own leadership, since it is not easy to "learn to lead while needing to be led." They are aware of their inexperience when compared to other members of the treatment team. They will need to simply appreciate the competence of others, rely on their information, and try to create good working relationships while being aware of group dynamics. They are ill-advised to defend against their feelings of incompetence by trying to appear omnipotent [17–19].

Nurses who work with psychiatric residents will often complain that they are not using their professional nursing skills. Patients will press residents for more freedom while nurses press for more control. Nurses may tend to see psychiatric residents as younger siblings who seem to get preferential treatment from the administration. Male-female issues will also be prominent. Resolving staff conflicts usually result in therapeutic benefits for patients [20–21].

The staff member's normal temptation to shift blame also produces conflict. Colyar describes blame as going upward, if the staff member is on the lower end of the hierarchy and going downward if the staff member is at the higher end. When fixed work shifts exist, the night and swing shift staff blame the day shift for any problems, and the day shift in turn blames the administration. Colyar describes this as "problem inheritance." The day shift often sets the tone for the day, and the demands on this shift are such that there may be little opportunity to form a cohesive front to other work groups. Another type of blaming can come from avoiding the incongruity between the avowed therapeutic purposes of the treatment center and what actually happens. Blaming the leader may also represent the staff's attempt to deny serious conflicts or to protect its own need to perpetuate an authoritarian structure [22–24].

Bettelheim writes that when things go wrong, the temptation is always to reproach someone, but that doing so destroys staff unity. Bettelheim felt that it was the director's responsibility to prevent blaming and to demonstrate that it would not remedy the situation. He describes the normal jealousy that staff members have toward each other, and advises its frank acknowledgment. Knowing that each staff member does things differently and even celebrating those differences can lighten the feelings of envy [25].

The Direct Care Staff

It may seem impossible to remove resentment from the system. Direct care staff may in many cases be the primary therapeutic agent, or at least the group that spends the most therapeutic time with residents and has the strongest influence as role models. It may never be easy for direct care staff members to play a secondary role when they often feel more experienced, informed and experientially involved than the therapist. However, since it is generally believed that good treatment proceeds best with one primary therapist, direct care staff members must make their peace with this fact and restrain their own desires to take this role. Their function is to provide emotional support and encourage the patient to discuss more intimate problems with the therapist. They do carry a great deal of informal power, but it may be often be used as resistance, both overt and covert. Covert resistance often stems from countertransference, which is evident in possessive feelings, and strong opinions about what the patient really needs. Resistance is unconscious and may prevent rational planning and discussion. It can restrict treatment to the boundaries of a treatment philosophy and prevent productive disagreement. While countertransference resistances are stimulated by the patient, treatment resistance may occur because of the staff members' feelings about the therapist. There can also be a general resistance to change. When a new program is introduced, staff members may inevitably feel that it is a criticism of their previous way of doing things [26–27].

Treatment resistance often occurs in the direct care staff's response to the therapist or to the therapist's theories or techniques. Staff members, for example, may blame the patient's impulsive behaviors on the therapist's passivity. They may question the therapists' actions or fear that the therapist disagrees with the unit's treatment philosophy. Although it may seem that resistances result from intellectual disagreement, Blotcky and colleagues believe that they are primarily an emotional reaction. Piersma writes that the direct care staff and therapist must realize that they have different roles and that both are necessary to help the patient get well. The direct care staff must deal immediately with behavior. The therapist can serve as a more objective observer of what is happening and can provide a conceptual framework for understanding the patient. The therapist may often need to become a "cheerleader" for the staff when it becomes discouraged or gives up when progress is slow [27–28].

COMMUNICATION

Many staff problems can be avoided by improvement in communication. The communication network is an integral part of the therapeutic social structure. Communication problems inevitably occur among different shifts. The staff must be alert to such blockages and correct them, transmitting information at the right time and in the right way. Distortions must be corrected, contradictions and misunderstanding recognized and worked through. Communications should be clear and free-flowing [29–30].

At times there may simply be too much communication. Schwartz writes that the staff members can spend so much time in meetings that they can no longer carry out their primary functions. Communication can become an end in itself rather than mobilizing the therapeutic process. Schwartz recommends a careful selection of what is transmitted. Those who lead staff meetings should set a tone that discourages triviality or digressions from professional to personal issues. Although staff members must often work together to explore conflicts that often have to do with their own countertransference, Abroms and Sweeney find that focusing on conflict often disrupts patient care, if the two tasks are combined in the same meeting. Zeitlyn finds this group process toxic when efforts to discuss patient care are so seriously interrupted. Perinpanayagam agrees that the staff's pathology does arise in its meetings, sometimes in projected form, where an individual staff problem is somehow seen as a problem in the unit or in another staff member. If the meeting is defined as one of group process, then the leader must be able to interpret group distortions, hostility, or dependence [30–33].

The treatment center's hierarchy also influences communication. In a treatment center that operates on the medical model, directions are given and taken according to status. Social workers or nurses rarely give orders to physicians, although they may give advice, usually only when consulted. However, farther down the hierarchy, team members usually try to redefine the system. Osborne, writing in the 1970s, felt that the hierarchical communication system of the medical model seriously affected therapeutic programs. The people at the top of the hierarchy often developed programs without knowledge of the traditions and special contributions of lower-echelon team members. Such programs may privilege the traditions of only one profession and ignore interdisciplinary collaboration [33–34].

Staff meetings often carry a predominant message about the values of the treatment center. Openness, honesty and interpretations may be expected in meetings on units when this is expected of patients. Task-oriented meetings may be the rule for short-term units. Indeed, staff meetings can implicitly nurture those attitudes that will inform the staff's work with patients. The style of the meeting should therefore be congruent with the treatment philosophy as well as the social reality of the work. The staff meeting builds strength from shared purpose, clears up conflicts among the staff, and provides information for diagnosing the current state of the treatment unit. In designated meetings with an open agenda, staff members can be encouraged to freely discuss their own problems in interpersonal and group dynamics.

Support for the Staff

Staff members require extraordinary support in order to do their work. Their own anxiety in working with disturbed patients may finally affect the overall structure and functioning of the milieu. The staff's struggle against anxiety can imbed defense mechanisms into the structure, culture and functioning of the treatment center to the point that therapeutic effectiveness can disappear. Axelrod and Axelrod describe such defenses against anxiety as depersonalization, detachment, denial of feeling, and attempts to avoid decisions by ritualized task performance. Staff members may design their own protective defenses when vulnerable: strict interpretation of the rules without considering patient welfare, unquestioning compliance with orders, excessive use of paperwork or excuses to avoid patient or staff contact [35–37].

Main writes that objectivity itself can become a defense against pain, which then results in the loss of the capacity to truly experience another person. The hospital structure and rules often provide an organizational defense against close encounters with patients. Fragmenting the patient into various functions, with several departments taking care of the patient's family, recreation, and therapy may leave no one available to care for the whole person. If this division becomes rigid, the staff may feel bored without the interpersonal gratification that comes from helping. The emphasis on objectivity deprives the patient of the staff members' subjective understanding and empathy. Subjective responses can become tools for the understanding of patients and providing informed interventions, but their use requires skill and discipline. Main believes that the study of object relations may finally provide more guidance for working with patients than conventional diagnosis. He mentions, for example, that some depressed people who may have a great deal of self-hate can stimulate compassion while others seem to simply irritate [38].

There are many reasons why the staff needs defenses while working closely with severely disturbed patients. When not defended they may feel extremely helpless. The severity of the patient's psychopathology may cause staff members to doubt their own personal capacity for containment and self-control or the maintenance of their own ego boundaries. The depressed patients' feelings are both contagious and demoralizing. When staff members have low morale, when they feel hopeless, ineffective and uninspired, they will most likely keep patients ill. Staff members become attached to patients and the rapid patient turnover leaves them endlessly vulnerable to the pain of separation [38–39].

There are many sources of stress. Staff members must consciously set limits. They need to face patients who make them angry, without responding in kind. Patients choose favorites, love one day and hate the other, and make hurtful comparisons among staff. The patient's hostility puts self-esteem under constant attack. The staff member must deal with a sense of failure for not being able to realize therapeutic ambitions. Yet when trust and collaboration work, the staff can have high energy and confidence [40].

Stress is expressed in many ways: high absenteeism, forgotten messages, withdrawal, short-term solutions instead of long-term planning, making exceptions for patients. Both staff and patients will withdraw from each other during times of stress. Staff members can expect support from other staff and will withdraw if they are unsupported. Patients will withdraw from staff on occasions when they don't get the support they need. Cornfield and Fielding describe the patients' need to feel that the staff is omnipotent. When they begin not to feel safe, they will mobilize the staff with covert messages: criticism, signing out of the hospital, sexual acting out or drug use. Gray and Diers report that when staff members are upset, patients will often stabilize. The acting-out behaviors of patients seem to peak during times when staff is not under stress. Stanton and Schwartz believe that staff members can develop high morale or avoid low morale if given a chance to ventilate, develop insight and understand their anxiety and sources of demoralization. If feelings can be shared and accepted by others and if there is a true concern for needs and difficulties, the staff members can learn to handle stress and regain morale. Staff morale influences therapeutic effectiveness. When staff members have high morale, when they function with enthusiasm, have a spirit of inquiry about their patients and derive satisfaction from their work they will be of immense help to the patient. The restoration of morale begins with trust. The staff must first know that it is safe to discuss emotional responses to patients before learning to master them [41–43].

Staff cohesion strongly influences the treatment environment. Emotional bonds come from working together and from real or fantasized feelings of commonality. Bettelheim suggests that cohesion gives the staff members a sense of security that allows them to act in a more open and less authoritarian manner with residents. Without cohesion, staff must resort to structure, increased rule enforcement and control. Staff cohesion affects both autonomy and support. The emotional climate of the treatment center can provide staff members with the kind of support they need to work with the mentally ill. The staff member needs to receive from colleagues the gratifications that aren't always available from patients. Axelrod and Axelrod believe that the staff's interaction builds a matrix of relatedness and stability that becomes the group introject. This positive group introject sustains the work of the staff and integrates them in a common cause. This can lead to the patient's re-integration and the formation of a therapeutic alliance. The group introject provides stability for the staff, as patients come and go. It provides a collective sense of the unit's continuity across time. It contains a distillate of all experiences with patients that can serve as a template for understanding others. Axelrod and Axelrod believe that the introject develops through the staff's own interpersonal involvement and capacity for attachment. The leader, too, can come to personify a positive group introject or ideal for staff [44–46].

The Staff and the Patient

Human relationships can change patients' negative view of themselves and the world. Treatment will not be effective unless the staff's efforts are integrated around each patient. Bettelheim believes that professionalism and the division of the patient's life into departments or specialties pulls the patient in various directions. The integration around the patient finally depends on how seriously the staff attempts to integrate itself [45–46].

A shared ideology can produce high *esprit de corps* and a unity of belief can reduce stress. Yet differing professional roles, educational backgrounds, and power conflicts result in strong ideological differences. Wells cautions that the progress of one's profession in the hospital should never be at the patient's expense. Different professions will see the patient in varying ways. What is observed about the patient as well as the treatment may be primarily designed to validate the views of the profession rather than taking into account the patient's unique needs. Social workers often focus on the patient's social skills. Psychiatrists may focus on the patient's odd behaviors. Nurses make judgments on the severity of the patients' illness based on their disruptive behavior, which disturbs the nurses' primary task of managing the milieu. They may be the most sensitive to the patient's potential for dyscontrol and provide therapeutic intervention when disruption occurs. The team members often speak in different languages, based on a valid but idiosyncratic view of the patient. Colson and colleagues' work suggests ways in which professional training and roles affect clinical concepts [47–49].

Roskin and colleagues studied attitudes toward patients among different health professions. Psychiatrists scored higher on both a biological-organic and psychodynamic approach to the patient, while nurses scored higher on a biological-organic approach. The most surprising finding was that the nurses scored higher on distancing-detachment and lowest on nurturant-empathic attitudes. Since nurses performed the most intimate caregiving, they apparently needed to develop more psychological distance than others working with the patient who were typically more distant. While members from other professions may remain neutral and stress the understanding of pathological behavior, direct care staff who confront it daily may not have that luxury. Since they respond to the patient's immediate behavior, the response may have only a remote connection to understanding [50–51].

There are some arguments for multiple treatment paradigms or ideological diversity. Roskin and colleagues feel that multiple paradigms can be beneficial, both for patient care and the growth of knowledge in the field. Kotin and Sharaf believe that when different treatment methods and paradigms exist in an institution, there will a variety of available approaches to meet the needs of each patient. This is most likely a minority view. The development of treatment programs usually requires ideological assumptions and commitment. In a psychoanalytic framework, it may be the patient that determines the treatment stance. James recommends systematic scrutiny of the form and content of the patient's relation to the nurse, therapist, other patients and the community to make hypotheses about the psycho-biological history. This would develop the staff's awareness of the whole psychodynamic picture of the patient and a prediction where difficulties might occur and what changes are needed. This provides the staff a theoretical perspective of the patient and increases therapeutic effectiveness [50–54].

The security and integration the patient needs can be provided by a primary staff member for each patient. In residential treatment centers, this may be a child care worker, and in the hospital, the primary nurse. The person in this position will observe and integrate the work of each profession and coordinate the patient's care. This person is central to the development and carrying out of the treatment plan, has daily contact with the patient and shares information with the treatment team in daily rounds and case conferences. In some structures, the primary person might also be the therapist. This primary person also serves as the patient's advocate and is responsible for ensuring that the staff works, not only in congruence with the treatment plan, but also in the patient's best interest. Ryan and colleagues, comparing a primary nursing model to team nursing, found that the primary nursing model increased interdisciplinary communication, provided a higher level of staff satisfaction and greater staff satisfaction with nursing services. The team nursing model provided greater knowledge of the entire client milieu, more satisfaction with peers and supervision, but more role conflict and less overall satisfaction. The Orthogenic School program removed the departmental hierarchy and entrusted one person to serve the patient. Bettelheim writes that unity for the patient came from the person who provided this care and the unique relationship forged with the patient [55–58].

The primary staff member for each patient may create a type of parental interaction that not all patients will appreciate. Emrich finds that patients perceived their nurses' interactions with them as parental and thus discomfirming. This interactional style may be due to authoritarian and hierarchical practices and lack of support for patient autonomy. In addition to relationships, the environment presents the patient with models for identification. Rosen feels that the staff should also be able to identify with the residents. If residents feel that their feelings are understood, this creates trust [59–61].

Colyar notes that it is easier for a large group to influence the behavior of a small group than for the small group to influence the larger one. Because patients are actively engaged in recreating past deviant interactions that have worked for them, they are consequently working to shape the staff's behavior. If staff members are to continue being therapeutic, they must be aware of this and respond in a predictable and consistent way. When staff members work individually rather than as a team or without adequate support, they are even more vulnerable to shaping by patients. Those who spend the most time with patients may receive the least support and help in their relationships [62].

The mental health profession is based on a belief that relationships influence human growth. The trust, empathy, and communication that relationships provide can help to change behavior. Now that treatment is usually short term, even the process of establishing a connection with the patient needs to be speeded up. Heifner describes connectedness in the nurse-patient relationship. When connectedness exists, the staff member and patient can deal with sensitive issues more quickly, more often, and with less difficulty. The ability to be vulnerable and to share information honestly without guilt or shame makes the patient more accessible. Heifner found, however, that sharing was not mutual in the nurse/patient relationship and connectedness did not require reciprocity. While less experienced nurses were tempted to speak about their personal lives, more experienced nurses wanted to disclose less. The staff member's own ability to identify with the patient increases feelings of connectedness, particularly when both share similar values, beliefs, or life situations. Connectedness also implies an investment in the patient, with the staff members investing time and caring in the relationship. Here the investment can be mutual. Nurses in the Heifner study also describe connectedness as feeling valued by the patient. The more valued the nurses felt, the greater their readiness to invest in the patient. Connectedness can also imply empathy with the patient. Empathy is not sympathy, but rather experiencing the feelings of another person, feeling the same way. Empathy by definition is a feeling of connection, but without going beyond the boundaries of the self [63].

The staff member's degree of social distance from the patient affects the therapeutic climate. Some degree of social distance is necessary for effective functioning, but the challenge is in measuring it. Empathy, identification, connectedness, must also be appropriate. The staff member may simply "get lost" within the patient and can develop relationships that will become countertherapeutic. Coltrane and Pugh's article will help a staff member examine those situations that signal countertherapeutic aspects of relationships with patients. For example, the staff member who spends a disproportionate amount of time with a patient needs to examine the reasons why and should consider checking with other staff members for their impressions. When the staff member spends off-duty time with the patient or the patient stays up in order to see the staff member on the night shift or dresses in a special way there are hints of a relationship beyond a therapeutic staff/patient connectedness [64].

The staff member may feel that the rest of the staff is jealous or critical of a special relationship with the patient. Yet the staff member somehow is the only person who "understands" the patient. These may be signals that objectivity is eroding. At this point the staff member may be starting not to see the person as a patient and may become defensive when asked about their relationship. The staff member must always be willing to accept feedback and then act constructively. If the situation does not change, it can erode communication and teamwork and affect the patient's treatment. If the patient always turns to the staff member because others are "busy," this may be a sign that the staff member is providing special treatment. Going beyond standard procedures to allow the patient privileges, is another sign of a nontherapeutic relationship. If patients speak too freely or with sexual nuances, staff members must examine whether they may be thinking about a social or sexual relationship and what the staff may be doing to encourage it [64].

Coltrane and Pugh write that keeping secrets with the patient is unethically taking on the patient's full treatment and devaluing the treatment program. Possessiveness can be nontherapeutic and prevents the patient from learning to interact with others. Shamsie and Lang describe this as the myth of exclusive property, which often progresses to a belief that the patient can be cured by a single person. Patients who require inpatient treatment usually need the work of several professions and several staff members before they make improvement. Krohn and colleagues write that if a staff member's self-esteem rides on the patient's behavior, the patients will experience this as a repetition of their parents' use of them as narcissistic extensions of themselves. The degree of social distance that the staff establishes can affect patient outcome. Some degree of social distance from others, patients or staff co-workers, is necessary for effective social functioning, but finding the optimal distance for both relationships is always difficult [64–67].

Parallelism

Patients and staff are bound together in a system with permeable boundaries. Staff members will often treat patients in the same way that they are treated within the inpatient environment. The patient group can easily infect staff members with its feelings about authority. Conflicts among staff members may mirror the intrafamilial struggles of the patient.

Procedures or rituals for staff in the treatment center often resemble those designed for patients, even admission and departure of both patients and staff. An administration that works with patients will ultimately develop similar techniques for work with staff. There is often a parallel between the themes in patient community meetings and staff in their meetings. Unit supervisors may tend to work with both staff and patients in very similar ways. Supervisory staff in residential treatment centers often adopts parental roles toward the child care staff. Colyar finds that this attitude often makes them less objective about performance and more forgiving of deficiencies. There is an unwarranted transfer of procedures and many supervisors somehow aren't able to distinguish between good therapy and good management of staff. Supervisors in mental health settings are also more willing to accept staff members' excuses if they are expressed in psychological terms. The psychiatric staff often tends to make interpretations about staff members' behavior, using the same tools they use with patients, and often as a form of control. Stanton and Schwartz write about how serious misunderstandings occur when explicit meanings of what staff or patients say are ignored in favor of inferred meanings. Staff members may make "deep" interpretations when dealing with colleagues, ignoring what they say in favor of what they think is "really going on" [68–70].

Collins suggests that when milieu managers have difficulties explaining patient behavior that they examine possible staff contributions to the problem. Staff rivalries and disagreement between senior staff and workers often cause disturbances in the patients' behavior. Patients who identify with their therapist may develop destructive relationships with each other or they can be the ones who will act out their therapists' feelings about the administration [71–72].

Staff members must absorb patients' anger without retaliating. The process of absorbing the patients' pathology is stressful and can often stimulate repressed feelings or pathological behavior. The staff's feelings often provide clues to the patients' covert pathology. Staff members can often so identify with patients and find themselves covertly encouraging disturbed behavior or deriving some secret pleasure from hearing about it. This can often happen when staff members are angry at their own authority figures. This overidentification with patients can make a staff member feel that the staff is hurting or punishing a patient rather than helping. They may resent other staff members because they feel that only they know what is best for the patient. This can be true for the patient's therapist who will often find it difficult to act on feedback from other staff [73].

Indeed, the treatment environment should not be one that cares exclusively for the patient and not for the staff. Hyde writes that if the environment is to be therapeutic it must be therapeutic for all and provide growth for both patients and staff. When the staff member finds colleagues who understand and help, this experience can serve as a template for working with patients. Both staff and patients need someone they can trust and someone who can relieve their anxieties. If staff members are treated unfairly or in an authoritarian manner without real concern for them as persons, and if their opinion is not respected, they may come to treat the patient in a similar way. Their contribution to the patient's self-esteem will be minimal. If the administration seems remote and distant, the staff may adopt a similar distance from patients [74].

These parallel processes occur in the milieu because the two systems have significant relationships with each other that bring about resemblance in emotions, thinking, and behaviors. While some parallel processes are consciously established, such as providing the same good-bye rituals for both patients and staff, others are unconscious. Covert dynamics in one group can be played out in another group. Conflict can erupt in a location far from the source, transported from patients to staff [75].

Other Staff Matters

TECHNIQUES

So much attention is given to the creation of the emotional climate that the need for effective techniques may be forgotten. The belief that good intentions from good people will help the patient may obscure the need for specific training. Good intentions will simply not compensate for a lack of knowledge. Colyar writes that the function of residential treatment is to identify behavioral deficiencies and then apply intervention strategies to deal with them. Planning staff responses to noncompliance requires equal attention. To be effective, the milieu program must not only have a system of caring techniques but also planned responses to behavioral situations. Otherwise, the result will be a chaotic living environment that reacts to the patients' behaviors in an unpredictable, contradictory way [76].

Staffing Patterns

The absence of significant staff on weekends causes separation problems for patients and affects the cycle of the patients' week, often producing regression, conflict and destructive behavior. These oscillations become evident in community meetings and group therapy. Ritvo reports that group cohesion and an alliance with therapeutic goals peaked in the middle of the week and decreased by Friday when members faced the weekend's uncertainty. Each Monday brought uncertainty about relationships, anger or passivity, and themes about power and control. A good program of weekend activities and more weekend passes can help. Stable shift assignments are recommended; milieu interactions often reflect unpredictable shift assignments [77].

Staff Turnover and Stability

In a study of the patient's length of stay and outcome, Bauer notes length of stay is not the critical variable correlated with good outcome. Patients who stayed less than five months in the hospital sustained as much improvement two years after discharge as those who stayed longer than a year. Bauer suggests that it may be stable staff and leadership that provides a long term culture that promotes change. Still, each patient would require a minimum length of stay so that the change process could be internalized [78].

Staff-Patient Ratio

Sacks believes that there are no definitive findings on an optimal staff-patient ratio. More is not always better. A record of patient incidents is often used to analyze staffing. Depp's analysis found no relationship between staffing levels and violent incidents but suggested that violent incidents often occurred when staffing levels were high. Felicetti remarks on those times of tedium and slow change in the milieu, when staff members may unconsciously need to create excitement. Milieu work often involves waiting patiently for something to happen. Felicetti relates stories of administrators who may look forward to crises in order to ride in like the Lone Ranger. Many writers examining the staffing question recommend that more attention be given to factors other than patient-staff ratios, such as the skill and training of the staff, the severity of psychopathology on the unit and the physical environment [79–81].

Training the Direct Care Staff

The most discussed and yet the most insoluble staff problem has been how to provide status, training and job satisfaction for child care workers and psychiatric technicians. By far the most exciting solution is the post-baccalaureate training based on the European model of the educateur, a model developed to train persons to care for the great number of displaced children after the second World War. The educateur is a total life specialist who works with children. The word is derived from the Latin "educare," which means to lead, pull out, or encourage potential. The process has also been described as a re-education process that began with Jeannine Guindon's work with delinquent youth in France and later developed into a 4-year psychoeducateur program at the University of Montreal. This holistic program was based on an integrated conception of the person and the environment. Some of the principles of the model are that crisis provides opportunity, assessment should be ecological, that the relationship is primary, and that teaching is humanistic. The training program includes learning and developmental theory, diagnosis and remediation [82].

Barnes and Kelman describe an American educateur training program. Students in this program earn a master's degree in special education and there is an appropriate emphasis on teaching, both direct instruction and behavioral methods. Each student is assigned to a residential treatment team. The educateur's most essential curriculum is the daily events in the lives of the children. An aggressive outburst gives an opportunity for the group to work to convert acting out to talking out. The program teaches method of positive peer counseling as a predominant method for harnessing the powerful influences that young people exert on each other. In the program Barnes and Kelman describe, the educateur serves as the child's therapist as well as directing the daily realities of living. The merging of these two functions is significant since the person who knows the child's functioning in the life space can make the most effective interventions. The child can then use these insights immediately. Barnes and Kelman use the analogy of the orchestra. The educateur or conductor can produce a symphonic process with each person in harmony, integrating a wide range of professionals. Nicholau and McCauley also describe an American educateur training program [82–83].

References

1. Garfat T. Editorial: Voices that fit. Journal of Child & Youth Care 1993;8(2):v.
2. Hall BH. Vicissitudes of psychiatric ward personnel. In: Levinson DJ, Williams RH, eds. The Patient and the mental hospital. Glencoe, IL: Free Press, 1957, 317–23.
3. Keltner NL. Psychotherapeutic management: A model for nursing practice. Perspectives in Psychiatric Care 1985;23(4):125–38.
4. Bettelheim B. Home for the heart. New York: Knopf, 1974.
5. Jones M, Rapoport R. The absorption of new doctors into a therapeutic comunity. In: Greenblatt M. Levinson DJ, Williams RH, eds. The Patient and the mental hospital. Glencoe, IL: Free Press, 1957, 148–62.

6. Schwartz MS. What is a therapeutic milieu? In: Greenblatt M, Levinson DJ, Williams RH, eds. The Patient and the mental hospital. Glencoe, IL: Free Press, 1957, 130–44.
7. Wells LA. Relationships with colleagues. In: Wells LA, ed. A handbook of psychiatric nursing. St. Louis: Warren H. Green, 1989, 315–8.
8. Leeman CP. The therapeutic milieu and its role in clinical management. In: Sederer LI, ed. Inpatient Psychiatry: Diagnosis & treatment. 2nd ed. Baltimore: Williams & Wilkins, 1986, 219–39.
9. Greenblatt M. The psychiatrist as social system clinician. In: Greenblatt M, Levinson DJ, Williams RH, eds. The Patient and the Mental Hospital. Glencoe, IL: Free Press, 1957, 317–23.
10. Bettelheim B. Training the child care worker in a residential center. American Journal of Orthopsychiatry 1966 Jul;36(4):694–711.
11. Greben SE. The multi-dimensional inpatient treatment of severe character disorders. Canadian Journal of Psychiatry 1983;28:97–101.
12. Colyar DE. Ten laws of residential treatment: What can go wrong when you're not looking. Child Care Quarterly 1983 Sum;12(2):136–43.
13. Gleeson S, Metz E, McEachen I, Sklar R. The psychiatric technician: trespasser or welcomed ally? Journal of Psychosocial Nursing & Mental Health Services 1992 Dec;30(12):28–31.
14. Boyd BJ, Paisley BK. Role stress as a contributor to burnout in child care professionals. Child & Youth Care Quarterly 1989;18(4):243–58.
15. Hyde RW, Williams RH. What is therapy and who does it? In: Levinson DJ, Williams RH, eds. The Patient and the mental hospital. Glencoe, IL: Free Press.1957, 173–96.
16. Osborne OH. Issues in achieving effective professional alliances. Hospital & Community Psychiatry 1973 Jan;26(1):207–13.
17. Martin HW. Structural sources of strain in a small psychiatric hospital. Psychiatry 1968;25:347–53.
18. Brent DA. The residency as a developmental process. Journal of Medical Education 1981;56:417–22.
19. Klamen DL, Ornstein E, Scofield C. Overcoming obstacles to communication on a psychiatric training unit. Hospital & Community Psychiatry 1994 Jan;45(1):78–9.
20. Levine HB. The fantasy residue: an antitherapeutic force on the psychiatric inpatient service. Psychiatry 1982;45:262–70.
21. Abroms GM. Defining milieu therapy. Archives of General Psychiatry 1969;20:553–60.
22. See reference 12.
23. Sacks MH, Carpenter WT. The pseudotherapeutic community: An examination of anti-therapeutic forces on psychiatric units. Hospital & Community Psychiatry 1974;25:315–8.
24. Kernberg O. Leadership and organizational functioning: organizational regression. International Journal of Group Psychotherapy 1978;28:3–25.
25. See reference 4.
26. Milliner EK. An introduction to psychoanalytic theory. In: Wells LA, ed. A handbook of psychiatric nursing. St. Louis: Warren H. Green, 1989, 34–67.
27. Blotcky MJ, Wiggins KM, Sheinbein M, Forgotson JH. The development of a therapist-staff alliance on a children's inpatient unit. Acta Paedopsychiatrica 1978;43:233–41.

28. Piersma H. "Mom and Dad": Views on the relationship between direct-care staff and therapists in residential adolescent treatment center facilities. Adolescence 1985 Win;20(80):975–80.
29. Redl F. The concept of a "therapeutic milieu." American Journal of Orthopsychiatry 1959;29:721–36.
30. Abrams RC, Sweeney JA. A critique of the process-oriented approach to ward staff meetings, American Journal of Psychiatry 1982;139(6):769–72.
31. See reference 6.
32. Zeitlyn BB. The therapeutic community: fact or fantasy? British Journal of Psychiatry 1967;113:1083–6.
33. Perinpanayagam KS. Organization and management of an inpatient treatment unit for adolescents. Journal of Adolescence 1987;10:133–48.
34. See reference 16.
35. Menzies IEP. A Case-study in the functioning of social systems as a defence against anxiety. Human Relations 1960;13:95–121.
36. Axelrod SD, Axelrod JB. Staff interaction and therapeutic structure on a short-term psychiatric unit. Hillside Journal of Clinical Psychiatry 1987;9(2):184–94.
37. See reference 5.
38. Main T. Traditional psychiatric defences against close encounter with patients. Canadian Psychiatric Association Journal 1977;22:457–66.
39. Shershow JC. Disestablishing a therapeutic community. Current Concepts in Psychiatry 1977;3:8–11.
40. Sederer LI, Thorbeck J. Borderline character disorder. In: Sederer LI, ed. Inpatient psychiatry: Diagnosis & treatment. 2nd ed. Baltimore: Williams & Wilkins, 1986, 81–106.
41. Cornfield RB, Fielding SD. Impact of threatening patients on ward communication. American Journal of Psychiatry 1980 May;137(5):616–9.
42. Gray S, Diers D. The effect of staff stress on patient behavior. Archives of Psychiatric Nursing 1992;3(1):26–34.
43. Stanton AH, Schwartz MS. Medical opinion and the social context in the mental hospital. Psychiatry 1949;12:243–9.
44. Johnson SM. Staff cohesion in residential treatment. Journal of Youth & Adolescence 1981;10(3):221–2.
45. See reference 4.
46. See reference 36.
47. Kotin J, Sharaf M. Intrastaff controversy at a state mental hospital: an analysis of ideological issues. Psychiatry 1967;30:16–29.
48. See reference 7.
49. Colson DB, Allen JG, Coyne L, et al. Patterns of staff perception of difficult patients in a long-term psychiatric hospital. Hospital & Community Psychiatry 1985 Feb;36(2):168–72.
50. Roskin G, Carsen ML, Rabiner CJ, Marell SK. Attitudes toward patients among different mental health professional groups. Comprehensive Psychiatry 1988;29(2):188–94.
51. Benfer B. Defining the role and function of the psychiatric nurse as a member of the team. Perspectives in Psychiatric Care 1980;4:166–77.
52. See reference 40.

53. Stannard F. Ideological conflict on a psychiatric ward. Psychiatry 1981 May;44(2):150–70.
54. James O. The role of the nurse-therapist relationship in the therapeutic community. International Review of Pychoanalysis 1984;11(2):151–9.
55. Swartz MS, Hargett AB, Fraker WW, Noll BK, et al. The inpatient milieu: organizational and functional principles. Psychiatric Annals 1988 Feb;18(2):80-84.
56. Romoff V, Kane I. Primary nursing in psychiatry: an effective and functional model. Perspectives in Psychiatric Care 1982 Apr-Jun;20(2):73–8.
57. Ryan JA, Poster EC, Auger JR, Davis B, et al. A comparative study of primary and team nursing models in the psychiatric care setting. Archives of Psychiatric Nursing 1988;2(1):3–13.
58. See reference 4.
59. Emrich K. Helping or hurting? Interacting in the psychiatric milieu. Journal of Psychosocial Nursing & Mental Health Services 1989 Dec;27(12):26–9.
60. Murray RB, Baier M. Use of the therapeutic milieu in a community setting. Journal of Psychosocial Nursing & Mental Health Services 1993 Oct;31(10):10–6.
61. Rosen JL. Personality factors in reactions of child care workers to emotionally disturbed children. Psychiatry 1963;26(3):2:257–65
62. See reference 12.
63. Heifner C. Positive connectedness in the psychiatric nurse-patient relationship. Archives of Psychiatric Nursing 1993 Feb;7(1):11–5.
64. Coltrane F, Pugh CD. Danger signals in staff/patient relationships in the therapeutic milieu. Journal of Psychosocial Nursing & Mental Health Services 1978 Jun;16(6):34–6.
65. Shamsie J, Lang G. Staff attitudes and management styles in psychiatric hospitals. Canadian Journal of Psychiatry 1976;21:325–9.
66. Krohn A, Miller D, Looney J. Flight from autonomy: Problems of social change on an adolescent inpatient unit. Psychiatry 1974;37:360–71.
67. Leckwart JF. Social distance: an important variable in psychiatric settings. Psychiatry 1968;31:352–61.
68. See reference 12.
69. Durkin R. Social functions of psychological interpretations. American Journal of Orthopsychiatry 1967;37:956–62.
70. Stanton AM, Schwartz M. The Mental hospital: Study of institutional participation in psychiatric illness and treatment. New York: Basic Books, 1954.
71. Collins DT. Dynamic issues in staff/patient groups of a therapeutic community. International Journal Therapeutic Communities 1989;10(2):123–6.
72. Astrachan BM, McKee B. The impact of staff conflict on patient care and behaviour. British Journal of Medical Psychology 1965;38:313–21.
73. Rosnick L. Use of a long-term inpatient unit as a site for learning psychotherapy. Psychiatric Clinics of North America 1987;10(2):309–23.
75. Lego S, Pawlicki C. How does parallel process manifest itself in psychiatric nursing practice? Journal of Psychosocial Nursing & Mental Health Services 1993 Oct;31(10):41–4.
76. See reference 12.

77. Ritvo J. Staffing patterns and the weekly cycle of community meetings on an adult inpatient unit. Hospital & Community Psychiatry 1982 May;33(5):384–5.
78. Bauer SF. Intrapsychic structure, object relations and interpersonal interaction: treatment process and change in the psychiatric hospital. Journal American Academy of Psychoanalysis 1990;18(4):566–86.
79. Sacks M H. Considerations in determining staff-patient ratios. Hospital & Community Psychiatry 1992 Apr;43(4):309.
80. Depp F. Assaults in a public mental hospital. In: Lion JR, Reid WH, eds. Assaults within psychiatric facilities. New York: Grune & Stratton, 1983,
81. Felicetti TC. The manufacture of crisis in the residential setting. Residential Treatment for Children & Youth 1988;6(2):5–8.
82. Barnes FH, Kelman SM. From slogans to concepts: A basis for change in child care work. Child Care Quarterly 1974 Spr;3(1):7–23.
83. Nicholaou A, McCauley A. Training the American Educateur: An interagency approach. Child & Youth Care Forum 1991 Aug;20(4):275–90.

5. Studying the Characteristics of the Treatment Center: The Ward Atmosphere

The social climate of the treatment center can be studied to determine the relation of environmental factors to treatment results. Various social climates encourage different behaviors and may have differential effects upon patient populations. The interaction between the type of patient and type of treatment program may explain differences in patient behaviors and treatment outcome. The social climate can be studied by observational field study, objective indices, or systematic reports from all participants, both patients and staff. Although most of the significant work on ward atmosphere was completed in the 1970s, the instruments that measure it are still helpful today.

Moos was able to create a taxonomy of treatment environments to empirically investigate what characteristics are therapeutic for what type of patients. The Ward Atmosphere questionnaire covered ten characteristics of the atmosphere of psychiatric wards: involvement, support, spontaneity, autonomy, practical focus, personal focus, order, clarity, control, and expression of anger. These ten characteristics, when combined, described three dimensions of hospital treatment: the relationship dimension, the treatment program dimension and the system maintenance dimension. The relationship dimension included

- Involvement, which refers to how active patients are in social functioning.
- Support, which refers to how supportive patients are to each other and how supportive staff is to patients.

The treatment program dimension included

- Autonomy: The patients' independence, self-sufficiency, and self-direction.
- Spontaneity: The program's emphasis on open expression of feelings.
- Practical Focus: The orientation of the program on preparing for life after discharge.
- Personal Focus: The emphasis on helping patients to understand their feelings and problems.
- Anger and aggression: The measurement of how much patients are allowed to express their disagreement, anger, and other aggressive behavior.

The system maintenance dimension assesses the orderly function of the unit and includes an examination of

- Order and organization—the importance of neatness, scheduling, and planning on the ward.
- Program clarity measures patient's understanding of routine and rules.
- Staff control measures the staff's strictness in enforcing rules and its role in determining them [1].

Analysis of the social climate by the Ward Atmosphere Scale (WAS) serves many functions. It can analyze the differential impact of social atmospheres upon different types of patients and staff. It becomes a permanent instrument that can determine whether the social climate varies over time or how it varies with treatment ideologies, staffing patterns, or changes in unit policies. Moos was able to apply this taxonomy to hundreds of treatment environments [2].

There have been other attempts to assess unit characteristics and treatment outcomes. Ellsworth and colleagues found that wards that performed best on outcome measures were characterized by the absence of a separate TV room, a high percentage of long-stay patients, and a high percentage of unmarried patients. The least effective units were characterized as exactly opposite in those characteristics [3].

Although it may seem that everyone knows what constitutes an effective treatment environment, the relation to outcome can bring some surprises. Jackson formulated the Characteristics of the Environment (CTE) Scale, which measured the following:

1. Active treatment—concerned with the degree of staff activity directed toward patient welfare and improvement.
2. Socioemotional activity—the degree to which social and emotional activity is encouraged among members.
3. Patient Self-Management—the degree to which the environment permits or encourages responsibility for the management of self or other patients.
4. Behavior Modification—staff attempts to influence, demand or control specific behaviors of patients.

5. Instrumental activity—whether the environment permits or encourages normal choice or rational problem-solving activity by patients [4].

King and Smith used the CTE scale and found that both high patient-staff socioemotional interaction and high patient autonomy were detrimental to later adjustment. These somewhat surprising findings led them to conclude that the most "humanistic" treatment characteristics do not necessarily result in improved community adjustment and that these interactions may produce a dependence syndrome that is more suitable to staying in the hospital than returning to the community. Apparently the patients were socialized to improve their hospital way of life and were not really prepared to function after that. This study suggested that even more of the treatment should have been designed to help the patient adjust to community life, rather than to the hospital. Perhaps more stress on a therapeutic system based on the explanation of symptoms and behavior in respect to their acceptability would be more functional [5].

DIFFERING PERCEPTIONS OF WARD ATMOSPHERE

Despite a widespread belief that patients and staff members perceive events differently because of different roles, King and Smith's study found no difference between patient and staff perceptions of ward atmosphere. Differing perceptions can open up discussion of therapeutic issues, clarify roles and work toward sharing responsibility for the treatment environment [5–6].

The Ward Atmosphere Scale can also be useful as treatment centers work toward better serving a multicultural population. Flaherty and colleagues studied racial differences in the perception of ward atmosphere in a VA hospital; 5 of 10 subscales reflected significant racial differences. The 17 black patients rated the ward lower on the 10 subscales than the 17 white patients. Subscales rating autonomy, spontaneity and expression of anger and aggression were highly significant while other subscales revealed a negative opinion of the ward. Flaherty and colleagues considered many possible explanations, one being that white professionals had created an atmosphere that would meet white patients' expectations. The most serious question is whether this treatment environment was helpful to black patients [7].

WARD ATMOSPHERE AND PATIENT DIAGNOSIS

It would be helpful to determine the optimal ward atmosphere for specific populations. Friis and colleagues' study of ward atmosphere finds that a milieu for psychotic patients should have a high level of support, practical orientation, order and organization and a low level of anger and aggression. Wards for nonpsychotic patients should have a high level of spontaneity, involvement, autonomy, practical and personal orientation and program clarity. This study strongly suggests that psychotic and nonpsychotic patients are best treated in milieus with different ward atmospheres. At the same time, one might question the effect of a milieu composed entirely of psychotic patients. And, of course, it is true that both psychotic and nonpsychotic patients have improved in integrated units. Friis and colleagues recommend that the staff monitor the ward atmosphere and restrict the admission of patients to those most likely to benefit in that setting. They believe that if more than 1/3 of the patients require specific social climates, then their treatment would be compromised [8].

Friis recognizes that many factors affect the ward atmosphere, some of which are not under staff control. The predominant variables are the number of patients, their ages, the percentage of psychotic patients, and the staff turnover rate. In the Friis study, staff turnover was paralleled by changes unfavorable to both psychotic and nonpsychotic patients. Both an increased number of patients and a higher percentage of psychotic patients were associated with changes that were antitherapeutic for psychotic patients [8].

Changing the ward atmosphere

The results of the Ward Atmosphere Scale can be used to plan changes. The Friss study notes, however, that it is one thing to want a special ward atmosphere and quite another to make it happen. Changing the ward atmosphere is difficult. It may not be easy to discover the factors that most strongly influence it. Verinis advises that the staff compare its rating of the milieu against its view of an ideal one. She describes a staff that wanted to change the degree of involvement, support, spontaneity, order and organization, program clarity and staff control [8–9].

Moos also describes a method for changing the ward atmosphere. Both staff and residents were asked to provide information about their concept of the ideal social climate. Particular attention can be given to similarities and differences in their perceptions and agreements and disagreements about their values and goals. The similarities and differences between the real and ideal environments were studied and specific methods planned in order to make changes. Moos describes a milieu setting that required changes in autonomy and staff control. The staff also needed help in handling limit setting for acting-out behaviors. After the assessment, a committee reviewed community meetings in order to learn how to make them more meaningful in relation to the total ward program. Another committee studied how to increase patient and staff participation in ward activities. The community meetings were then redesigned to transmit the treatment center's norms and values, and in this process, define and explain community expectations. Resident government was established to increase autonomy. The position of crew-job chairman was created with responsibility for supervising work around the house and of checking to be sure residents did their jobs adequately. Moos describes how systematic feedback from the Ward Atmosphere Scale can help the staff to organize its current concerns and motivate residents and staff by involving them in defining issues and goals [10].

MEASURING THE EFFECTS OF CHANGE

Not only can the WAS provide an impetus for change, it can also demonstrate whether it has occurred. A retest in the unit that Moos describes found that the staff perceived significant increases in support, practical orientation and program clarity. Patients perceived significant increases in involvement and support. When external changes in structure are made the Ward Atmosphere Scale can be used to study their effects. By the use of the WAS, Corey and colleagues were able to show that planned environmental change favorably influenced staff and patients' perception of the social milieu [10–12].

WARD ATMOSPHERE AND STAFF MORALE

Certain factors as measured by the WAS influence staff morale, although this may vary with the professional discipline. Dorr and colleagues found that the perceived degree of practical orientation was related to the nurses' morale and that program clarity, order and organization, involvement, and support all affected morale [13].

WARD ATMOSPHERE AND THE TREATMENT MODEL

The profile produced by the Ward Atmosphere Scale might be predictive of the ward's theoretical model; it might also signal when the model isn't working or when it is merely a fiction. Lehman and Ritzler contrast the ward atmosphere of wards using the therapeutic community and medical model. Therapeutic community members perceived more involvement, autonomy, greater emphasis on practical orientation, and more anger and aggression. They concluded that therapeutic community programs sacrifice an orderly environment in order to increase involvement, self-expression, and a practical everyday life orientation. Although there was a higher expression of satisfaction with the therapeutic community approach, a follow-up study showed that it was not effective in preventing a recurrence of symptoms after discharge [14].

Bouras and colleagues also contrasted these two environments and found the therapeutic community ward was significantly more disturbed and the degree of disturbance varied by the day of the week. For this measurement they used derivatives of the WAS, such as the Ward Disturbed Behavior Record and the Ward Dissatisfaction Scale. This would suggest that the very freedom of a therapeutic community model can encourage misbehavior and that this behavior is indeed related to ward culture, standards, and expectations [16].

WARD ATMOSPHERE AND PATIENT IMPROVEMENT

The most important function of the WAS is to learn what factors of the social climate can lead to stable patient improvement. Alden found that patient perception of staff control and acceptance of anger related to patient improvement. Wards with more staff/patient interactions demonstrated more patient improvement. Using post-hospital adjustment as a criterion, Collins found that those wards that performed best were those in which the staff perceived less order and organization [17–18].

Moos used the Ward Atmosphere Scale to discover what correlations might exist between ward climate as perceived by both patients and staff and treatment outcome as defined by dropout rate. He found that certain items rated similarly by both staff and patients correlated significantly with these certain outcomes. Wards with high drop-out rates were low in personal involvement and in feelings of support and low in organization and program clarity. Wards with high (rapid) release rates were perceived as well organized and clear with moderately high staff control but with little emphasis on open, spontaneous expression of feelings and little sense of support. Wards most successful in helping patients remain out of the hospital were perceived as emphasizing patients' autonomy and independence, high in organization and clarity and encouraging open expressions of feelings such as anger [19].

Conclusions

Although the Ward Atmosphere Scale was formulated in the 1970s, it can still be useful today. It may be used less frequently because the information it provided has been incorporated into the structure of modern treatment centers. There are few references to its use in the 1980s and 1990s. In the 1980s, Steiner and colleagues used the WAS to study the relation of ward atmosphere to patient outcome in a children's psychosomatic unit. Wards characterized by a low rate of readmission emphasized autonomy, practical orientation, order and organization, and open expression of emotions, particularly aggression. Better patient outcome was associated with a high level of patient/staff contact. Patient/staff perceptions in their later study were closer to agreement, demonstrating what Steiner and colleagues describe as a maturational effect [20].

The systematic assessment provided by the WAS can bring about meaningful discussion about goals and values in the treatment milieu. It can verify whether staff members are doing what they think they are doing. The WAS, when used carefully, can direct, facilitate, and evaluate change. In addition, WAS scores have been compared from four different countries and it has been demonstrated to have excellent cross-cultural properties in measuring fairly stable aspects of the ward environment [20].

References

1. Moos RH. Evaluating treatment environments: a social ecological approach. New York: John Wiley, 1974.

2. Price RH, Moos RH. Toward a taxonomy of inpatient treatment environments. Journal of Abnormal Psychology 1975;84(10):181–8.
3. Ellsworth R, Maroney R, Klett W, Gordon H, et al. Some characteristics of effective psychiatric treatment programs. Journal of Consulting & Clinical psychology 1979;47(5):799–817.
4. Jackson J. Factors of the treatment environment. Archives of General Psychiatry 1969;21(10):39–45.
5. King JA, Smith CG. The treatment milieu and prediction of mental hospital effectiveness. Journal of Health & Social Behavior 1972;13(2):180–94.
6. Main S, McBride AB. Patient and staff perceptions of a psychiatric ward environment. Issues in Mental Health Nursing 1991;12:149–57.
7. Flaherty JA, Naidu J, Lawton R, Pathak D. Racial differences in perception of ward atmosphere. American Journal of Psychiatry 1981;131(10):815–7.
8. Friis S. Characteristics of a good ward atmosphere. Acta Psychiatrica Scandinavica 1986 Nov;74(5):469–73.
9. Verinis JS, Flaherty JA. Using the ward atmosphere scale to help change the treatment environment. Hospital & Community Psychiatry 1978 Apr;29(10):239–48.
10. Moos RH. Changing the social milieus of psychiatric treatment settings. Journal of Applied Behavioral Science 1973;9(10):575–93.
11. Eriksen L. Ward Atmosphere changes during restructuring of an alcohol treatment center: a quasi-experimental study. Addictive Behaviors 1987;12(1):33–42.
12. Corey LJ, Wallace MA, Harris SH, Casey B. Psychiatric ward atmosphere. Journal Psychosocial Nursing & Mental Health Services 1986 Oct;24(10):10–16.
13. Dorr D, Honea S, Pozner R. Ward atmosphere and psychiatric nurses' job satisfaction. American Journal of Community Psychology 1980 Aug;8(10):455–61.
15. Lehman A, Ritzler B. The therapeutic community inpatient ward: Does it really work? Comprehensive Psychiatry 1976;17(10):755–61.
16. Bouras IN, Trauer T, Watson JP. Ward environment and disturbed behavior. Psychological Medicine 1982;12(2):306–19.
17. Alden L. Treatment environment and patient improvement. Journal of Nervous & Mental Disease 1978;266:327–34.
18. Collins JF, Ellsworth RB, Casey NA, Hickey RB, et al.. Treatment characteristics of effective psychiatric programs. Hospital & Community Psychiatry 1984 Jun;35 (6):601–5.
19. Moos R, Shelton R, Petty C. Perceived ward climate and treatment outcome. Journal of Abnormal Psychology 1973;82:291–8.
20. Steiner H, Marx L, Walton C. The ward atmosphere of a child psychosomatic unit: a ten-year follow-up. General Hospital Psychiatry 1991;13:246–52.

6. Partial Hospitalization

Partial hospitalization programs have proved to be as effective or no less effective as traditional hospital programs and much more cost-effective. These programs should now be evaluated as independent treatment modalities, not as transitional services or low cost-versions of inpatient care. Partial hospitalization provides a therapeutic influence not available in traditional psychiatric hospitalization. A partial hospital is an ideal setting to study the diagnostic and therapeutic meaning of the person's interaction with the environment [1–5].

Partial hospitalization offers a blend of security and independence that the traditional psychiatric hospital cannot provide. Chronic patients, for example, learn to take charge of their own treatment by being responsible for medication and becoming aware of symptoms that precede a crisis. Well-developed activity programs in partial hospitalization can help patients feel productive and feel a stronger sense of purpose, as if they are going to school or work. Through social interaction patients discover that others suffer from the same problems. This sense of universality remains a significant therapeutic factor in group therapy, as it often does in daily life. Realizing the extent of others' problems can help patients feel less confused and hopeless about their own. By giving support to others, they can feel competent, gain a sense of belonging and increased self esteem. They have the opportunity for catharsis, being able to vent feelings in a protected environment. Group interaction also provides feedback to help change behavior and improve the person's functioning in the community. Partial hospitalization can discourage dependency and mobilize the patient's social resources. Patients naturally develop autonomy, not only because the staff will not do things for them that they can do for themselves, but also because they will have special responsibilities essential to the community's functioning. They will also have an immediate opportunity to practice many of the skills they learn in treatment at home and in the community [6–7].

Models of Partial Hospitalization Programs.

There are three predominant models for partial hospitalization, designed to serve different populations:

Day Hospitals

Day hospitals provide treatment for acutely ill patients. This is an intensive care model that is a valid alternative to inpatient hospitalization. The length of stay is usually from four to eight weeks. It can provide all the benefits of inpatient hospitalization with few disruptive and regressive effects. When necessary, such programs can also provide a supervised residence ("guesting") for patients without other stable living arrangements. Day hospitalization can be quite effective for motivated patients who have a social network to encourage their compliance and provide support on nights and weekends [7–8].

Day Treatment

Day treatment has the goal of symptom reduction and improved functioning with lengths of stay between 3 and 12 months. This form of treatment can also incorporate a rehabilitation model, helping to improve the patient's vocational and social functioning. Such programs can set high therapeutic goals and expectations and required attendance, with many similarities to a work environment [7–9].

Day Care

Day Care, the third model, is appropriate for patients who need daily structure and supervision to prevent relapse. There may be modest expectations for these patients, but many of these programs will use a rehabilitation model [7–9].

Certainly not all partial hospitalization programs are so distinct or so specific as to the population they serve. Indeed, a heterogeneous mix often promotes recovery and rehabilitation. Pang finds, however, that separating acute and chronic patients will help staff and patients clarify and focus on treatment goals. These three programs can employ varying theoretical models. Day hospitalization programs, with their resemblance to traditional inpatient hospitalization, often use the medical model. A systems model, which deals with the social context of the patient's problems is effective in partial hospitalization, particularly if it incorporates intensive work with the family. Partial hospitalization programs, in contrast to traditional hospital programs, can use an educational model, based on the belief that maladaptive behavior is learned and can be unlearned. The behavioral model can be of help to some chronic patients, but works best when feelings and thought are also taken into consideration. Many programs will use a rehabilitation model, which will focus on helping the patient to develop skills [7–9].

Partial hospitalization programs can be designed not only for day, but for evenings, nights, or weekends. Night centers can be helpful for former inpatients once they become employed, providing a temporary home during transition from discharge or initial separation from the family. Gudeman and colleagues describe a dormitory inn, which provides a good alternative to 24-hour hospitalization. Turner and Hoge describe a day treatment program that provides overnight hospitalization for those in crisis. The program was designed as an alternative to emergency hospitalization in order to protect the patient from regression, feelings of failure and the discontinuity of care when treatment responsibility must be shifted to the hospital. This system increases the patient's safety, assures medication compliance, and permits more intensive observation that can facilitate assessment. The patient may also benefit from a temporary but necessary distance from stressful situations and relationships that may have brought about the crisis. The back-up system provides a safety net for day hospital programs and helps staff and patients better tolerate the anxiety that occurs as patients struggle for recovery outside a traditional hospital environment. Turner and Hoge found that 73% of patients in this study who required overnight treatment were able to return to day hospitalization. However, the results indicated that only 50% of this group were able to complete it [10–11].

Grabowsky and Kubinski describe a successful evening program for adults divided into cycles or 12-week periods with each cycle offering basic group therapies as well as rotating groups and workshops. The group programming consists of workshops with an interpersonal focus, giving social skills training and those with an interpersonal focus concentrating on stress management, relaxation, or cognitive therapy. The program also provided support groups for adults with special problems. Because most of the adults had been socially and emotionally isolated, a social milieu that was not available in their regular lives is a significant healing factor. The milieu becomes a social support network with a healing atmosphere of acceptance and belonging. It also provides a "social laboratory," continually addressing interpersonal difficulties to help members interact in new ways, providing an atmosphere for experimentation, risk-taking, and a free expression of feelings. Glaser describes much of the activity that occurs in partial hospitalization as the social analysis of events [12–13].

Appropriate Populations for Partial Hospitalization

Partial hospitalization will not be extensively used until it can be determined what types of patients benefit most from it. As informed treatment develops, one needs to determine not only the optimal treatment for each diagnostic group or population but also the best setting for it.

Personality Disorders

There is evidence to suggest that partial hospitalization can be as effective as traditional inpatient hospitalization in alleviating symptoms of personality disorders and affective disorders. A randomized trial study by Piper and colleagues found that patients in a day treatment program showed better outcome than control patients in 7 of 17 outcome variables: mood level, interpersonal behavior, life satisfaction, self esteem, social function, family function, and severity of disturbance. Karterud and colleagues describe encouraging results from day hospital therapeutic community treatment for patients with personality disorders, despite prevailing beliefs that this population requires the containment provided by traditional inpatient treatment [14–15].

Day hospitalization for patients with borderline personality disorder can protect against the regression that occurs in inpatient treatment. The reality orientation, the ability to maintain contact with all elements of nonhospital life, and the requirement to leave treatment at the end of the day and weekends makes limit setting easier and more acceptable. A day hospital program can be effective if the patient with borderline personality disorder has a supportive living arrangement with at least one responsible person. The limits of day hospitalization must be made clear, and specific clear limits on any self-destructive behavior are mandatory [16].

Creed and colleagues also found that day treatment programs were effective for patients with long-standing personality and affective disorders. The program helped patients to understand themselves and make adaptive changes. Patients attend the 18-week program for 7 hours a day, 5 days a week. Each program day begins with a large psychotherapy group, its themes reflecting the ongoing emotional concerns of the treatment milieu. Each patient then attends smaller groups that focus on group therapy, role playing, communication, and life skills. The program also includes video feedback and patient government. The mix of groups allows each patient in the group of 50 to have daily contact with every other patient. Glaser describes these group processes in day hospitalization as multiple interlocking group therapy, which differs from traditional group therapy in intensity. Since the patient participates in several groups each day, there is a cumulative effect and the person becomes more and more responsive to group processes. Glaser reports that one of the primary tasks of the program is to assure that multiple groups do interlock and are not merely beneficial isolated experiences. One method for interlocking occurs when the difficulties that occur in the groups are later referred to the community meeting and vice-versa. The program that Glaser describes also has two day groups for staff, with the belief that if the group process is effective for patients, it will also be for staff [17–18].

CHILDREN

Day treatment rather than inpatient hospitalization for children is without question the treatment of choice. Their lives are less disrupted and they can remain with their families. Forbes and Maddron describe day treatment for children based on a systems therapy approach. The program views and treats the children's problems as part of the problems of the larger system and the family. The treatment context extends beyond the center, to include the school and community. Information management becomes a central team task. The team sees interaction as full of relational meanings. In every relationship in the milieu, there will be analogues to family relationships as well as resources for a solution. This information goes to the team and the team responds [19].

The team's hypotheses about the presenting problem lead to interventions. Feedback from these interventions generates new hypotheses. Forbes and Maddron provide an example of an intervention based on an hypothesis that the child had been placed in treatment to solve the family's problems. Since the placement had removed any reason for change, the team intervened to produce a minor crisis so that the family would once again focus on trying to solve its own problems. Since children continue interactions with their families, systems therapy can be more effective than traditional hospitalization. The team makes interventions to finally empower the family [19].

SCHIZOPHRENIA

Several large-scale studies have shown equivalent outcomes for day hospital and traditional programs for schizophrenic patients. Smith and Draper found that day patients with chronic psychiatric conditions demonstrated significant reduction in symptoms and improvement in functioning. They felt that such day hospital programs were effective because they could "mobilize affect" in the chronic patient. Day hospital treatment encourages less dependency and helps patients develop their own social resources [19–20].

Partial hospitalization compares favorably with inpatient treatment in symptom improvement, relapse reduction and family adjustment. Hoge and colleagues predict that day partial hospitalization may in the future be confined to day hospitalization for acutely ill patients. They report that day care patients are now being referred to more "normalized" programs such as goal-directed rehabilitation and social clubs, both of which offer support and structure without institutional dependency [21].

References

1. Washburn S, Vannicelli M, Longabaugh R, et al. A controlled comparison of psychiatric day treatment and inpatient hospitalization. Journal of Consulting & Clinical Psychology 1976;44:665–75.
2. Herz MI, Endicott J, Spitzer RL, et al. Day versus inpatient hospitalization: a controlled study. American Journal of Psychiatry 1971 Apr;127(4):1371–82.
3. Guillette W, Crowley B, Savitz SA, et al. Day hospitalization as a cost-effective alternative to inpatient care: a pilot study. Hospital & Community Psychiatry 1978;29:525–7.
4. Creed F, Black D, Anthony P. Day hospital and community treatment for acute psychiatric illness: a critical appraisal. British Journal of Psychiatry 1989 Mar;154:300–10.
5. Glaser FB. Our Place: Design for a day program. American Journal of Orthopsychistry 1969 (Oct);39(5):827–41.
6. Hoge MA, Farrell SP, Munchel ME, Strauss JS. Therapeutic factors in partial hospitalization. Psychiatry 1988 May;51:199–210.
7. Pang J. Partial hospitalization: an alternative to inpatient care. Psychiatric Clinics of North America 1985;8(3):587–93.
8. Parker S, Knoff JL III. Partial hospitalizaton: an update. American Journal of Psychiatry 1990(Feb);14(2):158–60.

9. Hoge MA, Davidson L, Hill WL, Turner VE, et al. The promise of partial hospitalization: A reassessment. Hospital & Community Psychiatry 1992 Apr;43(4):345–54.
10. Gudeman JE, Dickey B, Hellman S, Buffett W. From inpatient to inn status: a new residential model. Psychiatric Clinics of North America 1985;8(3):461–9.
11. Turner VE, Hoge MA. Overnight hospitalization of acutely ill day hospital patients. International Journal of Partial Hospitalization 1991;7:23–36.
12. Grabowsky F, Kubinski JA. Making an evening program work. International Journal of Partial Hospitalization 1988;5(3):273–86.
13. See reference 5.
14. Piper WE, Rosie JS, Hassan FA, Azim MB, et al. A randomized trial of psychiatric day treatment for patients with affective and personality disorders. Hospital & Community Psychiatry 1993 Aug;44(8):757–63.
15. Karterud S, Vaglum S, Friis S, Johns S, et al. Day hospital therapeutic community treatment for patients with personality disorders: An empirical evaluation of the containment function. Journal of Nervous & Mental Disease 1992;180:238–43.
16. Pildis MJ, Soverow GJ, Salzman C, Wolf JG. Day hospital treatment of borderline patients: a clinical perspective. American Journal of Psychiatry 1978 May;133(5):594–8.
17. Creed F, Black D, Anthony P. A randomized controlled trial of day patient versus inpatient psychiatric treatment. British Medical Journal 1990;300:1033–7.
18. See reference 5.
19. Forbes E, Maddron T. Systems therapy in a day-treatment setting. International Journal of Partial Hospitalization 1988;5(3):237–50.
20. See reference 12.
21. Smith WR, Draper K. Mobilizing affect: A possible effect of day hospital treatment for chronic psychiatric patients. International Journal of Partial Hospitalization 1992 Dec;8(2):119–26.
22. See reference 9.

CHAPTER VI

Working with Specific Populations in the Milieu

Should diagnosis make a difference in the way the patient is treated in the milieu? Both research and direct experience would suggest that it should. Intensive milieu treatment, while helpful for many patients, is harmful for the patient with schizophrenia and can cause the patient with borderline personality disorder to regress. Gradual social interaction will help the depressed patient; the person with a paranoid personality disorder should not be pushed to interact. The psychiatric hospital or residential treatment center usually treats patients of varying diagnoses within a single unit so that milieu treatment must be "omnitherapeutic." Milieu planning, however, should proceed from a complete understanding of the disorder or behavior to the design of treatment environment.

Those who work in the milieu must share a body of knowledge about how the patient's diagnosis should affect treatment. This will enable the milieu staff to better understand the patient and develop diagnostic-specific techniques. Publications such as the American Psychiatric Association's *Treatments of Mental Disorders* have shown that there is an established body of knowledge for diagnostic-specific treatment. Treatment guidelines for various diagnoses published in the *American Journal of Psychiatry* in the 1990s demonstrate the advantages of research-informed treatment. The information in this chapter about milieu treatment for specific populations is not always informed by research, but is informed primarily by clinical practice. This chapter discusses only milieu design and treatment and builds upon the reader's own clinical knowledge of diagnosis. It does not repeat material from the *Diagnostic and Statistical Manual.* Behaviors characteristic of the diagnosis are mentioned only as they affect milieu treatment. It is presumed that those who work in the milieu work with sufficient background information about each diagnosis.

The discussion of milieu treatment for each population may be more helpful in informing the milieu staff what not to do, rather than what to do. Those who work in the milieu must not only know how to work with varying diagnoses; they must also be aware of how patients with these diagnoses will affect the milieu and other patients. The staff must be prepared for the milieu impact of a patient with obsessive-compulsive disorder, or a person with multiple personality disorder, or even a patient with borderline personality disorder. Their imprint upon the psychiatric milieu will not be invisible.

The populations discussed are not limited to the diagnoses from the *Diagnostic and Statistical Manual.* Other groups also deserve special consideration. Adolescents and children will have varying diagnoses, but there are treatment guidelines that are more relevant to their developmental stage than to their illness. Homosexuality is not an illness, but the staff must create a welcome and comforting milieu for this population. We are only now beginning to create a culturally competent and responsive milieu for an expanding multicultural population. Some populations are considered in the chapter on Addressing Special Problems in the Milieu. Violent patients or suicidal patients or difficult patients do not necessarily constitute a homogeneous group, but they do constitute a problem that must be addressed. Patients with AIDS constitute both a population to be treated in the psychiatric milieu, and the danger of AIDS transmission for psychiatric patients is in turn, a very serious problem.

1. Adolescents

The inpatient stay for adolescent patients is usually only an interval in a continuum of care that may include outpatient therapy, residential treatment, day hospitalization, halfway houses or group homes. In response to the great change in therapeutic resources, Lewis recommends that programs for adolescents be designed according to their varying needs. He recommends a short-term crisis intervention program oriented toward adaptation, psychosocial skills treatment for psychotic and neurobiologically-impaired adolescents unable to tolerate intense treatment, and a long-term intensive/reconstructive treatment for those with severe personality disorders. Although these programs might be designed for individual units, treatment groups are more suitable for the smaller hospital. Treatment groups can specifically address the appropriate treatment needs, goals, and resources for each of these populations. Treatment groups within the same unit are preferable to division into separate units because longer term patients form a stable unit culture while a rapid turnover of patients constantly disrupts it [1–2].

Acute Crisis Intervention

This program is suitable for adolescents with adjustment disorders, personality disorders, major affective disorders and emerging psychotic disorders. It can provide a supportive psychotherapeutic approach that helps to contain overwhelming impulses and feelings, bolsters defenses, and begins working relationships with the family. The treatment may include behavioral, cognitive, reality-oriented, supportive and psychoeducational techniques. The staff actively confronts resistances to treatment and gives only minor attention to transference. Family therapy begins immediately and sessions are frequent. Focal inpatient treatment planning concentrates treatment primarily on the changes necessary to prepare the patient for discharge [1–3].

Gold and colleagues describe a short-term program for adolescents based on a family treatment model. The psychotherapist, who sees the adolescent four or five times a week, becomes the "comprehensive therapist" with full responsibility for family therapy and discharge planning. Therapy strengthens useful defenses. Milieu therapy is behaviorally based with individual point sheets coordinated with the patient's treatment goals. Time spent in the program, rather than point accumulation, determines privilege levels [4].

Intensive Treatment

Work in intensive treatment is directed toward personality disorders that have not responded to short-term treatment. It is supported by the belief that appropriate treatment can bring about deep and lasting personality change. Patients are helped to build reparative relationships with their therapist, treatment team, and with each other. They will undoubtedly express their own pathology in these relationships and the milieu staff will prepare for regressions. Family work attempts to change the family system and requires a strong alliance that will help family members bear the confrontation, stress and pain they will inevitably experience during the adolescent's treatment [5].

Psychosocial Rehabilitation

This program can provide an ego-building developmental treatment approach that includes psychoeducational, behavioral and social skills training. The treatment milieu must provide a positive and respecting atmosphere. Treatment goals are limited [5].

Stages of Adolescent Treatment

Many writers have outlined the stages of adolescent psychiatric treatment, although these stages may now be a luxury that inpatient treatment can no longer afford. Extreme resistance, conflicts, and testing of limits usually mark the first stage. Trust will be a major issue. The milieu must provide high levels of structure and control and hold the adolescent responsible for behavior. Rinsley believes that the adolescent is not capable of realizing the need for treatment or the staff's motivation to help. The patient's resistance behavior is heavily loaded with transference and reveals the ways the adolescent has controlled relationships with others in the past. Resistance can include leveling (making sibling or peer relationships with treatment staff), seductiveness, oversubmissiveness, persistent avoidance, rebelliousness, scapegoating, gang formation, somatization, and elopement. Rinsley also regards transference diffusion (i.e., staff splitting), playing favorites and manipulation of peers as resistance maneuvers. Adolescents use action-oriented defenses, both self-destructive and destructive to others. The protective functions of the milieu are pivotal to the therapeutic process. The staff's therapeutic stance during this first phase is primarily to build trust, but there is also a "countertransference pull" to become the patient's advocate and offer advice and interpretations [6–9].

In the middle stages, adolescents will gradually decrease their acting out and develop some internal controls forged in the alliance with the milieu staff and therapist. Although this attachment may at first seem extremely dependent it will become the nucleus for all treatment. Real therapy can begin when the patient uses action less frequently to communicate. In this stage, the adolescent also becomes aware of working through feelings. Therapeutic strategies include acknowledging these feelings, supporting exploration, and providing hope. The staff's countertransference feelings during this phase include anger as well as fear that the patient will become psychotic or suicidal [6–9].

In the definitive or integrative stages of treatment, the adolescent is able to discard dysfunctional behaviors and defenses and work toward independence. A process of individuation gradually develops and the adolescent can respond to interpretations and develop insight. Another task of this phase can be the integration of the bad/good self. The therapeutic stance should be one of consistent availability and patience for trial and error. Carter finds that rather than occurring once during treatment, the phases may recur several times. Working through these phases again and again builds a higher level of ego functioning and integration [6–10].

Control of Behavior

The first requirement for effective treatment of acting out adolescents is control of behavior and an immediate response to infractions. When limit setting is inconsistent, the adolescent will challenge even the most complex situations, converting them to delinquent advantage. Although behavioral control is crucial, the staff might make the issue of good or bad behavior an everyday matter rather than charging it with powerful emotions. The personality, mood, and morale of individual staff members often lead to an inconsistent application of the unit's rules. Varying shifts also produce an uneven response to behaviors. The separation between the staff's firm limit-setters and those who believe in understanding and nurturance often confuses the definition of acceptable behavior. There should be a rapid response to the breaking of rules. A reprimand given later, even in the spirit of teaching a lesson, will not be productive. It may even provoke the adolescent, who will see it as an unfair use of power, unrelated to the behavior [11–12].

Without a consistent and predictable structure, adolescents will replicate the turmoil of their earlier family life or transfer the chaos of their thoughts and emotions to the milieu. Bruggen and colleagues believe that reestablishing adult authority with adolescents becomes the most urgent therapeutic task. When it is absent, the adolescent and family remain so anxious that useful learning and understanding can't take place. In the program they describe, parents collaborate in decisions about admission, weekend leaves and discharge, reestablishing their own authority with the treatment team's help [12].

The Assaultive and Violent Adolescent

Management with the violent adolescent requires quick intervention before violence escalates to assault. When property is destroyed or graffiti is discovered, repairs should be immediate to clear the atmosphere of violence that it creates. Many adolescents may be violent because of traumatic overwhelming stimulation or even because of deep wishes for human contact. They desperately need the self-object relationships the milieu staff can give them. Many adolescents simply have no awareness of their inner psychological world or their own emotions, thoughts and feelings, and have no choice but to discharge them by violent actions. The staff can help to support the structurally deficient violent patient. Treatment must be able to help them experience these emotions as part of themselves and learn to express them verbally, to finally be able to convert this motor behavior into verbal behavior [13].

Staff members, too, may be vulnerable to aggression. Joy examined aggressive interactions between staff members and adolescents in a large residential center. The staff members' need to demonstrate competence as crisis managers often brought about physical confrontations. Joy recommends redefining the therapeutic role of the evening shift to provide sources for esteem that don't rely exclusively on maintaining order and control [14].

Stages in an Adolescent Milieu

There is something intrinsic to the treatment of adolescents that produces oscillations of tension. Adolescent milieus, like the adolescent patient, are especially vulnerable to mood swings. The adolescent treatment setting has cyclical stages of organization, with abrupt changes from harmony and openness to resistance and turmoil [15].

DYNAMIC HOMEOSTASIS

Rosenstock and McLaughlin examine the vacillations that often occur in an adolescent milieu. They describe the ideal stage as one of dynamic homeostasis, when the mix of patients is conducive to growth. (They recommend not more than one sociopathic patient for every 12 adolescents.) The patient-staff ratio is appropriate and both groups share mutually satisfying relationships. Lines of authority are clear. Everyone communicates effectively with few distortions and misunderstandings. Staff members meet daily and feel free to express their thoughts and feelings and feel bolstered by support. The adolescents have good role models in patients who have succeeded in the program and are ready for discharge. Patient government is working well, and there are many activities to absorb adolescent energy. The staff reviews the state of the milieu every week [15–16].

TRANSITIONAL STAGE

In this stage, there are signs of crisis. Some destructive aggression occurs and there are minor infractions. The staff feels pressured as patients begin to test the limits. Patient/staff boundaries become less clear and patients seem to long for intense parental care. Patient cliques form and create disruptions with the staff. Staff and patients begin to feel far apart. Staff members disagree on ways to manage patients. No staff member feels confident enough to take leadership [15–16].

CRISIS STAGE

A crisis is marked by acting out by a large number of patients, vandalism, and destruction of property. Rosenstock and McLaughlin describe ways of responding to a crisis. Control is a priority. Patients who are ringleaders in the acting out should be separated from the unit. Both staff and the patient representatives will need to analyze the situation. Following a threat to the community, the staff should increase the number of activities that adolescents enjoy: excursions, competitive athletics, games, and special gym programs. Group therapy techniques may also be helpful [15–16].

Making repairs quickly to the milieu can activate the return to homeostasis. Important day staff members can take other shifts to increase milieu communication and restore morale. A positive expectation that the milieu will be restored catalyzes the return to homeostasis. The milieu leaders will begin to voice community ideals. The resolution of the crisis can restore a communal mood. Changes in policies and procedures often announce the milieu's renewal [15–16].

Oscillations are often predictable. They can result from staff turnover, seasonal changes, frequent discharges with the loss of patient leaders, or staff's emotional withdrawal in the presence of new patients [15–16].

The milieu and group process in adolescent treatment

In object relations terms, the therapeutic goal of adolescent treatment is internalization of the milieu through treatment figures. There is an implicit hope that the difference between the milieu and the adolescent's earlier environment will help to cure. The milieu can be so important that all other modalities are merely ancillary. Barish and Schonfeld describe milieu therapy for adolescents, not as a separate modality but a vehicle for all other treatment modalities. Others believe that if the milieu is not therapeutic all other treatments will fail because the relationships that patients and staff develop are the nucleus of treatment. The milieu exerts a great deal of control over the patient's psychosocial environment so that it can be potentially therapeutic. It provides a new type of reality that is valid only for those willing to participate in it [16–18].

The staff must appreciate the overwhelming presence of adolescent sexuality and treat it with awe and full respect for its normality. Residents should participate in the normal adolescent rituals, dances, spring proms, and concerts. Adolescence, even in the psychiatric setting, should be about fun, and the infusion of fun greatly enhances the general climate [18].

The milieu staff may need to do its share of corrective parenting, helping withdrawn or isolated patients to interact, and enabling many adolescents learn to see themselves as others see them. All adolescents will need an emotionally private place or shelter within the milieu, a space clearly defined as theirs [18].

High staff-patient interaction is an influential factor in successful treatment. The milieu staff works to behave in ways that demonstrate the belief that all interactions have therapeutic potential: "purposeful interaction." Staff can't always avoid confrontations with adolescents and effectively confronting them requires experience, confidence, and conviction. Confrontations risk being angry or impulsive, authoritarian, defensive or self-serving, and are not necessarily therapeutic. Interventions are not just to stop an action but to help model decision making. In some treatment centers the role of psychotherapy can become so significant that all other treatment modalities suffer. Meeks has noted that if the milieu staff is treated as little more than glorified baby-sitters waiting for the therapist to arrive with the correct intervention that they will finally identify with the adolescents and act rebellious. Of the many therapeutic modalities available for adolescents, none demands more personal engagement with patients than milieu management. Everything that happens in the milieu influences the adolescent. Although milieu interactions should have therapeutic value, Amini and colleagues caution that an intense focus on dynamics may be too threatening for adolescents who may feel "overtherapized, naked and exposed." The group process is a powerful force in adolescent treatment and when the group is effective, a mutual system of interaction and dependency can develop among the patients and staff. A group identity develops with its own mood, norms, values, and behavior [18–21]

The adolescent gradually finds a place in the group, and identification with the group and its acceptance can lead to changes in behavior. Adolescents develop a sense of responsibility to the group by sharing activities as well as sharing the group's rewards and punishments. Rose writes that at Peper Harow the older peers demonstrate the accepted values in the gang/tribe/community through relationships with each other, with new residents and staff. The new resident will have many chances to learn whether the expressed values are real. The new resident longs for acceptance from the group and will make changes in behavior to earn it. Once the peer group and the environment are integrated, the resident relates to the community almost as if it were an actual person. The staff can strengthen the group by considering such questions as: What's happening to the group right now? What does the group think about this? Staff members might suggest that the adolescent bring up an individual problem because the group might be able to solve it [22–23].

If the milieu culture is not stable and strong, the destructive potential of the group process can take over. Patients can be scapegoated on the unit. Naive and "good" adolescents face destructive peer pressure. A large number of aggressive patients can create serious problems [24].

STAFF

Psychiatric treatment is an expression of human beings—the staff. The staff's ability to work together as a cohesive team is the milieu's most effective force. Problems in communication, unresolved anger, and anxieties can distract from a treatment focus on the adolescent. Relationships among staff members are almost as important as those with patients since the adolescent projects family conflicts onto the staff who need their own healthy interactions to allow successful working of family issues. Perinpanayagam indicates that treatment problems can often be unraveled and understood by understanding staff members' difficulties with each other. Further, while caring directly for patients can lead to difficulties, caring for the philosophy of treatment and for the staff can lead to a solution of most of the patients' problems and their mutual growth. The therapeutic results of the milieu should be measured by its effect on staff as well as patients. Staff satisfaction can be increased by full participation in clinical staff meetings, staff retreats, and the administration's openness to questioning and criticism [25–26].

THE ADOLESCENT AND THE FAMILY

Parental involvement is crucial in inpatient treatment. Waugh and Kjos compared outcomes of patients in adolescent day treatment and found that those with parents involved in the program showed greater improvements and were less likely to require further hospitalization. The staff should make every effort to empower parents and restore adult authority to prepare for family reconciliation. Many adolescents blame their parents for putting them in inpatient treatment, and this and other previous events may have left them chronically angry. Reconciliation can begin with the simple acknowledgment of the parents' and adolescent's attachment to each other. This reconciliation is an essential step following their normal separation and disengagement from each other [27–29].

Discharge and Discharge Regression

Adolescents are vulnerable to regression as discharge nears. Although discharge is similar to leaving home and family, adolescents will deny its sadness and attempt to sabotage it. The staff, too, may be reluctant to process termination. The adolescent who plans an active role in researching and making an aftercare plan has a better chance for a healthy transition. If the adolescent does regress, the staff should reframe it as old, nonproductive behavior and provide encouragement to draw on new coping patterns learned in the milieu [30].

References

1. Lewis JM III. The changing face of adolescent inpatient psychiatric treatment. Psychiatric Hospital 1991;22(4):161–3.
2. Gold IM, Heller C, Ritorto B. A short-term psychiatric inpatient program for adolescents. Hospital & Community Psychiatry 1992 Jan;43(1):58–64.
3. Harper G. Focal inpatient treatment planning. Journal of the American Academy of Child & Adolescent Psychiatry 1989;28:31–7.
4. See reference 2.
5. See reference 1.
6. Miskimim RW. A theoretical model for the practice of residential treatment. Adolescence 1990;25(100):867–90.
7. Rinsley DB. Theory and practice of intensive residential treatment of adolescents. Psychiatric Quarterly 1968;42(4):612–38.
8. Rinsley DB. Psychiatric hospital treatment of adolescents: Verbal and non-verbal resistance to treatment. Bulletin of the Menninger Clinic 1961;25:249–63.
9. Fritsch RC, Heinssen RK, Delga I, Goodrich W, et al. Predicting hospital adjustment of adolescent inpatients. Hospital & Community Psychiatry 1991 Jan;43(1):49–53.
10. Carter TN. Phases, therapeutic strategies and transference-countertransference paradigms in residential treatment. Residential Group Care & Treatment 1982;1(1):29–49.
11. Crabtree LH. Hospitalized adolescents who act out: a treatment approach. Psychiatry 1982 May;45(2):147–58.
12. Bruggen P, Byng-Hall J, Pitt-Aikens T. Reason for admission as a focus of work for an adolescent unit. British Journal of Psychiatry 1973;122:319–29.
13. Marohn RC. Management of the assaultive adolescent. Hospital & Community Psychiatry 1992 Jun; 43(6): 622–4.
14. Joy DS. The maintenance of order on an adolescent inpatient unit: an analysis of work on the evening shift. Psychiatry 1981;44:253–62.

15. Levinson DF, Crabtree LH. Ward tension and staff leadership in a therapeutic community for hospitalized adolescents. Psychiatry 1979;42:220–40.
16. Rosenstock HA, McLaughlin M. On the primary prevention of critical mass: a systems strategy for adolescent units. Journal National Association of Psychiatric Hospitals 1982;13(1):9–11.
17. Barish JI, Schonfeld WA. Comprehensive residential treatment of adolescents. Current Psychiatric Therapies 1971;12:9–17.
18. See reference 6.
19. Meeks JE. Hospital treatment of the psychiatrically disturbed adolescent. Clinical Update in Adolescent Psychiatry 1984;1(19):1–18.
20. Youngren VR. Opportunities hard knocks: clinical training in adolescent milieu therapy. Psychotherapy 1981;28:298–303.
21. Amini F, Burke EL, Edgerton R. Social structure of a psychiatric ward for adolescents and the therapeutic implications of patient-staff and intra-staff conflicts. Adolescence 1978;13(51):411–8.
22. Rose M. The design of atmosphere: Ego-nurture and psychic change in residential treatment. Journal of Adolescence 1986;9:49–62.
23. Rose M. The function of food in a residential treatment process. Residential Treatment for Children & Youth 1988;6(1):43–60.
24. Kahn DG, Boyer DN. Inpatient hospital treatment of adolescents. Psychiatric Clinics of North America 1980;3(3):513–45.
25. Perinpanayagam KS. Organization and management of an in-patient treatment unit for adolescents. Journal of Adolescence 1987;10:133–48.
26. Rasmussen GG. Commentary on Marc I. Ehrlich's "Adolescents in Transition: a look at a transitional treatment center." Journal of Community Psychology 1981;9:93–7.
27. Waugh TA, Kjos DL. Parental involvement and the effectiveness of an adolescent day treatment program. Adolescence 1992;21(4):487–97.
28. Byalin K. Patient empowerment: a treatment strategy for hospitalized adolescents. Hospital & Community Psychiatry 1990 Jan;41(1):89–90.
29. Levy L, Pokart J, List P. Reconciliation with parents as a treatment goal for adolescents in an acute care psychiatric hospital. Social Work in Health Care 1987;13(1):1–21.
30. Shields JD, Choras PT. Treatment of the hospitalized adolescent: Management of regression during discharge. Adolescent Psychiatry 1982;10:407–24.

2. Persons with AIDS; Persons who are HIV-Positive

The milieu staff will need preparation to care for the increasing number of AIDS and HIV-positive patients who require hospitalization for substance abuse or psychiatric illness. Not only can psychiatric illness develop as a direct result of HIV infection, it can also be the result of an emotional response to the illness. In order to work effectively with AIDS patients milieu staff members must come to terms with their own fears and feelings about the illness, homosexuality, substance abuse, and death. Staff discussion must be free enough to enable members to share their own fears with colleagues in the milieu. Once the staff members realize that there are no taboo topics, they will be able to receive support by sharing feelings. Their work will be difficult [1–2].

The HIV virus can attack brain cells as well as T-cells. AIDS Dementia Complex creates disturbances of emotion, behavior, and cognition. Patients can become socially withdrawn, apathetic and forgetful. Personality changes often result. The staff may misinterpret many neuropsychiatric symptoms of AIDS as symptoms of a psychiatric disorder. In early stages AIDS-related dementia may present as a major depressive disorder. An experienced staff member can help patients understand these organic complications of AIDS, and teach them ways to compensate. Patients with AIDS often suffer anxiety and depression. As many as 15 to 20% of AIDS patients meet the established criteria for major depression [1–3].

In addition to treating the patient's psychiatric disorders, inpatient care should include counseling on risk-reduction measures and education about medical treatment. Psychoeducational groups for HIV-positive inpatients can decrease feelings of isolation, offer patients information about their condition, and help them develop responsibility to take precautions to prevent the spread of the disease. The group is an appropriate therapeutic format to address patients' fears and concerns about the disease and provide support [3–5].

Confidentiality

The staff should clarify the limits of confidentiality before the patient's admission. Disclosure of HIV status should be limited to the staff directly involved in the patient's care, and then when it is necessary for management and treatment. Disclosure to other staff is not appropriate. If there is not a psychiatric unit specifically for AIDS patients, the staff needs to learn whether the patient plans to keep the illness confidential and act accordingly. Even if the patient tells others, the staff's inability to openly discuss AIDS or sexuality may create walls around the topic and the patient's own feelings about it. If the patient does wish it to be confidential, staff members can still provide comfort through private talks with the patient about the illness and the patient's own anxieties. Patients who do tell others can often receive a great deal of support, but all of the after-effects of such a revelation should be planned for in treatment [3–6].

Some Crucial Guidelines

The staff should consult the most current American Psychiatric Association AIDS policy as well as their own professional guidelines before admitting a patient with AIDS. Guidance about informing sexual partners of the HIV-positive patient now state that it is ethically permissible to notify sexual partners at risk if the patient refuses to inform them or is unable to cease or change behaviors that put others at risk. Either the psychiatrist or public health authorities can inform. Since sex and the sharing of needles can occur in psychiatric settings, patients need protection from these high risk behaviors. Certain vulnerable populations such as the young, the chronically mentally ill and the developmentally disabled require even more protection [7].

PROTECTION OF PATIENTS AND STAFF

The hospital has the responsibility to reduce the risk of HIV transmission between patients and between patients and staff. All hospital members should be considered potentially at risk. There should be appropriate implementing and monitoring of infection control procedures, appropriate management of behavioral disturbances to reduce the risk and appropriate supportive and education services for the patients, their families, and the staff. Supervision must ensure that patients do not engage in behavior likely to transmit HIV in the hospital [7].

COUNTERTRANSFERENCE

Countertransference will be inevitable in working with patients with AIDS. Their despair and helplessness will produce similar feelings in the staff. Acceptance by the staff will help to alleviate their feelings of rejection and abandonment. Interdisciplinary collaboration will help staff members overcome feelings of helplessness [8].

AIDS AND HIV-POSITIVE PATIENTS IN CHEMICAL DEPENDENCY TREATMENT

Patients who are HIV-positive and patients with AIDS have particular difficulties in chemical dependency treatment. Since they believe that being HIV-positive will eventually lead to death, they will question the need to work toward sobriety. Their response to their diagnosis overwhelms other treatment issues and distracts from work to recover from chemical dependency. Since secrets are the enemy of recovery, keeping the HIV-positive status confidential will provide a serious challenge [9].

Pohl discusses the chemical dependency treatment of HIV-positive patients and reports that the traditional confronting of denial is not extended to challenging the denial of the infection. It may be years before the person will have to deal with its serious implications. When possible, a single focus on chemical dependency is preferred. The person is best treated in a community that can provide emotional support for those who are HIV-positive. Staff and resident education will be of help, but it may not be sufficient to change negative attitudes [9].

Spirituality can be significant in the lives of these patients. AIDS or an HIV-positive diagnosis forces the person to think seriously about questions of life and death. A spiritual foundation can help build a more positive response and better prognosis for HIV-positive patients who are chemically dependent [9].

THE NEEDS OF THE PATIENT

Therapeutic tasks for the staff will include helping patients deal with social stigma and their fears about AIDS, as well as preparing to face progressive mental and medical disabilities. Support is crucial for the AIDS patient, and the staff should make every effort to decrease the patient's isolation from the milieu, from normal staff contacts, and from other patients. Although the depressed AIDS patient may seek isolation, slowly increasing interaction with others will decrease the painful feelings of abandonment. Physically touching the patient may become an essential part of staff care. Staff members can feel deeply satisfied by offering their own companionship and their desire to share the patient's experience. There will also be times that the patient will need to withdraw; patients who are facing death may be withdrawing their emotional investment in others, and the milieu staff can help the family understand this process [10–11]

Patients with AIDS may be dealing with anger, decreased self-esteem, feelings of loss and abandonment. A milieu staff that can help them explore these feelings may accompany them along their way to resolution. Staff members experienced in the care of AIDS can assure them that all of these reactions are not abnormal. Patients may need to explore their own feelings of guilt, or they may feel that they are being punished for homosexuality and drug abuse. Staff members concerned about what they can do for the patient with AIDS often find that a good first step is to simply ask the patient what would be helpful [12].

Staff members can help AIDS patients begin to reminisce about their own lives, often by asking the right questions and by being interested. Some reflections upon the meaning and importance of the patient's life and kind affirmations may take on great significance. The work will be difficult and full of sorrow but staff members will never again need to question their own ability to be of help [12].

References

1. Levenson AI. Psychiatric aspects of AIDS. Psychiatric Hospital 1988;19(3):109–13.
2. Critchley DL. Commentary on Ellis. Archives of Psychiatric Nursing 1987;1(6): 441–3.
3. Grant SM. The hospitalized AIDS patient and the psychiatric liaison nurse. Archives of Psychiatric Nursing 1988;2(1):35–9.
4. American Psychiatric Association. Commission on AIDS. AIDS policy: Position Statement on Confidentiality, Disclosure, and Protection of Others. American Journal of Psychiatry 1993 May;150(5):705–12.
5. Lauer-Listhaus B, Watterson J. A psychoeducational group for HIV- positive patients on a psychiatric service. Hospital & Community psychiatry 1988 Jul;39(7):776–7.
6. Forstein M, Baer J HIV Infection. In: Sederer LI, ed. Inpatient psychiatry: Diagnosis and treatment. 3rd. ed. Baltimore: Williams and Wilkins, 1991: 189–211.
7. See reference 4.
8. Chachkes E, Kaufer S, Primack S, Ullah E. Countertransference in professionals working with chemically dependent clients with HIV. Journal of Chemical Dependency Treatment 1991;4(2):159–70.
9. Pohl MI. Residential treatment for chemically dependent clients with HIV. Journal of Chemical Dependency Treatment 1991;4(2):79–90.

10. Amchin J, Polan HJ. A longitudinal account of staff adaptation to AIDS patients on a psychiatric unit. Hospital & Community Psychiatry 1986 Dec;37(12):1235–8.
11. Ellis NK, Krch-Cole E. Providing a therapeutic milieu experience for a patient diagnosed with Acquired Immune Deficiency Syndrome. Archives of Psychiatric Nursing 1987;1(6): 436–40.
12. See reference 3.

3. Alcoholism

Inpatient alcoholism programs have not demonstrated greater effectiveness than outpatient programs. Because inpatient treatment usually has patients who are more seriously ill, it is not possible to compare outcomes. Moreover, it is not known which programs are best for which patients. Inpatient treatment provides a secure environment with close medical supervision, educational sessions, group therapy and positive peer influence. Alcoholics Anonymous and the 12-Step program is usually a significant component. Inpatient care attempts a total immersion in a recovering milieu to overcome the alcoholic's strong denial system. The impact of an inpatient experience can be profound and many patients have reported their inpatient stay as one of the most powerful and enduring emotional experiences of their lives. Due to the high early dropout rate of many programs, engaging the patient is a critical part of any effective therapy. The more comprehensive the treatment plan, the greater improvement for those patients who remain engaged [1–3].

Adelman and Weiss's meta-analysis of empirical studies finds that positive outcome in alcoholism treatment is associated with some of the following characteristics: counselors with good interpersonal skills, good peer support and many group-oriented treatment modalities, such as the group intake interview and group therapies. What they term "constructive coercion" by referring parties also led to positive outcome. The patient benefits from having a significant other person committed to support and help recovery. Other helpful factors were the employer's involvement in hospitalization as well as vocational assessment and rehabilitation [4].

THE MINNESOTA PLAN

Many inpatient treatment programs for alcoholism are based on the Minnesota Plan, which combines the philosophies of the self-help movement of Alcoholics Anonymous with milieu therapy in a caring community. One of the Minnesota plan's contributions was the concept of the multidisciplinary team approach that includes paraprofessional recovering people, physicians, nurses, psychologists, social workers and certified addiction counselors. The Minnesota-inspired programs usually involve a fixed period of hospitalization, usually 28 days [5].

Group Treatment

A strong group orientation in the milieu is more effective than an intensive individualized approach. Stinson and colleagues compare the results of two inpatient programs for alcoholics. One program had a high staff-patient ratio with the operating assumption that intensive staff-patient interaction produces good patient outcome. The other, peer-oriented care, had low staff density with the belief that patient-patient interaction is significant in recovery. The peer-oriented program proved to be superior to the intensive care approach in changing drinking behavior. This unit had 40% less staff and was run by a small self-governing group of patients helped by a professional consultant. Although Stinson and colleagues could find no explanation, they speculate that greater patient engagement and responsibility produced the better outcome [6].

The group setting is ideal for interventions that combat the problems of denial and poor motivation. The isolation of addiction begins to erode and defensive barriers crumble. Denial loosens its hold when the group rewards members for their openness. Acceptance and understanding soothe the pains of guilt and shame. The group sharing of experiences can overcome denial, self-hatred, self-pity and guilt. This experience becomes a bridge reconstructing honest human relationships that can also provide a spiritual experience that brings about change. Patients can identify strongly with this peer group and form a community of mutual assistance. Machell studied the importance of fellowship and belongingness in the residential treatment of 200 chronic, recidivistic adult male alcoholics. Data from the study of the 90-day program indicated that clients' perceived belongingness is an important factor in successful treatment outcome. Wilson and Kennard find that while alcoholics admitted to treatment received MMPI scores in the introverted range, those who stayed in treatment more than 6 months and more than 12 months showed consecutive increases in extroversion. This change was most likely an important factor in treatment success. There is apparently something curative about the fellowship of the group [7–11].

There are many group therapeutic approaches that are effective in treating alcoholism: focus groups that attempt to increase assertiveness and self-control, social skills, and relaxation/desensitization groups. Other examples include groups to cope with the denial of alcoholism, groups where the alcoholic tells a life story and the listeners respond, problem-solving groups where patients learn to cope with the urge to drink and learn methods of problem solving in order to overcome difficulties. Therapeutically the patients must be able to recognize the distorted feelings that alcoholism has produced, their self-pity, resentment, guilt and shame. These feelings have enabled them to excuse their continued abuse and even continue with more deviant behavior. It is only when alcoholics look at this behavior do they realize that it has distorted the true person. They can then begin to restore their own self-esteem [12–13].

EDUCATIONAL COMPONENTS

Inpatient alcoholism treatment milieus that use psychoeducational techniques and meetings have more favorable outcomes than milieus that don't. Educational materials can also instruct in ways that reduce drinking [14].

BEHAVIORAL TECHNIQUES

Olson and colleagues randomly assigned 113 alcoholic patients to 4 groups with varying treatments: behavioral groups stressing covert desensitization and relaxation, transactional analysis groups, groups combining behavioral and transactional techniques, and a milieu treatment control group. After four years of follow-up, they found that patients in the behavioral group consumed less alcohol, were abstinent longer, and had better clinical adjustment [15].

O'Farrell and Langenbucher describe a comprehensive behavioral approach for inpatient treatment. The treatment has three major goals: to facilitate a commitment to change, stabilize the change in drinking and plan aftercare and post-discharge life to maintain the changes. Individual and group behavioral therapy in this program consisted of 90-minute sessions devoted to relaxation training, problem-solving skills, alternatives to drinking in problem situations, training in assertiveness and drink refusal, instructions in self-control skills and the use of a contract with significant others to keep taking Antabuse [16].

An assessment for each patient investigates the individual, cultural and social antecedents to drinking. An investigation of consequences of drinking should also be part of the assessment. This should include: neuropsychological, medical, personality and social consequences. This assessment should lead to the patient's increased awareness of the extent of the alcohol problem and its consequences and strengthen commitment to a change in drinking behavior. Reasons for not drinking should be made explicit [16].

Stabilizing the patient requires teaching skills to deal with high-risk situations that could bring on drinking and strengthening the behaviors incompatible with abusive drinking. The program used aversion therapy to decrease desire for alcohol. Alcoholic beverages were repeatedly paired with either a drug that produced nausea or aversive mental imagery. Since many patients had used alcohol to cope with stress, tension and anxiety, they needed to develop alternative skills for dealing with these situations. This will include relaxation training and systematic desensitization as well as social skills training [16].

Social skills training for alcoholics usually involves a number of techniques designed to teach skills for interacting with people, including the ability to be converse with others, how to refuse drinks, and how to be assertive. Social skills training takes place in a group format. Patients learn to handle problem situations. For example, they will need to practice an effective response to requests or pressure to drink. The components of an effective response are modeled: eye contact, convincing affect, facial expression, gestures, posture, refusal of the request, changing the subject or suggesting another activity. Each person will have a chance to practice this response. Social skills training can be effective for alcoholic patients. A one-year follow-up of 24 residents assigned either to a conventional discussion group or social skills training group in alcoholism treatment revealed that those who received social skills training were sober and employed for twice the number of days as residents who attended the discussion group [16–17].

Vocational assistance and the improvement of marital and family relationships will also help to strengthen behaviors incompatible with alcohol abuse. Many patients will need training in how to find and keep a job and how to deal with work-related problems that can lead to drinking. Marital and family therapy are used to get the spouse and family to support the patient's decision to stop drinking and explore family behavioral changes needed to maintain sobriety. Specific plans for aftercare with the alcoholic are one of the staff's most important tasks. Plans may include continued use of Antabuse, Alcoholics Anonymous, alcoholism counseling, and marital or family therapy. Life style analysis and planned modification help patients left with a great deal of unstructured time explore pleasurable and meaningful activities that are incompatible with drinking behavior This modification may involve the addition of physical exercise, meditation, or what are called "positive addictions" [16–17].

McCrady describes two behavioral treatment models, the Community Reinforcement Approach (CRA), and Behavioral Self-Control Training (BCST). The CRA model increases access to a variety of positive reinforcers, but with continued access contingent on abstinence. Clients were helped to find jobs and a place to live, were helped to contact their families, and given membership in a social club that did not allow drinking. They were given social skills training to improve their communication with families and prepare for job interviews. Their abstinence was monitored each day. If they drank and went to work or missed work, they received no pay for the day. Family visits were canceled if they drank. They contracted with another person who supervised their taking disulfiram. This treatment produced good outcomes for inpatients who had been alcoholic for a long time [17].

Behavioral Self-Control Training is helpful for the heavy drinker who is not addicted. This program, based on the behavioral principles of self-management, teaches people to monitor their urges to drink, their drinking, and set goals to reduce it. Clients learn techniques for avoiding drinking companions and drinking environments [17].

Staff

Consultation and coordination among alcoholism treatment staff can uncover redundant endeavors and provide constructive input from all disciplines. Manipulative, drug-seeking behaviors may repel some staff members while the neediness and constant crises that chemically dependent patients experience may overwhelm others [18].

JOINT ADMISSION OF FAMILY MEMBERS IN ALCOHOLISM TREATMENT

Some alcoholism treatment programs have experimented with the admission of family members. A program that admitted chemically dependent women and their children under 12 provided a family-structured living environment, psychotherapy, education, and an AA program. The treatment included parenting and vocational rehabilitation components. Results from the program have been promising, with 49 of 65 participants over a 5-year period remaining sober and employed after completing the program. McCrady and colleagues reported on the promising results of joint hospitalized admission for alcoholic patients and their spouses [19–21].

THE TWELVE-STEP PROGRAM AND ALCOHOLICS ANONYMOUS

Alcoholics Anonymous, Narcotics Anonymous, and the 12-Step Program have been incorporated into inpatient alcoholism and substance abuse treatment and have proven to be the most effective way to maintain sobriety. Recovery from addiction in Alcoholics Anonymous is based on a spiritual, cognitive, and behavioral way of life that is able to provide interpersonal well-being and a value system based on honesty and humility. Participants find strong role models among an experienced membership. Continuing the 12 steps and attending Alcoholics or Narcotics Anonymous meetings provide the bridge to aftercare. AA meetings are often described as medication, with meetings to be taken daily for the first three months of sobriety. Most treatment programs prescribe 90 meetings in 90 days because of the high risk of relapse in the first three months and the need for an intensive experience to break through denial. Alcoholics Anonymous and 12-step programs are easily available and help from others is available 24 hours a day. In most cases if substance abusers stop attending meetings they run serious risks of returning to addictive behavior [22–23].

The AA group process becomes the catalyst for acculturation. Two processes are prominent: uncovering and universalization. Emotions and thoughts previously blurred by substance abuse arise dramatically in the uncovering process. Universalization, the mutual identification with others in the group and the sharing of emotions, gives the group a healing power. These emotions come to be recognized as part of the human experience. Peer concern energizes the treatment and prevents members from giving up. As they share their lives, group members in 12-step programs become attached to each other and to their group. When residents confront each other and force each other to change, their acting out in the milieu will correspondingly decrease [24].

The acceptance of a higher power has been difficult for those who do not share a religious and spiritual orientation. Agnostic AA members have provided another name for God: Good Orderly Direction. Galanter and colleagues describe another self-help process for substance abusers. Rational Recovery has a cognitive orientation and does not share the spiritual basis of AA. The approach is based on the assumption that psychological difficulties are caused by irrational beliefs which can be understood and overcome. Rational Recovery uses certain cognitive devices such as a conceptualization of "The Beast," to personify the compulsive thoughts that make one drink. Recovery rejects the belief that the person is powerless over alcohol. Rational Recovery uses a group process managed by those who have conquered addiction. Group cohesion helps to alleviate distress and reinforces continuing compliance [24–25].

Membership in Alcoholics Anonymous can help the person become more open and honest and more willing to learn. Many will grow through the honest acceptance they receive from the members, and others will be helped in achieving abstinence with the help of the spiritual dimension that it provides. The fellowship with others establishes hope and erects a support system of stable individual and group relationships, based initially on a shared experience. Working the 12 Steps involves humility. Many who join become more compassionate and eager to help others who are struggling with alcoholism and the problems of living [26].

Alcoholics Anonymous and the 12 steps also provide members with a comprehensive ideology which can help them evaluate, understand and overcome alcohol dependence. This ideology helps unite members in ways of understanding their problems and ways to overcome them. The group ideology helps to correct cognitive distortions that characterize alcoholism. The ideological bond among members who share the same problem helps to build group cohesion and trust, creating a basis for further change. The endpoint of the 12 steps is a higher sense of community. The AA ideology can give a new awareness and acceptance of limitations and powerlessness. The fact that members share the same problem gives them an ideological bond which in turn builds cohesiveness and trust, setting the conditions for the beginning of change [27–28].

References

1. Collins GB. Contemporary issues in the treatment of alcohol dependence. Psychiatric Clinics of North America 1993 Mar;16(1):33–48.
2. Goodwin DW. Inpatient treatment of alcoholism—new life for the Minneapolis Plan. New England Journal of Medicine 1991;325(11): 804–6.
3. Goldsmith RJ. The essential features of alcohol and drug treatment. Psychiatric Annals 1992;22(8):419–24.
4. Adelman SA, Weiss RD. What is therapeutic about inpatient alcoholism treatment? Hospital & Community Psychiatry 1989 May;40(5):515–19.

5. Ditzler JM, Ditzler JR. Treatment at Farm Place. British Journal of Addiction 1989;84:493–7.
6. Stinson DJ, Smith WG, Amidjaya J, Kaplan JM. Systems of care and treatment outcomes for alcoholic patients. Archives of General Psychiatry 1979;36(5):535–9.
7. See reference 3.
8. See reference 5.
9. Galanter M. Cult and zealous self-help movements: a psychiatric perspective. American Journal of Psychiatry 1990;145(5):543–52.
10. Machell D. Fellowship as an important factor in alcoholism residential treatment. Journal of Alcohol & Drug Education 1987; 32(2): 56–8.
11. Wilson S, Kennard D. The extraverting effect of treatment in a therapeutic community for drug abusers. British Journal of Psychiatry 1978; 132:296–9.
12. Michaely N, Eldar P, Weiss S. The Israeli residential center for alcoholics 1982–87. Journal of Substance Abuse Treatment 1989;6:59–75.
13. See reference 5.
14. Finney JW, Moos RH, Chan D. Length of stay and program component effects in the treatment of alcoholism. Journal of Studies in Alcohol 1975;36:88–108.
15. Olson RP, Ganley R, Devine VT, et al. Long-term effects of behavioral versus insight-oriented therapy with inpatient alcoholics. Journal of Consulting & Clinical Psychology 1991;49:866–77.
16. O'Farrell TJ, Langenbucher J. Inpatient treatment of alcoholism: a behavioral approach. Journal of Substance Abuse Treatment 1987;4(3–4):215–31.
17. Eriksen L, Bjornstad S, Gotestam KG. Social skills training in groups for alcoholics: one-year treatment outcome for groups and individuals. Addictive Behaviors 1986;11:309–29.
18. McCrady BS. Promising but underutilized treatment approaches. Alcohol Health & Research World 1991;15(3):215–18.
19. Mendelson JH. Inpatient Programs. American Association Task Force on Treatments of Psychiatric Disorders. Treatments of psychiatric disorders. v. 2. Washington DC: American Psychiatric Press, 1989, 1137–42.
20. Brow J, Cripps R. The Austin Family House Program. Journal of Substance Abuse Treatment 1985;2(1):63–7.
21. McCrady BS, Paolino TJ, Longabough R, Rossi J. Effects of joint hospital admission and couples treatment for hospitalized alcoholics: a pilot study. Addictive Behaviors 1979;4:155–65.
22. Chappel JN. Effective use of Alcoholics Anonymous and Narcotics Anonymous in treating patients. Psychiatric Annals 1982;22(18): 409–418.
23. Brock TF. In Lawson GW, Lawson AW, eds. Adolescent substance abuse: etiology, treatment and prevention. Gaithersburg MD: Aspen, 1992, 105–119.
24. Kemker SS, Kibel HD, Mahler JC. On becoming oriented to inpatient addiction treatment: Inducting new professionals to the recovery movement. International Journal of Group Psychotherapy 1993;43(3):285–301.
25. Galanter M, Egelko S, Edwards H. Rational Recovery: Alternative to AA for addiction? American Journal of Drug & Alcohol Abuse 1993;19(4):499–518.
26. Khantzian EJ, Mack JE Alcoholics Anonymous and contemporary psychodynamic theory. Recent Developments in Alcoholism 1989;7:67–89.

27. See reference 24.
28. Kassel JD, Wagner EP. Processes of change in Alcoholics Anonymous: a review of possible mechanisms. Psychotherapy 1993 Sum;30(2):222–34.

4. Bipolar Disorder, Manic Type

Persons with a bipolar disorder have both manic and depressive episodes. The patient with a depressive episode can be treated in the milieu with the same guidelines as those that apply to the depressed patient, but the staff should be aware that the bipolar depression may be more severe, with delusions and a stronger psychotic flavor. The euphoric person in the manic phase of a bipolar disorder is not someone who will willingly seek admission to the hospital. Hospitalization is usually at the request of family or community members.

Although lithium therapy is the predominant treatment of choice for the manic patient, hospitalization can also have a dramatic effect. Cohen and colleagues' study of 31 patients with acute mania in a psychiatric intensive care unit demonstrated considerable improvement with only moderate doses of antipsychotic medication. Although not much attention has been given to milieu management since the advent of lithium, the authors found that firm and unambivalent setting of limits can decrease manic symptoms. They recommend an intensive care unit as the most effective treatment environment [1].

Stages of Mania

The milieu staff should be aware of the progressive stages of mania. The staff can be caught up in the patient's charisma in the early stages and then be totally unprepared for stages 2 and 3. The initial stage is characterized by rapid speech and physical activity, and a euphoric mood with some grandiosity. The person is friendly and outgoing. In the second stage, both speech and physical activity speed up, sleep patterns are interrupted and the grandiose thinking may have a paranoid flavor. While stage 2 may be difficult, in the final stage the person is closer to a state of panic with incoherent thoughts and bizarre behaviors, barely able to respond to any staff verbal intervention. There may be hallucinations, delusions and disorientation to places and people. The person is equally responsive to all stimuli. Sleep becomes rare, and physiological exhaustion is the result. This final stage occurs in 70% of patients. As the episode remits, the person proceeds through these stages in reverse order. The staff should not confuse severity with prognosis, since this apparently has no effect on the patient's chance to improve [2–4].

Persons in a manic state are totally disruptive to the milieu and can quickly create interpersonal havoc, feeling euphoric, powerful, extremely confident and near to grandiosity. Their strong interactional skills often control communications and relationships. (Unfortunately, these remarkable skills deteriorate as the manic episode progresses and are lost when the episode remits.) Manic patients can involve all members in the unit in their causes or complaints, storm against injustice and organize patients against staff [4–5].

The staff should be highly visible on the unit when there is a patient in a manic episode, communicating with patients and with each other to assure that the person in a manic state is understood. The staff must be prepared to prevent articulate and argumentative manic patients from pursuing dangerous goals, particularly the exploitation of others. They may also become scapegoats on the unit, a source of amusement or hostility. The manic patient can not only exploit other patients but also can divide the staff. Staff members should meet frequently to explore their own conflicts. Community meetings are a helpful forum for both staff and patients. The staff can allay the anxiety of the unit by carefully explaining what happens during a manic episode and help other patients by getting them away from the person's very engaging appeals. The patient's peers must also be counseled as to what behaviors will be tolerated, which will not, and the consequences that will follow [4–6].

Goals and Techniques

The goal of treatment for manic patients may be simply helping them get through the episode with no danger to themselves or others. Manic patients will have difficulty sleeping. They may need quiet activities at night to channel their energy without disturbing others. They will need help with hygiene and with orientation to reality. Self-care skills will deteriorate and they may forget to eat. Brief, simple explanations will be more effective than long discussions or arguments. The staff should avoid power struggles whenever possible and respond positively to any reasonable request. Manic patients can sometimes be diverted from disruptive behavior since their attention span is short. Their agitation, pacing and irritability can often magnify the anxiety level of the unit. A decrease in stimulation should be planned as an intervention when needed. There will be times during the illness to restrict visitors and give the patient time alone. Seclusion should be avoided when possible, since it can lead to panic and agitation. If manic patients can be given single rooms in quiet areas on the unit, they may be able to retreat to their rooms when they feel agitation coming on [6–7].

Consistent limit-setting is essential. Limit-setting and consistent expectations can bring about feelings of safety and help to decrease manipulation. When the staff can make the patients feel that they are responsible for their own behavior, they will then see limit-setting as less controlling or parental. Gunderson warns that when the manic patient is pressing for privileges, there is then no doubt that restrictions are needed. He cautions that judgments about manic patients should be based on what they do, not what they say. When the manic patient is restricted, the restriction should be consistently enforced without ambivalence or conditions. Gunderson reports that when patients begin to deal with real life issues, they are no longer manic [6–7].

VIOLENCE AND DANGEROUSNESS

Bipolar patients are likely to be assaultive since they are often quite psychotic in the third stage of the episode. The staff can best prevent violence by being aware of cues. Huelskoetter notes the following signs of potential violence: demandingness, antagonistic behavior, abusive language, motor restlessness or pacing, antagonistic behavior, posturing as if ready for a fight. The presence of delusions or hallucinations also portends violence. These signs call for staff behaviors that will calm, support and provide security. Manic patients can be sexually provocative. They may bring alcohol or drugs to the unit. Gunderson warns of the danger of firesetting. Huelskoetter believes that the aggressive manic patient fears destructiveness and wants limits set to control behavior. She suggests removal to quiet room for 30 or more minutes away from the stimuli of other patients in the company of a staff member, who is calm and not fearful. This may be enough to calm the patient and gain control [7–8].

Work with the manic patient should address the illness, not the behaviors. If, for example, the patient gives away possessions, the staff should not address the behavior but let the person know how the illness has affected judgement. If treatment concentrates on behavior as illness the patient can develop understanding. Patients can eventually benefit from group therapy in diagnostically-homogeneous groups to help them to understand their illness and relate to others. Inpatient family interventions with psychoeducation can help the family identify precipitating stresses and will improve family functioning. In contrast to work with patients who have other psychiatric disorders, interventions and limit setting with manic patients will have no permanent effect. The interventions will not help in the person's future or development or provide inner controls. They are simply steps that must be taken [9–14].

References

1. Cohen S, Khan A, Clark A, Goldner M, et al. Hospitalization effect in acute mania. General Hospital Psychiatry 1988;138–41.
2. Duda D, Ulsaffer-van Lanen J. Milieu intervention for mania. In: Rogers C, Ulsafer-Van Lanen J, eds. Nursing intervention in depression. New York: Grune & Stratton, 1985, 181–93.
3. Carlson GA, Goodwin FK. The stages of mania. Archives of General Psychiatry 1973;28:221–8.
4. Aranow RB, Sederer LI. Mania. In: Sederer LI. Inpatient psychiatry: diagnosis and treatment. 3rd ed. Baltimore: Williams and Wilkins, 1991, 46–69.

5. Janowsky DS, El-Yousef MK, Davis JM. Interpersonal maneuvers of manic patients. American Journal of Psychiatry 1974 Mar;131(3):250–5.
6. Justic M. Nursing care for the hospitalized patient with psychotic symptoms. In: Wells, LA , ed. A handbook of psychiatric nursing. St. Louis: Warren H. Green, 1989, 245–87.
7. Gunderson JG. Management of manic states: the problem of fire setting. Psychiatry 1974; 37:137–146.
8. Huelskoetter MMW. The person with an affective disorder: depression or elation. In: Murray RB, Huelskoetter MMW, eds. Psychiatric mental health nursing: giving emotional care. East Norwalk, CT: Appleton & Lange, 1991, 493–534.
9. Pollac LE. How do inpatients with bipolar disorder evaluate diagnostically homogeneous groups? Journal of Psychosocial Nursing & Mental Health Services 1993 Oct;31(10):26–32.
10. See reference 2.
11. Haas Gl, Glick ID, Clarkin JF, Spencer JH, et al. Inpatient family intervention : a randomized clinical trial. II. Results at hospital discharge. Archives of General Psychiatry 1988;45:217–24
12. Clarkin JF, Glick ID, Haas GL, Spencer JH, et al. A randomized clinical trial of inpatient family intervention. V. Results for affective disorders. Journal Affective Disorders 1990;18:17–28.
13. Miller JW, Keinter GI, Epstein NE, Bishop DS, et al. Families of bipolar patients: dysfunction, course of illness and pilot treatment study. In: Proceedings of the meeting of the Society for Psychotherapy Research. Pittsburgh, Society for Psychotherapy Research, 1991.
14. American Psychiatric Association. Practice Guideline for the treatment of patients with bipolar disorder. American Journal of Psychiatry 1994 Dec; supplement:1541.

5. Borderline Personality Disorder

One of the most important things to remember about borderline personality disorder is that many persons who are called "borderline" may not meet the full criteria for the diagnosis. It is a term loosely employed by even the most amateur of diagnosticians once a patient proves troublesome. Even if the diagnosis is accurate, it has become a negative stereotype that can set the tone for all future interactions [1].

We now know that many of the "special patients" described in earlier literature were probably persons with borderline personality disorder. Main described the special patient as creating a serious loss of objectivity in the milieu, forming intense, exclusive and mutually harmful relationships. It was the borderline patient who quickly taught the mental health profession that psychiatric treatment should be more diagnosis-specific, that the treatment designed for the depressed patient could be destructive to the person with a borderline personality disorder. Mismanagement of the borderline patient, even in short-term treatment, can have serious long-term consequences. The borderline patient seemed to "cry out for a new social order." Gallop cautions that the borderline patient can easily threaten the nurse's long-established therapeutic competency and pride in being compassionate and nonjudgmental [1–4].

The person with a borderline personality disorder often seems to have a good grasp on reality and would seem to be capable of controlling behavior, more disturbing than emotionally disturbed. Such persons may seem to have incredible power and competency, but their talents are executed in quite the wrong direction. For example, they may have a unique ability to detect and manipulate the vulnerable areas in the hospital power structure. The staff may feel safer distancing themselves from these patients because they fear their manipulation. The rewards seem few since these patients are rarely cooperative or grateful [5–6].

The most predominant feature of borderline patients is instability: in self-image, emotions, behavior and in relationships. They may mark their time in the hospital with angry outbursts, falling in or out of love, sexual promiscuity, repeated suicide attempts or wrist-cutting, and numerous elopements. Johansen describes some of the effects of having too many such patients on the unit at any one time: behavior contagion, staff regression and role reversal, with the staff seeking positive reinforcement from patients or patient leaders, and competition for staff attention. He warns that so much energy is taken up with containment that other milieu functions are lost [7–8].

Treatment Paradigms

There are two basic paradigms for treatment of the patient with borderline personality disorder. The "empathic" or "structural" paradigm is designed to effect structural change through long hospitalization with psychotherapy. The second paradigm, the adaptational approach, depends upon the patient taking much more responsibility in controlling and containing behavior.

The Structural Approach

The structural approach attempts to bring about basic structural personality change. Even regression is potentially valuable, as a key to the interpretation of the transference. The structural approach emphasizes therapeutic attachment and a holding environment that can absorb the patient's rage and distress without retaliation. The relationship between therapist and patient, patient and milieu, will be the strongest therapeutic factor. Fenton and McGlashan seem to be describing a structural approach, when they advise that the patient's symptoms should be regarded as communications that might be better expressed as words. They see the milieu as a laboratory within which the patient can create an interpersonal world that reflects the difficulties experienced before hospitalization. Maladaptive patterns are allowed to be recreated and then presented to the patient for contemplation. They write about the distinct personal imprint that each person leaves in the social field. Borderline patients quickly transform the intrapsychic into the interpersonal. This process, when contained in the milieu, can lead to a progressive integration of more realistic experiences of the self and others [9–10].

THE ADAPTATIONAL APPROACH

The adaptational approach was designed to prevent regression. The approach clearly outlines limit-setting from the very beginning, making the patient responsible for controlling behavior. Taking responsibility may begin as early as a pre-admission contract, or a written contract soon after admission that sets out a negotiated set of expectations and consequences. The understanding that certain actions on the patient's part will make it impossible to continue work is an important feature of this approach [11].

Setting a discharge date at admission strengthens the adaptational approach and establishes a concerned, neutral, and reality-oriented atmosphere. When this is decided upon before treatment, patients will not see it as punitive. Nurnberg and Suh suggest that there be a clear statement that if patients are not ready to leave the hospital at that time, they can transfer to a state or custodial-type setting [12].

The adaptational approach has many proponents. Most would not see the period of hospitalization as ultimately curative, but expect treatment to continue in outpatient therapy. They believe that hospitalization should concentrate on pure treatment issues rather than focusing on building good relationships. This does not mean that a good therapeutic alliance and understanding do not contribute to treatment but that the elements of a corrective atmosphere should be magnified. The patient's motivation for change should have the highest priority.

Goals of Treatment

STRUCTURAL APPROACH

The ultimate goal of structural treatment would be for the patient to achieve a better integrated internal world (sense of self, relationships with others) and become a person who no longer needs to resort to maladaptive defenses such as projective identification or splitting to control aggression or mood. Kernberg and Haran write that treatment with borderline patients will be effective if they can become aware of their own inconsistencies, are less inclined to act out, and can become self-observant enough to control their behavior. This supports Nurnberg and Suh's description of borderline patients as persons who are unable to keep their egos available for self-observation, and whose primitive projective defense mechanisms prevent them from understanding their effect on others. If the staff employs the structural approach, it can help the patient to recognize life patterns in an alliance that would explore and anticipate repetitions during hospitalization. In the milieu the staff can facilitate a new kind of experience that will help the patient to tolerate delays and put feelings into words rather than acting them out. Eppel describes the final treatment goal as establishing a new object relationship or secure base for the patient, yet shaping it over time so that the patient can finally develop an ability to separate and be autonomous. Eppel, who writes about day treatment for the borderline patient, can afford to contemplate such long-term goals since they may be accomplished by a continuum of care from hospitalization to day treatment to outpatient treatment [12–15].

Adaptational Approach

The goal of acute hospitalization adheres to an adaptational approach, which should help the patient establish a more stable environment outside the hospital so that external reality will not reinforces inner chaos. Patients with borderline personality disorder are often not hospitalized unless they are suicidal. Then the goal of hospitalization should be to gain information that will help the patient and therapist forestall future attempts. Patients should remain in the hospital long enough so that observation and interactions can reveal this information [16–17].

Mixing of Paradigms

Fort indicates that many therapists and some treatment teams don't know which underlying paradigm they are following. Milieu staff instruction about the paradigm is necessary since the adaptational and structural paradigms cannot be combined; when they conflict, patients are at risk of becoming dangerously worse. Conflicts may occur when outpatient therapists have a different treatment philosophy than the unit or when the hospital staff unknowingly combine two approaches. Splitting can occur between the therapist and the milieu staff. The situation becomes even worse if the conflicts remain covert. Gordon and Beresin believe that this can happen because outpatient therapists and hospital staff neither view themselves nor represent themselves to others as exclusively selecting an adaptational or structural change in borderline patients. They caution against simply trying to fit the borderline patient into the "standard" hospital treatment, such as assigning all patients to individual and group therapy. Before the admission of a borderline patient, the staff should assure a goodness of fit between the outpatient therapist and the unit philosophy [17–18].

Problems in Treating the Borderline Patient

Regression

Inpatient treatment of the borderline patient has been reformulated through the years because so many patients seriously regressed with conventional psychodynamic hospital treatment. Regression was caused by the hospitalization experience itself. With a 24-hour nurturing environment available to meet every need, the milieu can dramatically evoke the patient's longings for nurturance. The patient may begin to exhibit clinging and demanding behavior, a great deal of anger, depression, suicidal ideation, and other forms of acting out. Eppel finds that these behavioral regressions are self-perpetuating and difficult to arrest. Lerner attributes these regressions to the staff member's excessive need to treat and calls for a redefinition of treatment to include therapeutic nonintervention. Braden finds that similar regressions occur with borderline adolescents when the milieu provides an opportunity for multiple and intense relationships. Braden describes a radical solution in the "supportive containment approach." Patients remain in their small private rooms for a large part of the day and involvement in the unit is titrated according to their ability to manage interaction without destructive regression. This containment makes the patient rely completely on the staff and develop negotiation within the context of stable relationships rather than through regression with intense relationships with peers [19–21].

COUNTERTRANSFERENCE—PROJECTIVE IDENTIFICATION AND SPLITTING

The most serious staff problem in the treatment of the borderline patient occurs because of the staff's countertransference and the inevitable splitting that occurs as a result. Much of this is a result of the patient's projective identification. McCready uses the term milieu countertransference to describe this collective countertransference phenomenon. Adler finds that staff members who receive the cruel and punishing projections from the patient find themselves feeling punitive and cruel. Those who received a loving or idealized projection can feel parental love and protection. The idealized staff members assume that they are the only ones who truly understand the patient. The "punished" staff finds the patient manipulative and impossible to like. When patients project different parts of their inner selves upon staff members, the patient's internal drama becomes the staff's battleground. Staff members play their own parts in the drama. If staff members present themselves as all good, unconditionally loving persons, they contribute to further splitting. Book and colleagues describe meetings in response to borderline patients where staff members spent their time complaining about each other. After they realized that these intense feelings were a result of the patient's own projections, they were then able to discuss their opposing views. Another countertransference response is hopelessness [22–25].

If staff members do become suspicious of each other and undermine each other's work, they will replicate the patients' own confusion and will simply reconfirm their projections. They will forfeit the opportunity to provide new healthy models for identification. Countertransference should be addressed, not denied or criticized. It is the staff members' sensitivity and concern that makes them vulnerable to countertransference and if they were not emotionally engaged, they would probably not experience it. Frequent staff meetings are necessary to prevent splitting. Staff members can work hard in meetings to air differences of opinion so that they can finally see the patient as coherent and whole. The staff member who feels proud about special knowledge of the patient quickly learns that others, too, have been chosen for secrets [25–26].

Suicidal Behaviors

The staff must help the patient to feel free to talk about feelings, even if such feelings are about self-destructive and suicidal actions. A clear distinction should be made between suicidal ideation and suicidal threats. Sederer and Thorbeck believe that if the patient cannot assure the staff that these impulses can be controlled, it will regard the patient as a suicidal threat. The suicide threat can transform the patient from a helpless victim to being in complete control and able to manipulate others. When the staff must turn all energies to security measures to prevent patients from suicide, it cannot really treat them. Sederer and Thorbeck recommend a locked unit for these circumstances. Viner indicates that the staff has no option in this situation other than 1:1 monitoring, and this results in a stalemate or deterioration in treatment since all treatment shifts to behavior control. Viner believes that it would be more effective for the staff to communicate that it cannot fully protect the patient and that meaningful treatment may carry with it a suicide risk. Then the family, the patient, and the hospital administration may need to agree to continue treatment with full recognition of this risk. The patient's chart must record this agreement. The staff then has a collaborative agreement to help the patient identify the emotional states associated with suicidal ideation and actions, and turn again to treatment rather than monitoring [27–28].

Techniques of Treatment

Many who write about a structural approach to the borderline patient find the concept of the holding environment to be helpful. The holding environment provides structure and self-regulation. It can block the maladaptive use of people and other sources, such as drugs, for self soothing and self-regulation. The successful treatment of the patient with a borderline personality disorder depends on the treatment team's skill in maintaining a careful emotional boundary, neither indulging the patient too much nor withholding. Team members cannot afford to be vague or ambivalent when they talk with the patient. Therefore, a treatment philosophy that meets everyone's approval will provide stronger definition. It not only provides structure but will help to maintain staff morale, boundaries, and direction. The team philosophy should clearly define roles for team members, define behavioral interventions and consistent limit-setting. One cannot overemphasize the team members' need to trust each other completely [29].

The role of the team leader has never been so central. The leader must be caring, honest and completely respectful of staff members, helping them understand the intensity of their emotions and the strong temptation to regress in response to the patient. Friedman advises the team leader to look at the danger signals that can hint of emotional over-involvement: when different staff members view the patient in opposite ways and the leader believes that only one is correct or when the staff criticizes the therapist and the leader agrees. Friedman believes that the therapist should not focus on the transference relationship while the patient is in the hospital, and advises that the therapist should help the patient formulate goals for the hospitalization beyond the strengthening of a therapeutic relationship [29–30].

Setting limits is vital. A major requirement is the unit's capacity to set limits empathically and not punitively. The therapeutic approach should recognize the patient's inability to gain sufficient distance for self-observation or from problems when overwhelmed. Gordon and Beresin advise that the staff tell patients at the beginning of their hospitalization that they, not the milieu staff, are in charge of controlling their own behavior and that acting out may bring about transfer or even discharge. The patient, family and staff must know that early discharge might happen. Adler indicates that the staff's attitude at discharge will influence future treatment. If the patient needs to be prematurely discharged, the staff should clearly outline the reason for it and offer readmission at a later time when the patient is ready. The patient's feelings of abandonment can be assuaged, and many patients will return. Adler notes, however, that these patients often may require many readmissions before they are ready to work. However, the patient's internalization of a caring, nonpunitive staff that can be respected may give sustenance until the next attempt at hospitalization [31–33].

Lewis warns against confrontation and interpretation during the early phases of treatment since the patient may experience them as cruel assaults. He argues for a style of respectful intervention. Confrontations that come from peers work better. They will be more effective if directed toward the behavior, not the person. McCready notes that when the milieu severely restricts the patients' behavior it deprives them of their primary means of discharging anxiety. This increases the danger of aggressive or self-destructive actions, or interpersonal difficulties. Lewis believes that the staff must be ready and tolerant of massive verbal assaults from patients, since the unit must serve as a holding environment for their projections. Pardes and colleagues, in describing efforts to manage patients in a therapeutic milieu, report that firm handling was intermittent rather than consistent, since the patient response was so very difficult to bear. Many patients when confronted, fell into rages, seemed to fall apart, and resorted to wrist-cutting or elopement. Pardes and colleagues believe, however, that a unified position that will not tolerate regressive behavior will eventually help the patient to gain control. Lewis suggests that in order to avoid confrontation, the staff might consider having the patients monitor their own behavior—by setting up a daily chart to record the dominating emotion of the day—lonely, sad, angry, feeling good. Across from this the patient can write several sentences describing the interpersonal experiences of that period. The patient can then begin to develop a rough understanding of the relationship between emotional states and relationships with others. Lewis also suggests that the patients define the levels of their anger and the response from the staff and others. Both these techniques should provide the patient with a way to observe the self in action and to develop an "observing ego "[34–36].

Gallop provides an even more specific treatment process derived from Linehan's work on dialectal-behavior therapy. Contrasted with other approaches, it is proactive rather than reactive. This model reframes the patient's destructive behaviors as an habitual response to overwhelming emotions. The staff must then help the patient explore alternative behavioral responses to intense stress. The staff trains the patient to: develop interpersonal skills when encountering conflict, regulate unwanted emotion, develop skills to tolerate high emotional stress, and learn self-management skills. When nurses can themselves reframe self-destructive behaviors as habitual responses, they become more tolerant and understanding. The patient's behavior somehow begins to make some sense. The staff can help the patient identify what triggers emotional and repetitive patterns and to recognize cues. Linehan's treatment, successfully employed in outpatient therapy, uses cognitive and behavioral techniques, provides support, education and construction of alternatives. Patients are supported in making a commitment to stopping self-destructive behaviors and educated about the self-defeating nature of these behaviors, which arc now referred to as habits [37–41].

Barley and colleagues describe an adaptation of Linehan's outpatient model to the inpatient setting. Patients are given intensive training in cognitive and behavioral skills and support to practice them in the hospital setting. Dialectical-Behavior Therapy (DBT) is not inconsistent with psychodynamic understanding of the borderline personality, which can continue to inform the treatment and the milieu. DBT provides ways to translate insights into behavioral habits that will help regulate emotions and handle interpersonal problems. Ways to cope with emotional stress and interpersonal problems can be taught and implemented by the inpatient staff at all levels [38–42].

In the setting that Barley and colleagues describe, DBT is introduced in a skills-training group and then supplemented by "homework groups" that focus on the actual application of techniques. DBT is applied in the wider milieu at morning rounds. Patients are asked to examine and problem-solve any self-destructive behaviors or behaviors that interfered with therapy during the previous 24 hours [42].

These skills training and homework groups usually take place in 3-month cycles. The skills include attentional training, emotional regulation, distress tolerance, reality acceptance, and interpersonal effectiveness. The learning of skills will focus on the patient's individual difficulties. The patients are each given homework assignments to be reviewed in the homework group. Assignments might include: observing and describing emotions, using self-soothing techniques in crisis, protecting self-respect in interpersonal interactions, and practicing non-judgmental thinking. The patient's participation in DBT work determines privilege levels. Barley and colleagues believe that both patients and staff can more easily understand and accept DBT principles than psychodynamic ones. The techniques provide a supportive understanding of the patient's maladaptive behaviors while still promoting adaptive change [42].

What then are the primary tasks for milieu staff members in working with these very difficult patients? They must fight against negative stereotypes when they have faced a series of difficulties from patients with borderline personality disorder. They must often withhold the satisfaction of establishing a therapeutic relationship because of the dangers of manipulation and splitting. Their need to contain their own anger and strong emotions may make them feel distant from the patient, a feeling that seems uncomfortable, given their training. Boundaries must be well established. Miller notes that even when they are clear, the therapeutic milieu can undermine them. Boundaries must also be defined around responsibility. Miller describes this as "holding without overcontaining." In the day treatment program that Miller describes, it is made clear that primary therapists will not be available for crises after hours. Instead, a crisis specialist is available for acute emergencies. Every attempt is made to shift responsibility to the patient. Miller believes that even holding medications or dangerous items for patients, mandatory group attendance or unnecessary rules, divert responsibility from patient to staff [43].

Despite all difficulties, working with these patients brings new satisfactions. There is the challenge of working together for the patient as a team, since team effort has never been so challenging and so crucial. There is a strength that comes from further self-definition, to be able to say: "Here is where I end and the patient begins. Here are my vulnerabilities and my strengths." There is a greater mental challenge than with most patients, in analyzing the internal drama as it unfolds in present relationships. There can be full admiration of the patient's powers with the hope that they can be molded in healthy directions.

References

1. Gallop R, Lancee WJ, Garfinkel P. How nursing staff respond to the label "Borderline Personality Disorder." Hospital & Community Psychiatry 1989 Aug;40(8):815–9.
2. Main TF. The ailment. British Journal of Medical Psychology 1957;30:129–45

3. Peters CP. The inpatient treatment of severe personality disorders: the borderline spectrum. New Directions for Mental Health Services 1990 Fall;47:65–86.
4. Fort JP. A unit for borderlines in a psychiatric hospital. Psychiatric Hospital 1990;21(2):61–4.
5. Nurnberg HG, Suh R. Limits: Short-term treatment of borderline patients. Comprehensive Psychiatry 1980;21(1):70–88.
6. Gunderson JG, Kolb JE. Discriminating features of borderline patients. American Journal of Psychiatry 1978;135:792–6.
7. Hartocollis P. Long term hospital treatment for adult patients with borderline and narcissistic disorders. Bulletin Menninger Clinic 1980;44:212–24.
8. Johansen KH. The impact of patients with chronic character pathology on a hospital inpatient unit. Hospital & Community Psychiatry 1983 Sep;34(9):842–6.
9. Fenton WS, McGlashan TH. Long-term residential care: treatment of choice for refractory character disorder? Psychiatric Annals 1990;20(1):44–9.
10. Tucker L, Bauer SF, Wagner S, Harlam D, et al. Specialized extended hospital treatment for borderline patients. Bulletin Menninger Clinic 1992 Fall; 56(4):465–78.
11. Gordon C, Beresin E. Conflicting treatment models for the inpatient management of borderline patients. American Journal of Psychiatry 1983 Aug;140(8):979–83.
12. See reference 5.
13. See reference 7.
14. Kernberg O, Haran C. Interview: Milieu treatment with borderline patienta: the nurse's role. Journal of Psychosocial Nursing & Mental Health Services 1984;22(4):31–6.
15. Eppel AB. Inpatient and day hospital treatment of the borderline: an integrated approach. Canadian Journal of Psychiatry 1988;33(5): 360–3.
16. Marcus E. Use of the acute hospital unit in the early phase of long-term treatment of borderline psychotic patients. Psychiatric Clinics of North America 1981;4(1):133–43.
17. See reference 4.
18. See reference 11.
19. See reference 15.
20. Lerner S. The excessive need to treat: a countertherapeutic force in psychiatric hospital treatment. Bulletin Menninger Clinic 1979;43(5), 463–71.
21. Braden E. Supportive containment in the hospital care of treatment-resistant borderline adolescents. Psychiatry 1984;47:315–22.
22. McCready KF. Milieu countertransference in treatment of borderline patients. Psychotherapy 1987 Win;24(4):720–8.
23. Adler G. Hospital treatment of borderline patients. American Journal of Psychiatry 1973 Jan;13(1):32–6.
24. Gabbard GP. Patients who hate. Psychiatry 1988;52(1):96–106.
25. Book HE, Sadavoy J, Silver D. Staff countertransference to borderline patients on an inpatient unit. American Journal of Psychotherapy 1978;32(4):521–32.
26. Sansome RA, Madakasira S. Borderline personality disorder: guidelines for evaluation and brief inpatient management. Psychiatric Hospital 1990 Spr;21(2):65–9.
27. Sederer LI, Thorbeck J. Borderline character disorder. In: Sederer LI, ed. Inpatient psychiatry: Diagnosis and treatment. 3rd ed. Baltimore: Williams & Wilkins, 1991, 108–40.

28. Viner J. Milieu concepts for short-term hospital treatment for borderline patients. Psychiatric Quarterly 1985 Sum;57:127–33.
29. Friedman H. Some problems of inpatient management with borderline patients. American Journal of Psychiatry 1969 Mar;126(3):299–304.
30. See reference 24.
31. See reference 14.
32. See reference 11.
33. Adler G. The borderline patient in the general hospital. General Hospital Psychiatry 1981;3:297–300.
34. Lewis JM. Early treatment planning for hospitalized severe borderline patients. Occupational Therapy in Mental Health 1983; 3(3):67–81.
35. See reference 22.
36. Pardes H, Van Putten T, Bjork D, Kaufman M. Failures on a therapeutic milieu. Psychiatric Quarterly 1972;46:29–48.
37. Gallop R. Self-destructive and impulsive behavior in the patient with a borderline personality disorder: Rethinking hospital treatment and management. Archives of Psychiatric Nursing 1992;6(3):178–82.
38. Linehan MM. Cognitive-behavioral treatment of borderline personality disorder. New York: Guilford, 1993.
39. Linehan M. Dialectal behavioral therapy. Journal of Personality Disorders 1987 Win;1(4):328–33.
40. Linehan MM. Dialectal behavior therapy for borderline personality disorder: Theory and method. Bulletin Menninger Clinic 1987;51:261–76.
41. Linehan MM, Armstrong HE, Suarez A, Allmon D, et al. Cognitive-behavioral treatment of chronically parasuicidal borderline patients. Archives of General Psychiatry 1991;48:1060–4.
42. Barley WD, Buie SE, Peterson EW, Hollingsworth AS, et al. Development of an inpatient cognitive-behavioral treatment program for borderlne personality disorder. Journal of Personality Disorders 1993;7(3):232–40.
43. Miller BC. Characteristics of effective day treatment programming for persons with borderline personality disorder. Psychiatric Services 1995 Jun;46(6):605–8.

6. Children

There has been a great deal of excellent writing on the psychiatric treatment of children in residential treatment centers and hospitals. The current emphasis and need for short-term treatment has made this fine writing somewhat irrelevant to programs today. Despite the shortened length of stay, psychiatric inpatient treatment for children can be successful. Follow-up studies have demonstrated positive treatment outcomes. Good prognosis has been associated with an adequate length of stay for children with nonpsychotic and nonorganic diagnoses, the absence of antisocial features and bizarre symptoms, adequate intelligence, healthy family functioning, and aftercare treatment [1].

The psychiatric hospitalization of children presents many difficulties. It interrupts the child's family, school and community relationships and creates a dependent attachment to another institution, which can only be temporary. However, children will require hospitalization when parents cannot manage their disturbance at home or when the family environment is such that it seriously interferes with their development. Placing the child in inpatient treatment is a serious decision. The clear message is that the treatment center can do better than the family, school or community. Hospitalization restricts natural living and brings the child together with other troubled children with the risk of quickly learning other maladaptive behaviors [2–3].

The Role of the Milieu in the Child's Treatment

The well functioning milieu should have the same healing properties as a well functioning family, providing a secure base that will encourage the child to explore healthier patterns of behavior and new relationships. The ideal task of inpatient treatment is to promote the internalization of the milieu's holding and attuning functions and provide the opportunity for the child to practice living skills. Simple interventions can often bring about effective internalization [2–5].

Goldsmith and colleagues describe the psychiatric milieu for children as an integration of clinical processes with planned living experiences, creating a psychodynamic environment in which the complete living experience is integrated with psychotherapy. The child's classes, recreation, relationships with staff and other children become part of the therapeutic technique. The management of daily life is based on sound psychiatric principles. This is perhaps the absolute ideal for the psychoanalytic model, and their article reflects its time. David Wineman, in a discussion of the article, sees the authors as describing an optimal clinical microcosm for each child in which the need for nurturance as well as for control can be assessed and acted upon [6–7].

This earlier writing about the function of the milieu may be only a template that informs our thinking, but it seems important not to forget the more idealistic and inspirational work. Jemerin and Phillips describe great changes in the psychiatric inpatient treatment of children in the last 25 years. While the emphasis for staff members was once to build relationships with children over extended time periods, control of aggression and self-destructive behaviors are now often the predominant focus. As economic factors demand shorter stays, hospitals for children have become diagnostic and acute treatment centers rather than stable therapeutic communities [8].

The milieu must be designed around the child's developmental needs with the day's activities designed for the varying abilities of particular age groups of children who may have developmental deficits in cognitive, sensory-motor, social or interpersonal areas that are reflected in their psychopathology. The staff should not require more than the child is capable of developmentally, but should not gear the program so low that the child does not learn to try [9].

BUILDING A TRUSTWORTHY MILIEU

Berlin and Hendren write that the staff can build trusting relationships in the inpatient milieu if some essential ingredients are present. They recommend that the milieu be structured by a level system, with simple and clear behavioral expectations at each level. Milieu staff members can prepare for the new child by learning about the problems and behaviors that led to admission as well as the contribution of environmental factors. From this information, they can write a tentative milieu treatment plan that they will continue to test and evaluate [10].

They recommend that each admitted patient be briefed by two staff members about the milieu rules. In addition to describing the level system and how points are made or lost, the staff members should clearly describe how the kinds of behavior the child had exhibited prior to admission might now be handled in the milieu. The child's primary milieu staff member should offer to help the child deal with such behaviors if they occur and be alert for signs of increased tension and anxiety so that the child can avoid them[10].

Berlin and Hendren believe that the more the children learn about their problems and behaviors and the more their positive behaviors are emphasized, the more quickly they will find the milieu a helpful place. They will come to see staff members as trustworthy allies, who will intervene to help them control disturbing behaviors. Children will feel understood if the staff empathizes with their problems. The feeling of closeness that follows helps to build trusting relationships [10].

The children will constantly test staff members in the milieu for their reliability and trustworthiness. An unusual degree of sensitivity is needed in handling daily life events in order to make the milieu experience a corrective one. Eiskovits and Guttman describe children in treatment as creating streams of events, a continuous flow of happenings over which the staff feels little control. Each new event seems to happen before the previous one has ended. The experienced child care worker learns to differentiate among the events, separating them, and acting as each situation occurs. Milieu staff members must insist on acceptable behaviors even when they fear the child's aggressive response [10–12].

The management of even trivial items of physical care must consistently reflect affection and concern and a willingness to continue to offer them despite the child's distrust. Proper attention to self care and grooming can alter the child's self-concept. The simple tasks of making beds and taking care of their rooms, becoming responsible for their hygiene and grooming help children learn that they can do things for themselves. The level system that positively reinforces completion of chores and cooperation and negatively reinforces inappropriate behavior can be very important in teaching. Dalton and colleagues believe that when the privilege level system is applied to the living situation the child's entire day can become an accretion of therapeutic experiences [10–13].

The milieu should be structured by a consistent routine for getting up, meals, school, therapy and bedtime. All of the children should be aware of the rules and the consequences, and these should be applied consistently. It should be possible to maintain compliance without the use of seclusion, but time-outs, such as sitting in the corner of the room, may be necessary to control impulses and process interactions [13].

The Child's Engagement in Treatment and Treatment Planning

Children should be told the truth, be taken seriously and participate in decisions that affect their lives. They are capable of learning why they are in the hospital, and hospitalization can help them learn more about their problems and how to deal with them. Given this knowledge they can take a more active role in planning their treatment. Although it may not happen at first, children are able to take a progressively more meaningful role. Beginning with admission, the child should be told what will happen in the hospital—including physical examinations, psychological tests, sharing rooms, point systems, therapy interventions, when they can and can't see their families. They should be quietly asked about their concerns and these should be addressed. The more concretely the staff can describe what happens in the hospital, the more likely the child's uncertainty and fears can be allayed [14].

The goals for the child's treatment should not be vague or indefinite. If the staff does not know precisely what it is trying to achieve, the chances of doing it are nil. Children should be able to discuss decisions made in treatment planning. Meeting with the staff to discuss their expectations and establish treatment contracts can keep them in treatment. They can make many choices, even to the point of choosing their therapist or the group they will attend. The child's direct knowledge about treatment removes many of its deep mysteries and counters passivity [15–16].

The Staff

While some milieu staff can work successfully with a wide variety of children, others have particular therapeutic abilities that allow them to be very effective with regressed and disturbed psychotic children or adolescents. Others can't work effectively with angry, aggressive or manipulative children. Often the staff can help identify the individual milieu staff members who can work effectively with particular children and families. Severely disturbed children do not easily acknowledge their willingness to work with staff members but they can sense that some aspect of their real lives can be shared. They can then use specific persons for support or limit setting or comfort. Progress is made when the staff member can encourage the child to begin to share private experiences [17–18].

Competitive feelings naturally arise between milieu staff members or between milieu and teaching staff. Senior staff can help treatment team members to work cooperatively and to acknowledge their varying contributions to the child's treatment. Berlin and colleagues describe the staff's covert effort to assign responsibility and credit to its members for success or failure of the child's treatment. Work with children eventually brings close relationships between children and staff, but it often results in feelings of possessiveness. These possessive feelings can produce problems in the staff's relationships with other staff members, the children, and their families [17–18].

Milieu staff members will inevitably disagree about how firm limit setting should be. Some will believe that being very strict is necessary to reduce difficult behavior. Other staff may feel that the child requires a close and permissive relationship that can still provide clear expectations for behavior. Such conflicts need to be examined in staff meetings and in discussions with the unit coordinator and the child's psychotherapist. The effort to clarify staff roles with a difficult patient is delicate [17–19].

A poorly maintained unit environment that ignores staff and patient feelings can be destructive. Effective supervision monitors staff reactions to patients and to each other to prevent untherapeutic interactions. When staff members are criticized for their interactions with children, they may feel vulnerable, as if their very being or way of life is under attack. They must be aware of how easily they can over-identify with a child and how easy it is then to make mistakes. Working with children brings a kind of permeability, which, although it brings closeness, can erode personal boundaries. This over-identification can easily lead to authority struggles or defensiveness. As therapists and staff work together they soon learn that an intervention is therapeutic when it results in reducing conflict, a growth in self-esteem or a change in behavior. Many nonverbal children will take a long time to make progress in psychotherapy, so that initial treatment gains will rely on the milieu staff's behavioral and interpersonal interventions. As staff helps the child to cope with tasks of daily living, trusting relationships develop in the school and milieu—enabling the child to better use the psychotherapeutic relationship [17–20].

MANAGING THE CHILD'S AGGRESSION

Aggression is a persistent problem in the treatment of children. Aggressive children use immediate action to solve their problems and seem not to benefit from experience. Aggression wards off their feelings of panic or disintegration. If in such circumstances, the milieu staff member can join in the child's defense, aggression can be channeled into some form of a game. Verbal support can relieve anxiety. However, when the child uses aggression to control others, it seems more effective to move swiftly to penetrate the defense by interpretation or physical limits when necessary [20].

Staff members may handle this aggression in the same way as they might handle an infant—by using nonverbal techniques such as direct action to stop the children from destroying the relationships they need so desperately. The aggressive child is greatly in need of an observing ego, and the goal is to strengthen these ego "wings." They will not grow stronger every day. These children must repeatedly test the trustworthiness of others. Staff members must remain vigilant for the signs of tension, irritability, restlessness, and loud-voiced complaints that often come before an impulsive aggressive act. They quickly learn that their own conflicts with each other often stimulate disturbed behavior in the children. Whenever possible, children should be helped to see how their underlying feelings relate to their disturbed behaviors. They should be rewarded when they communicate their distress in words rather than actions. Even the use of loud abusive language may need to be recognized as a progressive retreat from aggressive behaviors [20–21].

Experienced milieu staff appreciates the need to respond quickly when a child behaves aggressively to avoid group contagion. Removing the child quickly from a potentially disorganizing activity is often calming. In a quieter setting, the child may be able to use the relationship with a helpful adult to talk through distress. The effectiveness of isolation and removal depends on its timeliness and duration. If it lasts too long and the child experiences it as punishment, anger and aggression will escalate. When the child calms down, the staff member should offer symbolic gestures of support, a glass of water or a chance to wash up as a way of letting the child know that the adult is not angry or and does not wish to get even [21].

The staff should review all aggressive incidents that required isolation, holding, or medication to identify early warning signs and share reactions. Staff members who have participated in holding a child need to communicate their own upset feelings and their efforts not to feel punishing despite fears that the child would hurt them. There are times when they can convey this directly to the child. Disturbed children have seldom experienced this kind of honesty. They may feel closer and more trusting of adults who can admit their fears and discuss their efforts to avoid retaliation when confronted with the child's aggression. When reviewing an incident, the staff can also assess how well it has worked together so it can prepare for the next one. It should also consider how to inform the other children about what happened in order to decrease their anxiety [21].

Countertransference

If adult staff members overestimate the strength and permanence of their relationship with the child, they may be left disappointed and feel helpless and defeated. Children in inpatient treatment have many fears and little trust. They will transfer the anger they hae stored up from earlier experiences of disappointment and rejection. A child that is kind and loving at one moment can quickly turn when frustrated to accuse the staff of being punitive and not caring. Those who believe behavior should be predictable are puzzled by the child's shifting perceptions. As staff members struggle with feeling hurt, anxious and angry, it is helpful to remind them that the childrens' past experience has made them perceive adults as unpredictable and inconsistent. This will help them cope more effectively with their own labile emotional reactions [21]

The staff must also explore and resolve the transference and countertransference reactions from parents. Parents may transfer their own feelings of hopelessness or incompetence to staff members and perceive them as critical and judgmental. Their feelings of hurt and vulnerability lie beneath their efforts to blame staff for the child's problems. These transference and countertransference reactions, while painful for the staff to bear and explore, often provide a tool for appreciating the patient's previous experience [21].

Working with Families

Child psychiatric treatment without parental involvement does not lead to permanent change. Children can no longer be treated in isolation from their families and community. Inpatient programs now function as family support systems. Parents should clearly understand their role in treatment, and the staff should explain the treatment program clearly, without the use of jargon. Beginning with admission, parents should know that family therapy will be integrated with the child's treatment. They should have scheduled times to visit the unit and to talk with the milieu staff about the treatment program and how it is progressing, and come to understand how the hospital, milieu and school work together for the patient [22].

By the time the child reaches the hospital, parents will feel guilty, incompetent and waiting to be blamed. It will be helpful if family members can begin to see themselves as caught in a system that has problems but is capable of change rather than making them feel responsible for everything that has happened to the child. The evaluation with parents will center on the behavior changes that will need to be made before the child can come home. The parents will be able to learn from the milieu staff how these changes can be made [23–24].

PARTICIPATION IN THE MILIEU

Critchley and Berlin describe a progressive program of parental involvement. Parents contract for participation in the life of the milieu, weekly parent group sessions and family therapy. Milieu participation should begin in a nonthreatening atmosphere, and the child's classroom is a good beginning. Parents can watch teachers interacting with their child and later join in activities and recreation. At first the parents will have difficulty interacting with their children in front of staff members, feeling tested to see if they really are "bad parents." Participating with staff members in enjoyable activities with the children can help them relax and not feel under scrutiny. After the parents become comfortable and feel that they can benefit from instruction, they may be asked to play simple games with the child in a room with a one-way mirror and a tiny earphone so the staff can encourage them with new ways of interacting. Critchley and Berlin report that parents of psychotic children need special encouragement since they often feel "frozen" and unable to play spontaneously. Parents also benefit from knowing that the staff does not have all the answers. When staff members let parents know about problems that they, too, encounter with the child, it narrows the gap between the "competent staff" and the "inadequate parent" [25].

Parent Group Meetings

Parent groups reinforce the message that even though they can learn from staff, parents are still the experts on their own children. Parents can share their problems and experiences. They quickly learn that all parents seem to blame themselves and feel blamed by the staff for the child's illness. Somehow they also learn that this really isn't true. The parents group should set their own agenda for discussion after the first few meetings. They will want to share complaints about the staff, about the center's demands, and about the milieu, gaining courage to raise these issues later with the treatment team. The staff members must then be open to new ideas the parents offer, follow up and report back on their investigation of complaints. These groups can become the nucleus of future parent support groups, providing a forum for parents to help each other gain insight, confidence and support [26].

The Laboratory for Family Members

Carlo has described the children's residential treatment center as a living laboratory for family members. Families should be able to discuss ways to discipline and be able to learn the skills of behavioral management by participation in the milieu. Learning these skills will help the parent feel more competent when the child is discharged. The staff will serve as significant role models for many. An ecological perspective places the child care worker as a central person in the parents' environment, helping them discover their own strengths and assets. They can help parents identify and engage their own extended family, neighbors and friends to help support them in crises. The ecological perspective sees clients as inherently capable of helping themselves once they develop the capacity to influence their own environment [27–28].

THE FAMILY'S CULTURAL ORIGINS

Porter and Blackwell discuss work with families of different cultural origins. They warn that if the staff begins to consider itself better able to parent the child, the family will not feel competent enough to improve. The greater the economic or cultural differences between the family and staff, the more the family will feel blamed. If the staff tends to take all the credit for the child's progress, this leaves the family in an uncomfortable bind. Either they must credit the staff for success or they must resist change so they can prove that the staff is no more competent than they are.

The family may feel undermined by the child-centered environment. The child's relationships with staff can make parents feel powerless. The staff often labels the very strengths that help the family function well outside the hospital as resistance. For example, staff may label families as troublemakers when they serve as advocates for their children, give advice, or disagree with the treatment team [29].

Preschool Children

Preschool children are usually hospitalized when their symptoms are so severe that they can't be treated or contained within the family setting or managed in less restrictive out-of-home settings. A major problem with this age group is that the remission of psychiatric symptoms is usually dependent upon a stable primary relationship, but the time needed to develop a relationship with an adult will exceed the time limits of the hospitalization. Without this relationship, even the child's social and communication skills cannot be expected to improve [30].

Preschool children will need a special program to meet both developmental and psychiatric needs. They will need the reassurance of an extended hospitalization with plans for discharge based on the resolution of the psychiatric symptoms and the development of the child's primary relationship with a staff member. The child's discharge plan must also allow sufficient time for a healthy separation from the hospital [30].

Mansheim describes an innovative program for preschool children. A parent or primary caretaker comes to the unit and works with the staff to develop successful ways of limit setting and meeting the individual child's developmental and emotional needs. This is done in three one-hour sessions, scheduled at the parent's convenience. The parent participates with the child in activities, and the staff supervises the parent in making interventions. Mansheim also describes the problems encountered with this arrangement. The parents often criticized these suggested interventions and were skeptical that they would work or be effective at home. Staff members remained open to their criticisms but maintained their hope for establishing therapeutic relationships with them. This was of course not easy. The parents often felt competitive with the nurses. Mothers who worked with female staff members felt threatened. The nurses were sometimes included in formal psychotherapy sessions so that they could become aware of the parents' own perceptions of reality. A family recreational group was also helpful and often illuminated family dynamics [31].

Despite all of these difficulties, the children were able to make progress within several weeks and their behavior disturbances were not so frequent. In addition to the parental involvement, Mansheim attributes the improvement to establishing a structure, setting consistent limits and offering consistent social rewards. Once the behavior was under control, the child was given a therapeutic pass in order to practice with parents some of the new behaviors at home. The average length of stay was 77 days [31].

Adaptations for Short-Term Hospitalization

Recent changes in psychiatric care have called for the development of short-term units for children that direct their resources toward treatment and discharge within 90 days. Dalton and colleagues describe specific features of a nine-bed short-term program for children. Problem-oriented treatment plans with clearly detailed goals and objectives specify the team members responsible for particular treatment approaches. Goals realistically describe what the child might be expected to accomplish in the limited time, clearly directing unit resources. Parents learn successful ways to reinforce positive behaviors and extinguish negative behaviors. They focus on what they must do to maintain reasonable limits in their household as well as the outpatient therapies required to continue the child's developmental growth. Milieu therapy teaches appropriate interactional skills and discourages inappropriate ones. Positive and negative reinforcements provide motivation, and work is focused on building a therapeutic alliance between the staff and parents. Nurturance and control are the keys to the program's success [32].

Ponton divides short-term treatment into two categories, brief hospitalization (longer than a week and less than a month) and crisis hospitalization, typically offering treatment from one week to a month. Crisis units provide a safe environment, insuring that children or adolescents do not harm themselves. The treatment team defines a main problem to focus on during treatment. It may be as simple as stabilizing the child, preparing for a less restrictive level of care, and forming a liaison for the patient for longer term, day treatment, and outpatient facilities. Inpatient psychotherapy and milieu therapy focus on the admitting problem. Children who are acutely disorganized can make best use of frequent brief meetings, perhaps several 10-minute sessions each day [33].

For children close to adolescence, group therapies remain an effective treatment modality. In the short term setting the daily community meeting can provide a place to introduce new patients, promote discussion about how the unit is functioning, and give a community farewell to patients being discharged. Small group therapy allows more focused exchange [33].

Irwin and colleagues argue for realistic treatment goals. Although the children's problems are serious and complex, not all of them can be resolved during short-term hospitalization. The child can integrate only so much information at any one time. They suggest that the clinical staff create a focused treatment, since the child cannot integrate many goals at once. The team selects one or two therapeutic messages to deliver consistently and repetitively to the child. These messages can be developed by analyzing the individual and family dynamics and relating them to the problems the child presents. Issues that can't be related to these themes should be put aside in order to achieve the impact necessary to make changes. The themes and issues chosen relate to the reason for admission and focus on those problems that need to be solved before a child can be safely discharged [34].

The Child and the Staff in Short-Term Hospitalization

In writing about the necessary changes that must be made for short-term hospitalization, Irwin and colleagues outline a thoughtful plan to safeguard the primacy of therapeutic relationships in milieu therapy for children. They believe that children simply can't improve in briefer hospitalizations unless the environment strategically builds attachments. They use the concept of discriminate attachments—an affectional tie that the child forms with a selected staff member. Soon after admission, the children choose staff members to help them get settled into the room and introduced to the unit. They may also choose a staff member to accompany them to appointments. They are also encouraged to interact with the rest of the unit community. The staff member the child finally selects will be the one who comes when the child is upset or acts out, and this person will be the one who helps to transform these everyday situations into a therapeutic interaction. This plan is in contrast to the expected therapeutic situation, where the most available staff member would be the one to provide comfort or instruction. Irwin and colleagues report that to encourage the child to connect with every staff may limit the chances of connecting with any staff at all. The adult staff member is the one chosen by the child, a special person who can establish a relationship. This is further reinforced in community meetings, where the children are told that they can sit with their favorite adult. The incidents that are brought to the community meeting are reframed in terms of attachment and relationship [34].

The milieu is structured to actively develop many shared positive experiences between the adult and the child, building the foundation for discriminate attachments. The attachments, as they become stronger, are used therapeutically so that the child can work through behavioral difficulties and negative emotions. Obviously, these relationships do not always remain positive. The adult must be able to absorb the children's anger and aggression, helping them to learn that those they are closest to can tolerate and deal with their anger and that they will be cared for even when out of control. The children in turn, can learn to tolerate the good and bad in themselves and in others. The authors believe that if children can master difficulties with a person with whom they feel close, then they have taken the first step toward other relationships [34].

The staff also uses limit setting to strengthen attachments. Limits and consequences are directed to the person but applied in the context of the adult-child relationship. The intervention should not be just to control behavior but to work through underlying dynamics. The adult staff member who selects the consequence is also the one who enforces it. The intervention must remain within the crucible of the interpersonal relationships. In order to do this, there must be a distinction between the interventions that are individual and those that are group-based. Consequences for unit problems are given through unit restrictions, allowing the group to work through its shared difficulties [34].

Family therapists also participate fully in unit life and attend community meetings. They help guide the interactions on the unit and formulate the treatment model for direct care staff in order to integrate individual and family goals into the therapeutic work [34].

The pain of abandonment after termination is softened by designating the favored staff member as the outpatient therapist. The children are encouraged to visit after discharge and they may call the unit to talk to their favorite staff. Irwin and colleagues caution that theirs is a conceptual model, not an empirical model. It establishes a framework for understanding and integrating the child's experience during hospitalization [34].

The Transactional Risk Model

Woolston introduces the transactional risk model as a way to meet the challenge of short-term treatment and the need for family involvement. The transactional view interprets childhood psychopathology as a result of the interplay between the child's inner life and environment. The transactional risk model idoes not try to change or fix the child or family but rather tries to change the fit of the child and environmental transactions so that positive developments occur. Hospitalization then becomes a catalyst for the child, family, and environment. The hospital staff become consultants, not the healing agent. What is special in this model is the engagement of the child's family (and if possible, members of the child's community) as active members of the treatment team. Staff members come to understand that they are the least permanent group who will work with the child and that the work is only started, not completed in the hospital [35].

The first step is for the parents to observe the child's strengths, weaknesses, and environment, to learn how the child perceives and misperceives self and environment, and how significant others view the child. Then they are able to link these perceptions with the interpersonal behaviors that perpetuate the process. In the second stage, the parents try new strategies to help to diminish the child's anxiety and lack of control. They begin to experience the child's perceptions of their control. At the same time, the hospital must provide a catalytic environment to help the child to interact positively with the environment. These positive experiences set the stage for new relationships with the family. The third stage is the generalization of new understandings and behaviors following hospital discharge. The parents are taught how to organize various community resources to help maintain the progress made in the hospital [35].

Parents participate in all aspects of unit living, from helping with the work to implementing behavioral protocols. After the evaluation period, they become full members of the treatment team, helping to design a specific treatment model for assessing the child's strengths and weaknesses and how they should be addressed during hospitalization. They can learn from the milieu therapist, teachers, the family and child therapist. Their own hospital tasks are assigned for the implementation of treatment goals. Their tasks usually focus on the areas of greatest parent-child difficulties. For example, when trying to set limits they may find that they often switch between excessive permissiveness and punishment. When parents join the team they become less self-blaming and more focused on solving problems. Once they are able to practice limit setting with success both they and the child feel relieved. They have a more adaptive solution to the chronic, self-sustaining cycle that often perpetuates the child's disturbance [35].

Staff and parents agree on a behavior protocol giving parents a prescribed role. The milieu staff can be actively consulted. Staff and parents examine their failures and successes. After parents master the protocols, the children may have longer passes away from the hospital. The goal is for the child to internalize what is learned in the hospital, and this internalization can provide a new image of self and interpersonal relationships. As members of the team, parents can see their child much more objectively and accurately, and are much less influenced by earlier history and distortions. Woolston believes that the transactional risk model provides a more realistic goal of hospitalization—that of changing the fit between the child's internal life and the interpersonal environment, rather than the model of "fixing the child" [35].

References

1. Blotcky MJ, Dimperio TL, Gossett JT. Follow-up of children treated in psychiatric hospitals: a review of studies. American Journal of Psychiatry 1984;141(12):1499–1507.
2. Dalton R, Muller B, Forman MA. Psychiatric hospitalization of children: an overview. Child Psychiatry & Human Development 1989;19(4):231–45.

3. Barker P. Residential treatment for disturbed children: its place in the '80s. Canadian Journal of Psychiatry 1982; 27:634–9.
4. Rowe J. Attachment theory and the milieu treatment of children. Journal of Child & Adolescent Psychiatric & Mental Health Nursing 1988;1(2):66–71.
5. Bleiberg E. The clinical challenge of children and adolescents with severe personality disorders. Bulletin Menninger Clinic 1990 Win;54(1):107–20.
6. Goldsmith JM, Schulman R, Grossbard H. Integrating clinical processes with planned living experiences. American Journal of Orthopsychiatry 1954;24(4):281–90.
7. Wineman D. Discussion. Goldsmith JM, Schulman R, Grossbard H. Integrating clinical processes with planned living experiences. American Journal of Orthopsychiatry 1954;24(4):290.
8. Jemerin MJ, Phillips I. Changes in inpatient child psychiatry: Consequences and recommendations. Journal American Academy Child & Adolescent Psychiatry 1988; 27:397–403.
9. Berlin IN. Developmental issues in the psychiatric hospitalization of children. American Journal of Psychiatry 1978 Sep;135(9):1044–8.
10. Berlin IN, Hendren RL. Effective treatment planning. In: Hendren RL, Berlin IN, eds. Psychiatric inpatient care of children and adolescents: A multicultural approach. New York: John Wiley, 1991, 67–87.
11. Eiskovits Z, Guttman E. Doing competent residential child and youth care work: the normative and experiential dimensions. Children & Youth Services Review 1987;9:271–90.
12. Kitchener H, Sweet B, Citrin E. Problems in the treatment of impulse disorder in children in a residential setting. Psychiatry 1961;23:347–54.
13. See reference 2.
14. Roth EA, Roth LH. Children's understanding of psychiatric hospitalization. American Journal of Psychiatry 1984 Sep;141(9):1066–70.
15. See reference 3.
16. Brewer T, Faitak MT. Ethical guidelines for the inpatient psychiatric care of children. Professional Psychology 1989;20(3):142–7.
17. Berlin IN, Critchley DL, Rossman PG. Current concepts in milieu treatment of seriously disturbed children and adolescents. Psychotherapy 1984 Spr;21(1):118–31.
18. See reference 5.
19. Finkelstein N. Family participation in residential treatment. Child Welfare 1974 Nov;53(9):570–5.
20. See reference 12.
21. See reference 17.
22. See reference 3.
23. See reference 19.
24. See reference 10.
25. Critchley DL, Berlin IN. Parent participation in milieu treatment of young psychotic children. American Journal of Orthopsychiatry 1981 Jan;5(1):149–55.
26. Whittaker JJ. Ecology of child treatment. Journal of Autism & Childhood Schizophrenia 1975 Sep;5(3):223–37.
27. Carlo P. The children's residential treatment center as a living laboratory for family

members: A review of the literature and its implications for practice. Child Care Quarterly 1985;14(3):156–71.
28. Rueveni U. The family therapist as a systems interventionist. International Journal Family Therapy 1979 Spr;1(1):63–75.
29. Porter N, Blackwell S. Working with resistance in families: A cross-cultural perspective. In: Hendren RL, Berlin IN, eds. Psychiatric inpatient care of children and adolescents: A multicultural approach. New York: John Wiley, 1991, 144–60.
30. Dalton R, Forman MA, Daul GC, Boulding D. Psychiatric hospitalization of preschool children: admission factors and discharge implications. Journal American Academy of Child & Adolescent Psychiatry 1987;26(3):308–12.
31. Mansheim P. Short term psychiatric inpatient treatment of preschool children. Hospital & Community Psychiatry 1990 Jul;41(7):670–2.
32. Dalton R, Bolding DD, Woods J, Daruna JH. Short-term psychiatric hospitalization of children. Hospital & Community Psychiatry 1987 Sep;38(9):973–6.
33. Ponton LE. Short term psychiatric hospitalization of children and adolescents. In: Hendren RL, Berlin IN, eds. Psychiatric inpatient care of children and adolescents: A multicultural approach. New York: John Wiley, 1991, 177–193.
34. Irwin M, Kline PM, Gordon M. Adapting milieu therapy to short-term psychiatric hospitalization of children. Child Psychiatry & Human Development 1991;21(3): 193–201.
35. Woolston, J. L. The transactional risk model for short and intermediate term psychiatric inpatient treatment of children. Journal American Academy Child & Adolescent Psychiatry 1989;28(1):38–40.

7. The Conduct-Disordered, Antisocial, and Delinquent Population

Although they may differ in age and in the severity of their disorders, many of the same principles apply in the treatment of the conduct-disordered, antisocial, and delinquent population. Therefore, these three populations will be discussed together. Although "delinquent" is not a psychiatric term, it is widely used in the literature to refer to persons with conduct disorders who have committed delinquent acts. Most of the literature reviewed will focus on the younger person with conduct disorder rather than those with antisocial personality disorders. The most common feature of the disorder is the presence of a persistent pattern of behavior that violates social standards and the rights of others. Violations include such behaviors as stealing, running away, violent acts or aggression. One of the hazards of working with these patients is that they can so transform the milieu that it is no longer experienced as humane and effective [1].

Many believe that conduct disorders represent a failure in ego development which leaves the person with a diminished capacity to repress socially unacceptable drives and urges. Persons with conduct disorder seem to have diminished internalized controls, a faulty defensive organization and a deficient super-ego.

Psychotherapeutic work requires that the emotional release they gain through acting out be blocked so that they become aware of their own internal dysphoria and conflict [1].

The Delinquent's Influence on the Milieu

Delinquents or adolescents with conduct disorder seriously disrupt the milieu, since they often seem unable to abide by the rules. The staff will be constantly concerned about sexuality, assaults, vandalism, and victimization of others. Attention devoted to handling disruptive behaviors often precludes the therapeutic teaching of any alternative prosocial behaviors. Within the peer group the delinquent has a strong investment in power and image and is very sensitive to any hint of humiliation and disrespect, especially from adults. The treatment team will continuously struggle to channel the delinquent's natural leadership ability into more productive behavior [1–2].

Unless the milieu is specifically designed for the treatment of delinquents, the staff must monitor the mix of patients. A large number of patients with conduct disorder may increase the need for more structure in the program, changes in group activities, creative and careful group living assignments and room changes [1–2].

The Delinquent's Effect on the Staff

When there are many delinquents in the unit, the staff becomes preoccupied with controlling aggression and violence. Violence becomes a milieu theme, resulting in an increased level of fear which, in turn, can increase acting out. There will be predictable power struggles since delinquents usually have a tremendous need to control others. The staff is denied its strongest leverage, the therapeutic relationship, since so few of these patients can bond with others, least of all, with adults [1–2].

Crabtree warns that the delinquent patients' disruptions often bring about the milieu staff's worst responses, with reactions ranging from callousness to cynicism and avoidance. While some become petty rule enforcers, others simply run away from setting limits. Some simply explode in anger and condemn the patient, sometimes openly, and at other times in the guise of confrontation. This kind of staff behavior is the perfect match for the delinquent's personality make-up and often found in the family of origin. When the staff acts this way, the delinquent feels very much at home again, with adults who are petty, hypocritical, arbitrary, unsympathetic and retaliatory. The delinquent learns no new lessons [1–2].

These patients desperately need a strong staff that adheres to its value system and cannot be manipulated. But delinquents are very talented in creating divisiveness. Teamwork was never so necessary. The team needs time to agree on treatment strategies. Colyar recommends that at times the staff might confer openly in front of the patient about the immediate problem behavior and possible consequences. This is preferred to retreating to an office to confer in private, since this makes the delinquent feel even more powerful. Working with delinquents requires a high level of trust among staff members and the confidence that support will be there when requested. More time may be needed for senior staff to be on the floor to model child care techniques [2–3].

ADMINISTRATIVE SUPPORT

Colyar advises that the child care staff will often need increased demonstrations of administrative support, including direct presence on the unit. The administration must not only solicit and welcome advice from the child care staff but also give it authority to make decisions. The staff will need flexibility and authority to make program changes when needed. Children and adolescents with conduct disorders may require rapid changes in behavior management plans in terms of rewards, penalties and the granting of privileges. The child care staff should have as much authority as is practical to make adjustments in behavior management [2–3].

Milieu staff members must not feel blamed for the patients' behavior. This will only cause them to increase controls, resulting in a cycle of destructive behavior followed by more controls. The administration should be careful to avoid the appearance of criticism where none is deserved [2–3].

COUNTERTRANSFERENCE

Gabbard and Coyne describe three staff reactions to adult antisocial patients: disbelief, collusion, and condemnation. These patients so contradict the staff's own view of the world and of humanity, that it simply won't believe that anyone is so ruthless or is so willing to exploit. Staff members will tend to view such behaviors benevolently as a cry for help and thus join with these patients in minimizing their pathology. They may also be fooled into believing that these patients can be successfully treated. But their own anger and frustration finally leads to condemnation. Staff meetings must continually address countertransference toward these patients. The staff should continually monitor its ability to treat them and recognize that transferring them may become the only acceptable treatment plan. Gabbard and Coyne believe that antisocial adult patients usually require a specialized treatment setting rather than a general psychiatric unit with mixed populations [4].

Treatment Strategies

Treatment requires effective staff teamwork with good communication and consistency. Not only should there be immediate consequences for present behavior but there should be a positive focus about future behavior. Gabbard and Coyne advise that the treatment plan for older antisocial persons provide a consistent and rigid structure with swift implementation of consequences. Marohn writes that treatment must not permit the gratification that comes from acting out, with the hope that motor behavior can eventually be converted into verbal behavior. The staff member's ability to support and guide the patient and a milieu where behavior can be understood will promote effective treatment. Ideally, the patient should internalize the structure of the hospital milieu [4–5].

Forming a Community

A positive peer influence model can be effective even with conduct-disordered children and adolescents. If an entire group is rewarded for improved behavior by certain of its members there will be stronger group pressure toward prosocial behavior and a greater interpersonal attraction among members as they share in the reward. The attraction to the group can lead to stronger pressures for conforming and more frequent sharing of rewards, which again reinforces the attraction to the group. Developing responsibility to others is a goal of treatment with adults in inpatient treatment. This might include a willingness to inform when others break a rule. It will include honesty with peers and when possible, restitution to victims [6].

Behavioral Treatment

Behavioral treatment for conduct-disordered children and adolescents will often include management training for parents, including operant conditioning techniques. Behaviors of many conduct-disordered children began in an environment with minimal prosocial reinforcement. Social skills training using such procedures as instruction, modeling, practice, feedback and reinforcement can help develop social skills. Kolko and colleagues compared the results of social skills training with social activities groups for conduct-disordered children and found that those in a social-cognitive skills program received higher sociometric ratings and developed more appropriate social skills. Social skills training improves social competence and reduces aggression with inpatient conduct-disordered children [7–8].

Level Systems

Level systems outline expectations and the corresponding level of privileges. A daily level system can be extremely effective. However, unless the treatment center can operate a level system with complete consistency, it should not be attempted since the behavior management problems will only become more pronounced. Colyar believes that these adolescents need an "immediate feedback loop," both positive and negative, and that consequences should be immediately applied [9].

Consequences

Consequences which are natural to the system seem to work best. However, the rapid addition of consequences for continued noncompliance is not effective. Since many of these persons have been punished all their lives, adding one more punishment just seems to reinforce their expectations of the abuse of power and perpetuate their negative behaviors. Power struggles can be avoided by having a program dictate the consequences of behavior. Staff members can then help the patient meet program expectations and follow through on consequences [9].

Staff must remove emotion from the process of applying negative consequences. When it is possible the resident should be given a choice. In addition, if the circumstances are right for the person to choose the consequence, then the staff should also allow the choice of its duration and intensity. Consequences should not be applied for a long period of time. After the consequences are met, a way should be provided for the resident to return to the community and experience positive feedback. Only positive attention has a real chance of changing behavior [9].

Although having the program dictate consequences of behavior dilutes power struggles, others recommend individualized rewards and consequences. This can be difficult since there is considerable effort to standardize behavior management responses, e.g., group living rules and penalties, point allocation. Colyar finds that youths with conduct-disorder seem more responsive to a program structure with individualized rewards and punishments. For example, time-outs have been effective with some conduct-disordered adolescents but not with others, so designing a cottage program that dictates time-outs for certain offenses may be counterproductive. Some other consequences must be thought about. Also, level systems and point economies that individualize rewards and penalties will tend to be more effective [9].

BUILDING RELATIONSHIPS

Staff members should be advised not to give up trying to build a relationship with these patients. The relationship may depend on the acceptance of the youth but not the behavior. A relationship with the staff member can often help to get the adolescent invested in the program. Some relationship work always needs to be done after consequences are applied. The staff member should follow up by showing support and helping the person to explore alternative behaviors [9].

Children with Conduct Disorders

Inpatient treatment of children with conduct disorders can result in significant improvements, although no treatment stands out as the definitive answer for this population. The milieu provides a well-developed routine with programmed therapeutic activities. The way the child interacts with staff and peers and responds to structure is potentially therapeutic. The staff has the opportunity to observe and provide interventions and mediate corrective feedback founded on their supportive relationships with the child. Peers provide a great deal of corrective feedback that will be helpful. [10].

The child care staff is usually responsible for the atmosphere of the milieu and for the fundamental details of treatment. Although children with conduct disorders have found interpersonal relationships difficult, relationships with the staff will play a central role. Staff relationships begin to develop naturally through general caretaking routines and later progress to discussing feelings and problems. The support, the emergence of the relationship, and the child's identification with the staff may help significantly. The children can develop a sense of belonging with others and a sense of responsibility. Close relationships are strengthened by the value system of the unit as well as the great amount of time spent together in close proximity [10].

The milieu must be prepared to handle problem behaviors. These might include using such behavioral techniques as time out from reinforcement. Milieu therapy might also include some forms of group decision making such as patient government and community meetings which provide feedback about interpersonal behaviors. The treatment program must also address the system in which the child normally functions. Parent management training is helpful. The family must participate in treatment to prepare for the child's care after hospitalization.

Successful Programs

No programs have proved successful with all delinquents and few programs have produced long-term definitive changes after discharge. Recidivism rates are high. Garrett integrated findings from multiple outcome studies on patients with delinquency and found that treatments based on behavioral theory produced the greatest amount of positive changes. Cognitive-behavioral interventions, family therapy, and Outward Bound programs also resulted in positive changes. By the use of these techniques, psychological adjustment, community adjustment and academic performance all showed improvement. Recidivism was modestly reduced [11].

Some examples of successful programs are discussed here with the hope that some of their features might be helpful when added to traditional therapeutic strategies for this group. The Achievement Place/Teaching Family Model has been replicated in many programs in the United States. Although it began as a model for a group home rather than residential treatment, it has much to offer [12].

The Achievement Place Model

The Achievement Place model has a motivation system based on points and a contractual agreement. This system is later systematically replaced by intensive social reinforcement and the development of self-government through the use of peer management and peer involvement techniques [13].

Group home programs based on the Achievement Place Model serve a small group of residents, usually six. The staff is also small, with two people, the Teaching Parents, usually psychologists or child care workers who design and carry out specific treatment procedures to correct problem behaviors. They supervise and monitor the activities of the young people in the home, school, and community and serve as a liaison for all parts of the child's life. They work out specific behavioral goals for each resident based on individual behavioral deficits and also on what members of family, school and community decide are a priority. Teaching Parents employ the teaching interaction which consists of initial praise, description of the inappropriate behavior, a negative consequence, followed by the description of the appropriate behavior, practice of the appropriate behavior, descriptive feedback, a positive consequence and final praise. The adolescents in the Achievement Place Program can make the rules, change them, change the motivation systems, review each other's behavior, and bestow various powers on an elected peer manager [14–15]. (For more information, see Chapter II on Treatment Models.)

A CANADIAN MODEL: "THE HOME"

Harris and colleagues describe a Canadian program which they found to be effective in treating disturbed delinquents. Despite a rich and varied program, the need for effective control over maladaptive behavior took precedence over all other therapeutic measures. There was a consistent core of staff providing a staff/adolescent ratio of nearly one to one. The director played a significant role, formulating policy and guiding the philosophy of treatment. He had a forceful personality and both staff and adolescents acknowledged his authority and leadership. He was consistently available to staff and adolescents in difficult times. The staff believed that even a brief lapse in leadership or structure quickly leads to disturbed behavior. They also assumed that the alternative to firm control is the rapid growth of a gang structure. Most staff worked 24 hours a day, with days off. This consistent contact permitted the staff to know the adolescents, their hour-by-hour and day-by-day progress and build strong relationships with them [16].

The program included a school, a farm which required animal care, horseback riding, woodworking shop, odd jobs and maintenance, recreation and sports. A few of the residents attended the community school. Some were able to work on nearby farms and in the village. The core of treatment was the living, working and learning environment which included predictable long-term relationships with staff, who provided role models for behavior and for identification. The need to live harmoniously in groups of 3 to 15 required the development of social skills. Key staff provided intensive psychotherapeutic experiences usually centered around crisis situations or family interventions. The staff related to the adolescent over a period of many hours to deal with behavioral difficulties. Living through a crisis with the help of staff who were important to them became the predominant psychotherapeutic process for the adolescents [16].

The "Home" resembled a pioneering community, with long hours of work each day. There was a practical orientation with clear structure of authority, responsibility, work assignments and standards of conduct, a work and learning ethic. The staff encouraged acceptable behavior, discouraged and quickly controlled unacceptable behavior. Relationships were caring and consistent. The director provided strong leadership. The adolescents had an opportunity to experience new models of relationships and behaviors and to identify with key people [16].

The adolescents admitted to the Home are usually aggressive and destructive, but finally develop control as they are made members of a structured and special community. The adolescent is told clearly and directly what must and must not be done. The work program helped to control behavior for many of these adolescents who had been used to days without structure or socialized activity. Hours were structured and filled with work and activities. The staff supervised recreation time and did not permit antisocial behavior. Good alternatives were offered to replace earlier social and behavior patterns. Only occasionally would an adolescent refuse to become involved in the hardworking, socialized lifestyle. Strenuous physical exertion changed mood, attitudes and behavior. Both athletics and hard work such as clearing rocks from fields could achieve this goal. Instead of merely supervising, staff often worked along with the adolescent. Hardworking, productive adults and peers served as models. In the most successful cases, adolescents internalized the work ethic. The ability to work often became a major source of strength and support to counteract social and personal problems. replacing idleness, antisocial activity and aggressive activity. It provided the possibility for personality growth and helped improve self-esteem. The authors believe that the concept of one's self as a worker can substitute for a self-concept as an unsuccessful and criminal person. The work situation helped build new relationships with adults and peers [16].

Harris and colleagues do not provide statistical long-term results of this program. It is discussed here as an example of a growth-producing culture for adolescents with conduct disorder. Program elements which can lead to success for conduct-disordered adolescents include: strong leadership, discipline and firmness, good relations among peers, among staff, and good staff-adolescent relationships. A work program, recreation program, and special education are also key to rehabilitation. The milieu should be characterized by warmth and harmony and high expectations [16].

Successful Programs in Correctional Hospital Settings

Reid writes about the principles of character restructuring in model correctional programs. The first principle is that the person is regarded as a human being with feelings and with a capacity to change. A second principle is the provision of a consistent setting immune to manipulation, with a level system that will eventually lead to release. Patients who have been in the program for a long time can prevent "con games" and serve as role models who have overcome an antisocial identity. There are firm rules for moving through the program with no room for bargaining and consistent, predictable responses to patient behavior [17].

Treatment continually addresses the patient's emotional deficits, fantasies, ability to learn from experience and trust self and others. In some programs, experienced participants are often encouraged to open up emotionally as a model for more highly defended patients. Aftercare is vital to the success of the program. The connection to the hospital is maintained to help patients handle the anxiety that arises in their new lives and to control impulses that could bring on more criminal behavior. Yochelson and Samenow describe treatment based upon the belief that the criminals are not fragile and willingly choose their own actions. The residential treatment they recommend is based on individual responsibility with immediate consequences for inappropriate actions (17–19).

Rutter found that the following factors correlate with a good outcome in residential treatment for delinquents: firmness, warmth, harmony, high expectations, good discipline, and a practical approach to training. Patients must come to realize that their present actions are not effective in getting what they want, either in hospital, society or in the community, and learn that there are healthy ways to reach their goals. The staff must be ready to help them learn how to do it. An idealistic view might postulate that if an unhealthy and disorganized background formed this delinquent adjustment, then a stable and healthy milieu can reverse it [20–21].

Kazdin proposes that it finally may be helpful to employ the chronic disease model in formulating treatment for this population. Treatment would be based on the assumption that the condition will need continued care, management, and treatment. The traditional model for a chronic disease is to administer an intervention for a specified time period and to hope for change to last as long as possible. Conduct disorder does resemble a chronic condition in its development and course [22].

Many therapeutic models have produced changes in antisocial behaviors. Social skills training and behavioral programs have changed aggressive behaviors. The Achievement Place model has been extremely effective during inpatient treatment although long term effects are simply not guaranteed. The chronic disease model would suggest that such successful treatments may need to be applied intermittently on a continuous or as-needed basis. Kazdin suggests that it might be reasonable to continue to monitor antisocial children and adolescents after discharge in order to plan subsequent treatments [22].

References

1. Crabtree LH. Hospitalized adolescents who act out: a treatment approach. Psychiatry 1982 May;45(2):147–58
2. Colyar DE. Residential care and treatment of youths with conduct disorders: conclusions of a conference of child care workers. Child & Youth Care Forum 1991 Jun;20:195–204.
3. Gralnick A. Management of character disorders in a hospital setting. American Journal of Psychotherapy 1979;33(1):54–66.
4. Gabbard GO, Coyne L. Predictors of antisocial patients to hospital treatment. Hospital & Community Psychiatry 1987 Nov;38(11):1181–5.

5. Marohn R. Assertiveness in the treatment of juvenile delinquents. Psychiatric Annals 1985 Oct;15(10):606–13.
6. Reid WH, Burke WJ. Antisocial personality disorder. In: American Psychiaric Association Task Force on Treatments of Psychiatric Disorders. Treatments of Psychiatric Disorders. v. 3. Washington, DC: American Psychiatric Association,1989, 2742–8.
7. Wodarski JS, Feldman RA, Flax IN. Social learning theory and group work practice with antisocial children. Clinical Social Work Journal 1973 Sum;1(2):78–93.
8. Kolko DJ, Loar LL, Sturnick D. Inpatient social-cognitive skills training groups with conduct disordered and attention deficit disordered children. Journal of Child Psychology & Psychiatry 1990;31(5):737–48.
9. See reference 2.
10. Kazdin AE. Hospitalization of antisocial children: clinical course, follow-up status, and prediction of outcome. Advances in Behavioral Research & Therapy 1989;2:1–67.
11. Garrett CJ. Meta-analysis of the effects of residential treatment on adjudicated delinquents. Journal of Research in Crime & Delinquency 1985;4:287–308.
12. Kirigin KA, Braukman CJ, Atwater JD, Wolf MM. An evaluation of Teaching-Family (Achievement Place) group homes for juvenile offenders. Journal of Applied Behavioral Analysis 1982;15:1–6.
13. Brown B. An application of social learning methods in a residential programme for young offenders. Journal of Adolescence 1986;8:321–31.
14. Blase KA, Fixsen DL, Freeborn K, Jaeger D. The Behavioral Model. In: Lyman RD, Prentice-Dunn S, Gabel S, eds. Residential and Inpatient Treatment of Children and Adolescents. New York: Plenum Press, 1989, 43–59.
15. Fixsen DL, Phillips EI, Wolf MM. Achievement Place: Experiments in self-government with pre-delinquents. Journal of Applied Behavior Analysis 1973 Spr;3(1):31–47.
16. Harris DP, Cote JE, Vipond EM. Residential treatment of disturbed delinquents: description of a centre and identification of therapeutic factors. Canadian Journal of Psychiatry 1987;32:579–83.
17. Reid WH. The Antisocial Personality: A Review. Hospital & Community Psychiatry 1985 Aug;36(8):831–7.
18. Yochelson S, Samenow SE. The Criminal personality. Vol. 1. A profile for change. New York: Aronson, 1976.
19. Yochelson S, Samenow SE. The Criminal personality. Vol. 2. The change process. New York: Aronson, 1977.
20. Rutter M, McGiller H. Juvenile delinquency. New York: Guilford Press, 1984.
21. See reference 3.
22. See reference 10.

8. Persons with Depression

Although depression is the most common psychiatric illness and the most common reason for psychiatric hospitalization, attention in the psychiatric literature to milieu techniques for the patient with depression has been sparse. This contrasts with the periodical literature about the inpatient treatment of multiple personality disorder, a relatively rare disorder which is now accompanied by specific well-focused writing on milieu management. There may be fewer guidelines because psychotropic medication for depression is quite effective. It also might be assumed that everyone has some intuitive knowledge about how to help the person who is depressed. The sources for information in this section will include books and psychiatric nursing texts, as well as some excellent periodical articles.

Depressed patients are hospitalized when they cannot cooperate with outpatient treatment, when they are at risk for suicide or homicide or when they lack psychosocial supports. The clinically depressed person feels sad and hopeless and has lost self-esteem and pleasure in life. The goal of treatment is to restore morale and to help the person learn and test more adaptive behaviors which will help to prevent a recurrence of depression [1–2].

RESTORING MORALE

Grady and Sederer define remoralization as the reexperiencing of confidence in the self. Increasing participation in the activities of the unit is a first step toward restoring morale. The milieu provides an escape from loneliness and isolation and interrupts the total self-concern that comes with depression. It provides belief that the person can improve while providing encouragement to be a part of the process. The milieu staff provides empathic listeners who help the patient tolerate despair and vent feelings. The staff encourages but does not force socialization with others [1–2].

An emotional atmosphere which promises security and acceptance can encourage communication and activity. The unit should operate in a spirit of belief in the person's ability to improve. This also helps to restore morale. In this atmosphere a person can eventually rediscover an ability to care for others and be cared about in turn [1–3].

RESTORING MOTIVATION

The very actions which might help alter depression—social interaction, getting back into operation, accomplishing daily tasks—are those which the depressed person has come to dread. The milieu must somehow motivate the withdrawn person for reentry into life, but the beginning steps are difficult. When the patient is awakened in the morning and doesn't want to get up and begin the day, the staff member can honestly provide assurance that the day will eventually get better. The depressed person benefits from an organized schedule to provide protection against a passive or vegetative state. The milieu staff provides expectations for personal hygiene, dressing, going to meals, and activities. An activity as conventional as a unit meeting can be helpful. It allows the person to experience social reintegration with others and creates another opportunity for peer group support. The patient can begin to feel a part of things. The depressed person needs an awakening of creative ability to interrupt the repetitive nature of depression. Small group activities and unit meetings help the person to feel productive; this would include such simple tasks as choosing an activity and helping to plan it [1–3].

Something as simple as the regular rhythm of unit activity seems to help. The patient may slowly emerge from preocccupation with self to rediscover the world of others with a stronger spirit. Hole and Wolfersdorf designed the Activation Program in a special unit for depressed patients. It includes sports, physical and occupational therapy, social and communicative experiences, concerts, and morning gymnastics. The activities are designed for varying degrees of encouragement, interest and commitment, but are not obligatory. Weiner refers to this as ego activation, the catalyst that makes patients give up their passivity and proceed to contend with ordinary life. Depressed persons feel helpless—not only in not being able to control their feelings but also in trying to cope with life. Beck and Young suggest activities that will include experiences of pleasure and mastery—activities that will counteract the person's ruminations and hopelessness [2–5].

While staff members must allow the depressed patient to be dependent in the beginning of treatment, they must prepare for more independent behaviors. It is important to begin by establishing short-term reachable goals. As the patient meets these, there may be associated changes in attitude and behaviors. More specific activities that will alter the patient's sense of personal effectiveness will be of value. Increased self-reliance can eventually increase control over emotional reactions. Brunnell recommends problem-solving skills training to help patients develop abilities to cope with the problems of daily life, such as facing tasks and handling disagreements. This training, done in a group format, helps the patients realize that problems are a normal part of life (not just something that happens to them), and that solving problems involves defining all the aspects, considering alternatives, and finding the most effective strategies. The person goes through the steps of solving problems, develops the strategy and then evaluates how effective it was. Weiner believes that if depressed persons can find new ways to solve problems they can learn to replace their ineffective cognitive, affective and interpersonal behaviors with more adaptive ones [5–7].

Physiological Regression

The seriously depressed person may regress to the point of needing to be fed and bathed. These services should be provided in a nurturing manner. The staff should investigate whether the inability to eat or sleep stems from delusional fears. This may be difficult if the person is not interacting. Insomnia may be severe, but if a staff member simply stays with the patient at bedtime it may help. The patient, even when not communicating, will need the security of a non-demanding and accepting presence. The vegetative signs of depression indicate that the person's body has slowed considerably so that monumental effort is required for the smallest task. As long as the body remains this still, the emotional state cannot be altered. Helping depressed persons start to move their bodies gives a chemical lift. When the body becomes more alive, the emotions also begin to respond [7–8].

COMMUNICATION WITH THE DEPRESSED PERSON

Seriously depressed persons may simply not talk at all. Although staff members should quietly encourage talking, they must also be willing to sit peacefully with the silent patient. This can be comforting, particularly if staff members are able to convey that they accept this silence and wish to sit with the patient. However, this conventional wisdom can be challenged by writers like Beck or Arieti who write that allowing long silences merely allows the person to continue rumination, and that being silent supports these hopeless feelings. Arieti argues that one should be more active and try to discuss other topics to prevent the focus on symptoms, at least in the early stages. Both of these writers are referring more to the psychotherapeutic session rather than specifically to milieu treatment [7–10]

The depressed person needs a new experience in communicating with others that can help release feelings and make a satisfying connection. An investment in new relationships can be the beginning of a reinvestment in living. Although withdrawn and seeming to be not interested in others, the depressed person desperately needs human companionship. Forming relationships will not be easy. Potts and colleagues describe depressed persons as "aversive for nondepressed others." In a research project, depressed subjects evoked significantly more depression, anxiety, hostility and rejection from a group than did nondepressed outpatients and controls. Kohut writes that the depressed person's lack of response to our efforts to "infect him with a minimum of joy" lowers our own self-esteem and can cause us to react with depression and/or rage [11–14].

Tudor discusses the ways to counter the mutual withdrawal that occurs between patient and staff. Nonverbal communication might be the easiest way to start. Staff members consider alternatives for responding to the person, try a number of these, and determine which are the most successful. Then it is important to share the most successful techniques with all staff members. This might be as simple as introducing a staff member who happens to share the patient's interests. But the staff must think about helping to widen the circle of communication since the patient may withdraw again. Hole and Wolfersdorf offer more specific and trained interactions to the staff and they cite elements of conversational and behavioral therapy which can be used in interaction with depressed patients. They emphasize an accepting and unconditional emotional attention, empathy, unconditional reinforcement as well as positive reinforcement of nondepressed behavior [15–16].

Kerr calls attention to the anger and aggression that may be present in depressed persons and reviews efforts to release this "frozen negativity." She reports previous findings that depressed patients in state hospitals often improved after scrubbing floors. Apparently the energetic activities helped to release their aggression. Activities that can help sublimate the aggressive drive are usually helpful, even when the person is not aware of the aggressive feelings simmering within [17].

Those who work with depressed persons must be able to accept sadness, not only in the patients but within themselves. If they haven't been able to do this they will find themselves avoiding depressed patients and trying to escape from their pain. They may be duplicating the family's reaction, which was to grow impatient and try to force the person to get rid of depressed feelings. Empathic communication helps the person to express this sadness. The empathic response involves not only understanding the person's feelings but also conveying that understanding to them [17].

The depressed person's self-esteem can be modified through interaction with caring others. The staff member has many opportunities to show that others see the patient in a positive way. Simple expressions of care such as calling the person by name and beginning a conversation can be helpful since the depressed patients' nonresponsiveness can make them seem invisible. The person's self-esteem can be modified through identification with another person's respect and treatment. Wells warns against cant in the self-esteem literature and says that it is ridiculous for a nurse to tell the patient how good she is five or ten times on each shift. The patient doesn't believe it and all the verbalizing will not change that. In fact, it may hurt the person's self esteem because there is nothing sincere about the statement. Nonverbal techniques that show genuine caring are far more effective. Self-esteem can also be modified if the patient can begin to feel competent in dealing with life's demands. When the staff can help the patient develop skills to gain greater independence, self-esteem increases [17–19].

Psychotic Depression

While depressed patients do not feel good about themselves, the person who is psychotically depressed feels worthless. The psychotically depressed person "lives in the illness" while the neurotically depressed person usually fights the problem. The person with a psychotic depression is not able to fight the engulfing pain and will ruminate about self-destruction. There may be delusions of sinfulness and punishment. The patient needs the strength of another person for support. The patient must finally be convinced that this guilt is unfounded. Staff interventions to help increase self-esteem may finally lead to the person to question these delusions of worthlessness. At the same time, the staff member should neither challenge nor agree with the delusion. Agreement with the delusion will confuse the patient. Instead, patients should be given positive interest when they talk about feelings and real experiences [17–20].

SUICIDE

Psychotic and delusionally depressed persons are at an even greater risk for suicide. Suicidal thoughts and threats should always be taken seriously. The person who talks about suicide is in danger of committing it. The staff must assess the suicidal potential of every depressed patient and establish measures for safety. The patient's belongings must be checked for all materials that could be used for suicide. Patients who are able should establish a contract which promises to inform a staff member about any impulse toward self-destruction. Those who cannot write such a contract should always be highly visible to the staff while in the community space and otherwise should always be in the presence of a staff member. Those who are extremely suicidal may require treatment in a closed ward to prevent their leaving the hospital. Others will need 1:1 supervision. Hole and Wolfersdorf recommend an intensification of the system of personal relatedness for these patients. In the special depression unit, when no other action seems possible, they advise that the staff can help solve the problem by temporarily locking the ward rather than removing the patient, a technique that they call interception, not isolation. The staff must not feel complacent or relaxed when depressed suicidal patients improves. It is only then that they may acquire the psychic or physical energy to commit a suicidal act [21–23].

SPECIFIC INTERVENTIONS

More specific interventions will also be of value for the patient with a depression. These include education, cognitive techniques, social skills and assertiveness training. Grady and Sederer describe the educational experience that the milieu can provide. The person with depression can learn that it is a highly treatable disorder that affects a large population. Realizing that treatment has been effective for so many may be a corrective cognitive experience. Brodaty and colleagues describe a more formal educational program which includes such topics as mood disorders in general, drug treatment, risks and effects of affective disorders. The unit established a library of self-help books on depression and patients and their families were helped to become well-informed about the illness [23–24].

SOCIAL SKILLS TRAINING

When the patient is on the unit there are many opportunities to become aware of ineffective ways of coping, communication style and negative self-concept. Constructive feedback from patients and staff can alter some of the depressed person's beliefs and behaviors. Behavior therapists find that deficits in the frequency or quality of social reinforcement is causally related to the development and maintenance of depression. The person prone to depression lacks the ability to elicit positive reactions from other people, and should learn the necessary skills to avoid or improve negative interpersonal exchanges. Social skills training can be an invaluable defense against a post-discharge relapse into depression [23–24]

Cognitive Techniques

Cognitive-behavioral interventions are based on the premise that the person's interpretation of experiences determines emotional responses. Habitual negative appraisals may cause depression. Although the patient's interpretations are taken seriously and should not be challenged in the beginning of treatment, the milieu staff can work with these negative cognitions on a daily basis. The interventions may begin, not with cognitive techniques, but with behavioral strategies to reactivate the depressed patient. The patient is asked to do things, small tasks at first. Following success in a variety of tasks, the staff can challenge the patient's beliefs about not being able to accomplish anything. Success may also bring some pleasure and self-esteem. Other strategies include making an activity schedule and a mastery and pleasure schedule. This schedule asks the patient to plan and report daily activities and rate the degree of mastery associated with each activity. The patient is then assigned graded tasks. Success may lead to more complex tasks which are more related to the patient's own sense of despair or inadequacy. The patient records progress and is rewarded by immediate positive reinforcement for trying. Patient and therapist then realistically evaluate the performance. The staff member can often identify the thoughts that reinforce the person's depression. When the staff member can help the patient change some of these irrational beliefs or thoughts, there is an opportunity to change the depressed feelings and behaviors associated with them. Renate de Jong and colleagues write about using specific cognitive techniques in inpatient treatment for severe and chronic depression [25–26].

The Specialized Unit

Much can be learned from a unit specifically for depressed patients. Hole and Wolfersdorf describe a special depression ward that provided an opportunity to test specific psychotherapeutic treatment strategies: reinforcement of non-depressed behavior, more effective ways of working with regression, study of underlying dynamics of depression and accumulated experience in dealing with suicidal and dependent patients [27].

There were also definite disadvantages. Such empathic conditions can create severe regression, and a large population of depressed persons can virtually paralyze therapeutic activity. However, the results of the work on this depression ward indicate that treating depressed patients on a unit specifically designed for them contributes to the effectiveness of therapy. The day's activities, for example, can be structured to fit the more typical patterns of depressive behavior. In wards centered around crisis intervention, the more agreeable and passive depressed patient may compete poorly for therapeutic attention. The authors recommend selecting workers motivated to work with depressed patients and a team nucleus that can develop continuity over the years. Every patient is provided not only with a personal therapist but also with a person in charge of the patient's total care, who is already present at the admissions interview. They also recommend that both sexes be admitted to the ward and that patients be admitted with varying degrees of depression. Hole and Wolfersdorf warn that a ward cannot simply be transformed into a depression ward by admitting depressed patients. It must be well planned with specific use of staff members, space, and organization [27].

Brodaty and colleagues describe a mood disorders unit which provided not only a clinical service but also served as a research center and a resource for teaching. The policy of the unit was to withdraw patients from psychotropic drugs for at least two weeks since medication might be obscuring symptoms and independently causing depression. Treatment included cognitive therapy with homework assignments completed on the ward with staff support. Social skills and assertiveness training was a significant part of treatment. This was based on the premise that since depressed persons can't express negative feelings or reject demands placed on them, they tend to internalize their negative emotions. They often need help in developing interpersonal skills. Their social deficits have often been a factor in causing their depression, or in turn their depression has made learning such skills more difficult [28].

DEPRESSED CHILDREN

Rawson and Tabb report successful results from a short-term residential therapeutic intervention for depressed children (8–12) from deprived cultural and social backgrounds. The comparison group consisted of a similar group of depressed children from a traditional school setting. In comparison with the control group, the depression levels of the treatment group decreased significantly, as measured on the Reynolds Childhood Depression Scale. The 10-day treatment program was based on earlier findings that positive reinforcement in the child's environment had a direct effect on depression, while living in a rejecting environment which did not promote parental attachment or social skills could lower self-esteem and increase it [29].

The treatment program seems simple and might be one that any wise, loving and experienced staff member would provide, but what is significant is that the ingredients were clearly specified, included in a therapeutic ritual, and the results were measured. The first element of the program was frequent verbal praise for every part of the child's behavior which deserved it. The staff provided continual physical gestures of affection and approval such as hugs or handshakes toward each child for socially appropriate behavior. There were many opportunities for awarding participation in fun-filled activities as rewards for tasks that the child was capable of achieving. The staff was able to create situations where the peer group could recognize and congratulate the child for personal successes and successes in the program. In addition, there were community ceremonial awards (three times a day) for personal achievements [29].

This richly reinforcing environment was strengthened by a highly structured activity program which had 5- to 10-minute modules of instruction, frequent use of audiovisual teaching materials designed for children with behavior disorders, and modeling of appropriate behavior by both adults and peers. Each child also had two 20-minute tutoring sessions in school subjects where they were weak. A token economy allowed the children to earn "fun" activities in many ways: working up to ability level, behaving appropriately, acting as teachers to their peers when appropriate. There was also one long-term activity each day where the child worked with a group of same-age peers on a long-term project chosen by the group. Each child could experience success in working with others and achieving goals. There were also daily competitions among groups. Here the adult staff modeled appropriate ways of winning and losing [29].

A 1:2 staff/child ratio was maintained at all times. The treatment program provided a positive therapeutic environment where the children could succeed on their own by working together to achieve a common goal, or by competing within the security of their own unit. This program is a good example of informed treatment. Every feature of the program was based on earlier studies related to changing children's behavior and internal states often associated with depression. Many aspects were based on research on raising self-esteem, decreasing anxiety and increasing the internal locus of control [29].

Family Involvement

The literature on inpatient care of the depressed person has seriously neglected the treatment of the family, despite the fact that the family will play a continuous role in working with the patient's depression. Not only should there be psychosocial treatment and psychoeducation for the patient, but this should also be provided for the family. Glick and colleagues studied patient populations (24 patients with Major Affective Disorder) in three countries. The study demonstrated that only four of the 24 families had achieved a relatively successful resolution, and that the treatment alliance was almost twice as good with patients as with families. Very little was done to help families understand the patient's symptoms in a family context. Glick describes some of the family behaviors which can be countertherapeutic in working with the patient's depression. The family's lack of involvement can force the patient to rely exclusively on the hospital team for support. Fears of upsetting the patient can become so extreme that the family members are afraid to interact. The family can become "over-involved" and display high expressed emotion. During the patient's treatment, other family problems will be neglected and then erupt later when the patient recovers. The family that is uninvolved during hospitalization will be angry and not helpful if the patient relapses. Glick and colleagues believe that the greater the delivery of treatment to the family, the higher the achievement of treatment goals. The hospital will need to form a treatment alliance with the family and consider the family context of the patient's depression. Supportive family therapy and family psychoeducation will also be necessary. Some knowledge of the biological etiology of the illness will help alter the family's 'blaming" of the patient and alleviate the sense of helplessness. They should join the treatment team so that they can help work with the patient's illness from the beginning of inpatient work [30].

Conventional milieu wisdom about working with the depressed patient should continue to be scrutinized since interpersonal relationships are complex. Travelbee, for example, writes that when a depressed person begins to improve, it might be better for the nurse not to comment on the improvement since such comments may have a paradoxical effect. The person may go back to more severe depression [31].

References

1. American Psychiatric Association. Practice guideline for Major Depressive Disorder in adults. American Journal of Psychiatry 1993 Apr suppl;150(4):1–26.
2. Grady TA, Sederer LI. Depression. In: Sederer, LI, ed. Inpatient Psychiatry: Diagnosis and treatment. 3rd ed. Baltimore: Williams and Wilkins, 1991, 3–45.
3. Hole G, Wolfersdorf M. Advantages and disadvantages of special depression treatment and research wards. Psychopathology 1986;19, suppl. 2:184–93.
4. Weiner ML. Ego activation in the treatment of acutely depressed out-patients. Journal American Academy of Psychoanalysis 1982 Oct;10(4):493–513.
5. Beck AT, Young JE. Depression. In: Barlow D, ed. Clinical handbook of psychological disorders. New York: Guilford Press, 1985.
6. Brunnell LF. Mental hospital: Designing specific treatments for specific problems. Professional Psychology 1978;9(4):570–9.
7. Justic M. In: Wells, LA, ed. A handbook of psychiatric nursing. St Louis: Warren H. Green, 1989, 87–91.
8. Kerr NJ. Signs and symptoms of depression and principles of nursing interventions. Perspectives in Psychiatric Care 1977/78;24(2):48–63.
9. Beck AT, Rush AJ, Shaw BF, Emery G. Cognitive therapy of depression. New York: John Wiley, 1980.
10. Arieti S. Severe and mild depression: The Psychotherapeutic approach. London: Tavistock, 1980.
11. Pearce J, Newton S. The Conditions of human growth. New York: Citadel Press, 1963, 175.
12. Swanson AR. Communicating with depressed persons. Perspectives in Psychiatric Care 1975;13(2):63–7.
13. Potts T, Caron, Carson RC. The Affective disorders. In: Adams HE, Sutker PB eds. Comprehensive textbook of psychopathology. New York: Plenum, 1984, 349–81.
14. Kohut H. The restoration of the self. New York: International Universities Press, 1977.
15. Tudor GE. A sociopsychiatric nursing approach to intervention in a problem of mutual withdrawal on a mental hospital ward. Psychiatry 1953;15:193–217.

16. See reference 3.
17. See reference 8.
18. Wells LA. Affective Disorders. In: Wells, LA, ed. A handbook of psychiatric nursing. St Louis: Warren H. Green, 1989, 87–91.
19. Robinson L. Psychiatric nursing as a human experience. Philadelphia: Saunders, 1977, 147–79.
20. Rosenthal TT, McGuinness TM. Dealing with delusional patients: discovering the distorted truth. Issues in Mental Health Nursing 1986;8:143–54.
21. See reference 18.
22. See reference 3.
23. See reference 2.
24. Brodaty H, Boyce P, Wilhelm K, Mitchell P, et al. The establishment of a mood disorders unit. Australian & New Zealand Journal of Psychiatry 1987;21:375–81.
25. Helm SB. Nursing care of the depressed patient: A cognitive approach. Perspectives in Psychiatric Care 1984 Jul-Sep;23(3):100–7.
26. deJong R, Treiber R, Henrich G. Effectiveness of two psychological treatments for inpatients with severe and chronic depressions. Cognitive Therapy & Research 1986;20(6):645–63.
27. See reference 3.
28. See reference 24.
29. Rawson HE, Taub LC. Effects of therapeutic intervention on childhood depression. Child & Adolescent Social Work Journal 1993 Feb;10(1):39–61.
30. Glick ID, Burti L, Minakawa K, Maehara K, et al. Effectiveness in psychiatric care II. Outcome for the family after hospital treatment for Major Affective Disorder. Annals of Clinical Psychiatry 1991;3:187–98.
31. Travelbee J. Interpersonal Aspects of Nursing. 2nd ed. New York: F. A. Davis, 1971.

9. Persons with a Dual Diagnosis

Persons with a dual diagnosis suffer from the combined effects of two debilitating and chronic illnesses. The most common use of the term dual diagnosis is in reference to a diagnosis of substance abuse and mental illness. Recovery does not come quickly or easily. Both mental illness and substance abuse diagnoses carry with them social stigma, a risk for violence or suicide, a high relapse rate and impaired family and social relationships [1–2].

When alcoholism occurs in a patient who is also mentally ill it complicates the clinical picture. No matter which disorder is primary, each exacerbates the other. A person with schizophrenia may counteract psychotic anxiety with alcohol, become addicted and then when trying to withdraw, experience hallucinations, disordered thoughts and disorganization, a result of either the psychotic or addictive process. Drinking episodes can end compliance with antipsychotic medication [1–2].

There are at least three major substance abuse groups:

1. Those whose primary problem is a psychiatric disorder but who are also chemically dependent.
2. Those whose primary problem is chemical dependence but who also present a history of psychiatric disorder.
3. Those whose primary problem is chemical dependence who also have an Axis II personality disorder (usually borderline or antisocial) [1–2].

A dual problem requires a dual response. The challenge lies in creatively integrating relevant theories and treatment. Some promise lies in the fact that many dual-diagnoses patients improve dramatically when they stop abusing alcohol and other drugs. Those who make this commitment will at the very least be able to manage their psychiatric vulnerability. Although many psychiatric day treatment programs advocate abstinence, they don't identify it as the major goal or as the reason for the program. The client's ongoing need for treatment makes it impractical to refuse to treat persons who are using drugs or alcohol periodically and who will not or cannot undertake a commitment to total abstinence [1–3].

ESTABLISHING A PRIMARY DIAGNOSIS

The patient admitted to a psychiatric unit with symptoms of mental illness or alcoholism or both must be evaluated for both illnesses. Learning which came first is helpful because clinical management of primary alcoholism is different from addiction secondary to mental illness. Others have found, however, that unless a patient's primary diagnosis is immediately evident the question becomes almost irrelevant. In some cases the mental illness is clearly the primary problem and in others the substance abuse predominates. In either case the secondary problem sabotages treatment of the so-called primary disorder. These two illnesses are so entwined and mutually reinforcing that the question of primary diagnosis is no longer important [1–4].

Treating only the primary disorder makes a false promise that amelioration of the secondary disorder will follow. Treatment must focus on both illnesses since treating one does not automatically remove the other. For example, a person may develop a drinking problem while self-medicating for depression. Even if that person stops drinking and is totally involved in treatment the depression may not lift.

Denial for dually diagnosed patients may fluctuate as they bargain for which illness to accept. They may take advantage of this situation by claiming to be too fragile to confront issues during therapy and unable to attend self-help groups because they feel overwhelmed. If the psychiatrist proposes psychotropic medication, they refuse it because of "addiction." They will need to be convinced that they have two illnesses requiring medical attention [5].

Some Differences between Addiction and Psychiatric Treatment

Psychiatric treatment usually emphasizes differential diagnosis, psychotropic medication to treat the core disorder and therapies with the goal of uncovering its cause. Addiction treatment emphasizes personal responsibility in recovery and on staying in recovery on a day-to-day basis. The treatment center uses recovering staff who has personally experienced the problems the patient is experiencing. Standard addiction treatment often uses no-cost, nonprofessionally directed 12-step programs, with recovering patients assisting others, an aggressive confrontation of illness, more often eliminating rather than prescribing medications or drugs [6].

Models of Treatment

When treatment focuses on two illnesses, there will be several choices as to how it should be done.

Serial treatment model

In the serial treatment model, one treatment follows another. The schizophrenic patient with alcoholism would be first stabilized on a psychiatric unit, then transferred to an addiction unit or vice versa. The model permits the two systems to co-exist without requiring the staff to learn new skills or change basic treatment concepts. However, the system can fail to address individual patient needs. Patients can be given contradictory information, explanations and therapies. The sequential model works for psychiatric disorders and for mild to moderate substance abuse disorders. It does not work for major psychotic disorders or severe substance abuse. To make it more effective, both staffs should learn about the two types of treatment so they won't give conflicting messages and treatment directives. The addiction unit staff needs to know more about suicidal thoughts and management, psychiatric medications, how to distinguish drug-induced depression from major depression. Staff on psychiatric units needs to know more about working with denial [6].

The Parallel Model

The parallel model permits concurrent but separate treatment of both psychiatric and addiction disorder. The patient lives on a psychiatric unit but attends chemical dependency treatment groups in an adjoining addiction treatment unit. The patient has psychotherapeutic treatment but also attends Alcoholics Anonymous. The parallel model requires more therapists and system changes. Because the patient quickly notes conflicts in models in parallel treatment, therapists have had to become fully acquainted with both disciplines. So one benefit of this model is that it starts to force an integration of concepts [6].

Parallel treatment may be stressful because of the many hours of therapy that the patient must tolerate in a short period of time. Fragile patients may decompensate when transferred between units or groups. Parallel treatment works best for psychiatric disorders, stabilized bipolar and schizophrenic disorders, and some chronic patients who can go to concurrent AA meetings or addiction counseling. Patients with major depression can see a psychiatrist and an addiction counselor concurrently once each disorder is partially stabilized. When the patient has a major psychiatric illness such as schizophrenia, treatment may concentrate on preventing recurrence of psychosis by medication compliance, family education, and understanding psychosocial stressors. Group and individual psychotherapy may help patients with personality or anxiety disorders achieve insight and personality change [6].

Parallel treatment is more effective for addiction disorders once the person is stable. Spreading therapy across two systems may dilute treatment. Thus a highly addicted patient in denial may need the full intensity of an inpatient chemical dependency unit so that relapse will not occur. Many patients will never stabilize sufficiently from either a substance abuse or psychiatric condition to be able to profit from either the parallel or serial treatment models. For example, the alcohol-abusing person with schizophrenia may display behaviors too bizarre to allow participation in chemical dependency groups or work with an AA sponsor [6].

THE INTEGRATED MODEL

An integrated model simultaneously applies basic concepts and methods from both psychiatric and addiction treatment with integrated staff, concepts, and program in one facility. Ries writes that integrated treatment does not always work for persons with psychiatric and addictive disorders. Patients with stable psychiatric disorders whose primary problems are in getting and staying sober may not get the intensity of addiction treatment they need in an integrated program. They might respond better to a parallel treatment with minimal psychiatric care but focused addiction treatment. Moreover, patients with severe chronic psychiatric symptoms who episodically use substances but who have not developed dependent or compulsive use may not fit in well with severely addicted patients. Treatment with a relapse prevention model within standard psychiatric care might be more effective [6].

Minkoff describes an integrated model based on the Alcoholics Anonymous 12-step disease and recovery model and the standard biopsychosocial illness and rehabilitation model for treatment of serious psychiatric disorders. Both addiction and major psychosis are chronic, biological mental illnesses best treated through simultaneous applications of parallel concepts from both models.

Although they were not the only models for treatment, combining the addiction and psychiatric models meant treating them as equally valid. Developing an integrated framework justified focusing on parallels between the two models, rather than their differences. The disease concept of the addiction model and the illness concept in the psychiatric model are similar. In both, the patient is powerless over the primary disease and unable to cure it alone. Both diseases share loss of control of behavior and patterns of thought. The integrated model proposes that the disease of addiction is primary and becomes independent of whatever symptom relief was sought through initial substance use. Addiction will continue even after relief from psychiatric symptoms. The integrated model further states that the primary disease of addiction requires specific addiction treatment and finding alternative means of relieving underlying symptoms won't treat it sufficiently [7].

The 12-step program of recovery for addiction stresses the need to overcome denial and accept one's powerlessness to control substance use on one's own, admitting the need for help from others and actively using the treatment program to learn new skills to cope with life without substances. Factors that appear to help mentally ill patients recover are similar to those that contribute to recovery from addiction: acceptance of the illness, compliance with treatment, learning new coping skills and agreement to actively collaborate. Engaging the patient involves establishing a treatment relationship, educating about the illness, teaching the patient how to maintain stabilization through compliance with treatment. This will involve overcoming denial and other resistances in order to make a commitment to the ongoing treatment program [7].

Training the Staff for Integrated Treatment

Administrative splits in addiction and psychiatric care often make it difficult to train a staff. Continued separation of professional training in addictions and psychiatry, undertraining of medical doctors in addiction, separate and noncooperating certification of personnel and provision of funding for treatment may make integrated treatment seem impossible. Yet integrated programs rely on having either staff members from each discipline working together or individual staff cross-trained in both disciplines. Expanding cotraining is an ultimate goal. The staff needs to become cotrained and able to translate principles from one model to another harmoniously. Certain key concepts may initially seem to conflict [7].

Staffing must be as open-minded and as flexible as the treatment program. Counselors who believe that addicted persons should never receive medication or social workers who continually search for a family systems reason for chemical dependency are not ready for integrated treatment. If the staff and the treatment program are divided—with some groups focusing on addiction and others on psychiatric symptoms—patients will bargain away one illness. Countertransference feelings toward dually-diagnosed patients impede treatment. Staff members will inevitably feel frustrated, angry, impatient and helpless. Supervisory meetings should always leave time for sharing of countertransference feelings because treatment is extremely difficult.

Components of Treatment

There are many therapeutic components available in inpatient treatment: psychopharmacology, individual and family therapy, social skills training, therapeutic community meetings, substance abuse education, self-help groups, relapse-prevention groups, school and vocational training. Dually diagnosed patients require direction, structure, and support. Firm limit setting will help them to give up maladaptive behaviors for more responsible mature living. Structure is important because they often have difficulty solving problems or setting goals. The ability to set a schedule for the day and follow it becomes a helpful first step [8].

DRUG AND ALCOHOL EDUCATION

Drug and alcohol education is also helpful and must provide extensive opportunities to explore how the two illnesses affect each other. An educational format and approach has promise as a way to engage such clients in treatment. In this framework the client does not have to recognize or publicly acknowledge alcohol or drug use as a personal problem and can discuss it without confrontation. Luyster and Lowe describe a dual diagnosis program with afternoon lectures based on the 12 steps and morning lectures covering such topics as ego strengths, effects of the various addictions, grief and loss, and spirituality. Patients need education about the dual diagnosis concept, including the necessity for psychopharmacological treatment together with participation in recovery programs. Since they often accept only one disorder and deny the other, the treatment staff should focus on the reality of having two coexisting and interacting disorders [8].

ABSTINENCE AND TREATMENT

From the beginning of treatment patients should be encouraged to complete their own analysis of the costs and benefits of their chemical use. This self-examination process is crucial for dual diagnosis therapy. Providing information rather than confrontation and a climate in which the patients can evaluate and make decisions about their use can be very effective.

INDIVIDUALIZED TREATMENT FOR SPECIFIC PSYCHIATRIC DISORDERS

Despite the success of shared and combined programs, some dually diagnosed patients will require individual treatment. Many patients cannot deal with large group sessions, educational seminars or even 12-step programs. A slow but progressive involvement may work for some patients with psychiatric disorders not otherwise ready for standard treatment. Sheehan describes diagnosis-specific treatment of psychiatric illness during dual diagnosis treatment. Dually-diagnosed patients with anxiety will benefit from educational materials about anxiety disorders and their relation to dependence. The 12-step program may provide the support and structure these patients need to bind anxiety, although joining such a program will initially create anxiety of its own. The structure of AA meetings can be particularly helpful for patients with social phobias. Initial attendance is a difficult but manageable challenge, an exposure *in vivo* experience with graded desensitization. At first they should only attend the meeting, sit back and be silent. As their anxiety decreases, they can begin to participate. Other components of substance abuse treatment—codependency counseling, relaxation training, stress management, and assertiveness training—should be particularly beneficial to patients with anxiety disorders [9–10].

Bipolar patients may have a cyclic use of chemicals, especially when manic. They may use stimulants to stay high and alcohol as sedation to alleviate the manic phase. Sheehan finds that plotting drug use and mood swings reinforces the disease model of mood disorder and addiction. Sheehan describes the difficulty in distinguishing major depression from alcohol-induced depression. Moreover, many depressed patients experience self-pity. Helplessness and expectations that others will care for them may limit their recovery. Sheehan recommends helping them to assume personal responsibility for their own recovery [10].

Patients with substance abuse and schizophrenia frequently travel between psychiatric and addiction programs, not fitting into either. The staff can provide a safe environment for detoxification and work toward establishing honest and empathic relationships with the patient. They can present goals and expected behavior in simple and concrete terms. A behavior contract will prove less threatening than constant confrontation. The therapeutic process for the schizophrenic patient should include social skills training which emphasizes ways to refuse alcohol and drugs, communication training, and when possible, vocational rehabilitation. Treatment of dually diagnosed patients with cognitive disturbances should include praise and encouragement [10–11].

Relapse Prevention

The staff should maintain close involvement and positive regard even during relapse. Adolescent treatment should emphasize getting a commitment to abstinence, rather than making it the end goal. When adolescents verbally make this commitment this leads to emotional and behavioral reactions which often illuminate their own previous history. The 12-step model helps the adolescent prepare for relapse and learn how to deal with it.

DISTINGUISHING BETWEEN SUBSTANCE ABUSE AND DEPENDENCE

Study of the long term course of dual diagnosis patients with substance abuse disorders reveals that those with substance abuse have higher rates of change than those with substance dependence. Bartels and colleagues recommend that these different outcomes suggest the need for using different types of clinical interventions for these two groups. Distinguishing between abuse and dependence bears upon assessment, treatment and progrnosis of dual diagnosis patients [12].

Any dual diagnosis program, if it is to be effective, must have a clear commitment to work with frustrating and difficult patients and not suspend them when they become too troublesome. Substance abuse is a chronic disorder. The longitudinal perspective used in very severe psychiatric disorders such as schizophrenia applies equally to substance abuse. The treatment of the dually diagnosed patient may occur continuously over years, rather than episodically or during a crisis. Progress, too, is measured over years, not weeks or months. Stable recovery cannot usually be expected during the first year of treatment. Treatment of dual diagnosis must continually address demoralization, both of the patients and those who work with them [11–13].

References

1. McKevy MJ, Kane JS, Kelison K. Double trouble: substance abuse and mental illness. Journal of Psychosocial Nursing & Mental Health Services 1987 Jan;25(1):20–25.
2. Bean-Bayog MI. Inpatient treatment of the psychiatric patient with alcoholism. General Hospital Psychiatry 1987;9:203–9.
3. Brown VB, Ridgeley MS, Pepper B, Levine IS, et al. The dual crisis: mental illness and substance abuse. American Psychologist 1989 Mar;44(3);565–70.
4. El-Guebaly N. Substance abuse and mental disorder: the dual diagnosis concept. Canadian Journal of Psychiatry 1990 Apr;35(3):261–7.
5. Attia PR. Dual diagnosis: definition and treatment. Alcoholism Treatment Quarterly 1988;5(3/4):53–63.
6. Ries R. Clinical treatment matching models for dually diagnosed patients. Psychiatric Clinics of North America 1993 Mar;16(1):167–75.
7. Minkoff K. An integrated treatment model for dual diagnosis of psychosis and addiction. Hospital & Community Psychiatry 1989 Oct;40(10):1031–6.
8. Luyster G, Lowe R. Dual facilities: interprofessional collaboration in treating dual disorders. Journal of Chemical Dependency Treatment 1990;3(2):213–35.
9. Wallace M, Weiner H. The dually diagnosed patient in an inpatient chemical dependence program. Alcoholism Treatment Quarterly 1988;5(1–2):197–218.
10. Sheehan MF. Dual diagnosis. Psychiatric Quarterly 1993 Sum;64(2):107–34.
11. Morris JA, Wise RP. Identification and treatment of the dual diagnosis patient. Alcoholism Treatment Quarterly 1992;9(2):55–64.
12. Bartels SJ, Drake RE, Wallach MA. Long term course of substance abuse disorders among patients with severe mental illness. Psychiatric Services 1995 Mar;46(3):248–59.

13. Drake RE, Bartels SJ, Teague GB, Noorsdy DL, et al. Treatment of substance abuse in severely mentally ill patients. Journal of Nervous & Mental Disease 1993;181(6):6–11.

10. Eating Disorders

Patients with anorexia nervosa or bulimia nervosa usually begin treatment as outpatients. Inpatient treatment is necessary only if their condition cannot be controlled. An integrated treatment program can address varying levels of severity and may have as many as four interacting components; an outpatient clinic, inpatient treatment, a day hospital and an eating disorders information center. LaRocca describes a treatment program for anorexic and bulimic patients divided into varying levels of intensity. The program places anorectic patients into one of three levels: intensive, intermediate or convalescence. Bulimic patients have three treatment divisions: total dyscontrol, partial remission, and convalescent [1–2].

In addition to nutritional rehabilitation and weight restoration, most patients with eating disorders must come to understand and correct the role that dysfunctional thinking and impaired interpersonal relationships play in their lives. Treatment programs combine psychotherapy, behavioral interventions, and group methods. Interventions are first aimed at nutritional rehabilitation and restoring normal eating patterns, particularly the malnutrition that may perpetuate eating disordered behaviors. The long-term goal is to diagnose and help resolve the associated emotional, family, social, and behavioral problems to prevent future relapse [2].

Treatment methods: Individual Psychoanalysis and Group Therapy

Story describes treatment in a psychoanalytically oriented hospital for severely disturbed patients with eating disorders. The foundation of treatment rests upon the need for the psychotherapist and staff to be absolutely clear about the nature of the illness and how their theoretical conceptions relate to treatment. Anorexia in this severely disturbed population is interpreted within a developmental framework as "camouflaging" profound early difficulties. Treatment success rests upon a strong attachment and alliance with the therapist, who coordinates the treatment. Despite the attachment, the patient must in no way be seen as "belonging" to the psychotherapist. Staff integration with the patient's treatment is crucial. Boundaries between treatment modalities must remain clear and be monitored so that differences in opinion do not result in splitting [3].

Group therapy remains the most recommended treatment in both inpatient and outpatient settings. Piran and colleagues report that in the day hospital program primary treatment takes place in groups. In order to develop cohesion, patients enter the program in small groups. Therapy groups deal with destructive behaviors and attitudes about eating and weight. Other groups focus on body image, sexuality, relationships and assertiveness, with staff members in the program becoming group therapists in their special fields. Patients are expected to report both to the staff and to their group when they break the rules. Such confessions are the first step toward gaining control. Direct discussion of the impulsive actions that group members use to discharge tension can help prevent symptom substitution [4].

Roth respects the role that patients can play in each other's treatment, and the program he describes communicates this message from the beginning. All patients, with or without eating disorders, are expected to help each other develop healthy life patterns and to refrain from fasting, bingeing, or purging. The staff imposes restrictions both on those who break these rules and their peers who allow them to do so. The expectation that the community will reinforce adaptive behavior results in fewer splits between patients and staff and efforts to defeat the treatment program. When the patients confront denial in groups, this prevents behavior from becoming a staff control issue [4–5].

Vandereycken, who describes a leading European therapeutic center for anorexia nervosa, also argues for the power of group treatment. In this program, the anorexic patient's behavior is interpreted as a maladaptive solution of interpersonal problems, particularly attachment/autonomy conflicts and insecurity in heterosexual relationships. The program defines the core problem as a lack of self-esteem centered in a distrust of the body. The patient must become the active change agent in her own treatment as well as in the treatment of fellow group members. Although there is a contract system designed to change symptomatic behaviors, the entire treatment is organized around a group format. Even hospital programs that do not treat eating disorders exclusively rely upon group treatment [6].

Although specialized units and programs seem to be the norm, Strober and Bowen recommend hospitalization of the anorectic patient in a general adolescent psychiatric milieu, where peer group confrontation can help erode denial. Interaction with nonanorexic peers with "less restrictive models of coping" can help the patients to discover other ways to resolve conflicts and free their emotional expression. Group support combined with nonhostile confrontation can help the patient to "acquire more flexible and developmentally appropriate solutions for her maturational anxieties" [7–8].

Behavioral Approaches

Although programs may use a psychoanalytic or family-centered model, social learning theory is a foundation for many treatment techniques. Behavioral approaches are usually necessary in eating disorder programs to bring about weight gain and treat maladaptive eating patterns. Behavior therapy is based on the belief that eating behaviors are learned and can be changed by new learning experiences. This may include a planned system of positive reinforcement, which makes rewards contingent upon eating and weight gain. Simple positive reinforcers such as praise or negative reinforcers such as exercise restrictions influence the rates at which patients eat and gain weight. Although programs using behavior therapy often result in shorter hospitalization, the speed of weight gain during inpatient treatment does not predict long term outcome. Behavioral methods are central to many programs. Patients with bulimia nervosa who have out-of-control bingeing and purging have a treatment protocol that involves tasting their favorite bingeing food under supervised conditions. The initial acute anxiety response gradually decreases until the link between these foods and bingeing can be broken after 8 to 10 exposures [9–11].

Meals and Staff Attitudes toward Weight

Supervised meals are usually essential. Patients often participate in meal planning, and nutrition education is an important part of most programs. Mealtimes can become a social as well as a therapeutic experience, with patients remaining in the dining room for 45 minutes for social time after the meal. This prevents purging; otherwise, staff supervision in another setting is required. Talking at meals should be encouraged. Depending on the philosophy of the program, patients are encouraged to eat by using educational strategies, behavioral contingencies or by socialization that detracts from obsessive thinking about eating. Many treatment programs discourage talking about food itself during meals. In a post-treatment evaluation by Kennedy and Garfinkel, both bulimic and anorexic patients rated meal supervision and the fact that they did not select their own food as among the most helpful parts of the program [9–12].

Story cautions against a premature insistence on weight gain, believing that this would lead to the patient's mistaken belief that pounds gained are the crux of treatment and would repeat the anorexic family pattern of surface conformity. Unusual therapist and staff attention about details of weight and diet are contraindicated. Patients in the program Story describes share contractual responsibility for maintaining adequate weight and nutrition but failures to do so in this psychoanalytic program are "understood." In the program LaRocca describes, patients are weighed daily but not informed of their weight, in an attempt to deemphasize their preoccupation and correct some of their problems with controls. Since these patients have difficulty both keeping or giving up control, giving the control of their weight to the physician allows trust to develop [13–14].

Privilege Systems and Therapeutic Passes

Many program use privilege systems to help alter behavior. LaRocca advises that privileges must differ, since what is a privilege to one patient may not be to another. Therapeutic passes are often used as part of the privilege system after the patient has inspired staff confidence in her motivation and control. LaRocca finds that allowing patients to go home on pass helps to diagnose their continuing eating problems, their motivation to get well, and helps them prepare for life outside the hospital [14].

The Work of Milieu Staff

Regardless of the treatment setting, the milieu staff should be trained and knowledgeable about caring for persons with eating disorders. If the staff is inexperienced and untrained, qualified professionals must be available to train and supervise. Staff education and consultation are essential for treatment success.

MANAGEMENT MODELS

Tinker and Ramer describe staff subversion of treatment for anorexia nervosa in a pediatrics unit. The staff responded inappropriately to the patients' needs and interfered with behavior management. Conrad and colleagues describe a turf battle between the psychiatrist and nurse that seemed to reenact the power struggle of the patient and family. Some programs endorse a split management model of treatment with the therapist conducting psychotherapy and the psychiatrist concentrating on disturbed eating patterns and weight gain. This split model can be successful only if staff members work closely together, maintaining respect for each other and open communication. Another model places the medical providers in charge of all nutritional, eating, and weight management while psychiatrists address only psychodynamic issues [15–16].

THE APPROACH TO THE PATIENT

The milieu staff must work hard to establish trust. Patients with eating disorders will usually be very secretive, particularly early in their treatment before a trusting relationship can be established. The milieu staff must construct a safe environment that will make secretive behaviors logistically difficult. This would include such measures as having the person eat meals in the presence of others, recording the amount of food eaten, observation one hour after meals and regular room checks to assure that food is not hidden. One goal for the patient is to report transgressions to the therapist. Therapists will not chastise patients, but will ask them to explore the conditions antecedent to the eating behavior. Understanding these stresses becomes a learning experience. Power struggles and issues of control are inevitable. The eating disorder has been the patients' only way of achieving control, and it will not be easy to give up. Patients will see the milieu staff as punitive for making them eat and destroying their own sense of control [16].

Both patient and family must be engaged from the very beginning of treatment. They should receive the same education about eating disorders and be ready to consider all family matters that may be related to the condition. LaRocca shares testimonial letters from former patients in order to restore hope to families. Story recommends conveying to the patient that her difficulties are human, can be talked about and understood. She is told that she is in the hospital not only to be cared for by staff but also for the first time to learn or relearn as much as possible about caring for herself. Strober and Bowen believe that the hospital should hold out the promise of improved self-understanding and change [17–19].

Cognitive interventions will help the patient to identify problems of thinking and distorted and dysfunctional beliefs that perpetuate the eating disorder. Patients can learn to identify and express feelings, explore the thoughts that lead to symptomatic behavior, find new ways to deal with symptoms and learn relaxation techniques to decrease anxiety. Cognitive therapy has been shown to be even more effective than interpersonal psychotherapy and behavioral therapy in reducing binge-eating by altering the patient's disturbed attitudes toward body image, weight, dieting and the use of vomiting [20–21].

Story describes how difficult it is for the staff to work patiently and without anxiety in the midst of patients who are starving themselves and in life-or-death crises. Staff feelings about patients can become extreme. These patients will severely test all the resources of the therapeutic holding environment and the staff must often rely on its own cohesion. Story cautions the staff against "robbing" patients of their own responsibility and against taking over the management of their lives even though their behavior consistently invites it. Story's strongest message is that collusion between patient, family, and the treatment staff that they are treating weight and eating symptoms alone "trivializes" treatment. Vandereycken stresses integration and cohesion of the therapeutic team. The team he describes includes a central therapist who gathers information from all adjunctive therapies and a supervisor who acts as a participant observer without being actively involved in treatment. There is one clear therapeutic figure for the patient and family, one detailed treatment program made with the patient, and all decisions are made in weekly team meetings [22–23].

Manipulation

Schlemmer and Barnett describe manipulation as one of the most predominant problems in working with anorectic patients. Manipulative behaviors not only revolve around food but are a reaction to any setting of limits. More "lenient" behavioral programs that use initial bed rest and a protocol of returning the patient to bed if weight gain does not continue may be as effective and more efficient than more stringent programs in which caloric intake or daily weight precisely determine all privileges. Patients seem to struggle to show that they, not the staff, are in control. Irwin describes how patients in a behavior modification program can be even more manipulative than those in other programs since manipulation always occurred in reaction to limits. Staff were ill-prepared to deal with the "constant barrage of power struggles." Frequent meetings allowed them to safely ventilate their anger and frustration and prevented such feelings from being directed to patients. This helped them realize that these feelings were shared. They found that manipulative behaviors decreased if they tried to be consistent but accepted valid criticism and admitted their mistakes. This apparently established some trust. Their own consistency made their actions predictable, providing the patients with a feeling of control. Until the patients were assured that the staff would be consistent, they were extremely manipulative. Assertiveness training has become an essential component of many eating disorder programs, and anorectic patients have rated it as extremely valuable. The milieu staff must learn to distinguish between appropriate assertion and manipulation as they plan a response [24–28].

THE HOLDING ENVIRONMENT

D. W. Winnicott's concept of the holding environment has proved helpful in the design of many eating disorder programs. A holding environment provides a consistent and secure structure and routine that will help to organize the patient. It can provide an auxiliary ego so that the patient's full energy can be used to resolve developmental crises and discover alternative ways to manage tension. The concept of the holding environment is significant in the treatment of anorexia nervosa in a psychoanalytically oriented hospital. Piran and colleagues describe a day hospital program for eating disorders as providing a "containing and controlling" framework for therapeutic intervention. The staff explains all program rules and hospital routines before and after admission, emphasizing the "nonnegotiable" aspects of treatment—attendance in therapeutic groups and completion of all meals. In this program, the cumulative group attendance solidifies structure, control and commitment. Deering and Niziolek find both Winnicott's concepts of the "holding environment" and "good enough mothering" helpful to a program for eating disorders. The nursing staff can provide the structure for emotional and physical safety. The nurse's role can be that of the "good enough mother" who sets limits, encourages the patient and promotes independence. Stern and colleagues extend the holding environment to parents of the anorexic patient's family, providing the family with sufficient structure to support its own efforts. The entire therapeutic team provides this holding environment while conveying certain significant messages to the family: that it will not allow the patient to act self-destructively and that the treatment program will immediately involve the family. The family will continually test the structure and the team's ability to maintain authority and control over the therapeutic situation [29–32].

The milieu staff for eating-disordered patients must be guided by a shared theoretical formulation with a prescribed stance toward food, weight and weight monitoring. There should be appropriate safeguards against the patients' manipulation, dependence and regression. The staff can expect patients to continually test the holding environment. They will need to build staff cohesion and integration while maintaining clear boundaries between treatment modalities [33].

References

1. Gold Award. A multifaceted program for preventing and treating eating disorders: Programme for Eating Disorders, Department of Psychiatry. The Toronto Hospital. University of Toronto. Hospital and Community Psychiatry 1990 Oct;41(10):1120–3.
2. LaRocca FEF. An inpatient model for the treatment of eating disorders. Psychiatric Clinics of North America 1984;7(2):287–98.
3. Story I. Anorexia Nervosa and the psychotherapeutic hospital. International Journal of Psychoanalytic Psychotherapy 1982;9:267–302.
4. Piran N, Kaplan A, Kerr A, Shekter-Wolfson L, et al. A day hospital program for anorexia and bulimia. International Journal of Eating Disorders 1989;8(5):511–21.
5. Roth D. Treatment of the hospitalized eating disorder patient. Occupational Therapy in Mental Health 1986;6(1):67–87.
6. Vandereycken W. Organization and evaluation of an inpatient treatment program for eating disorders. Behavioral Residential Treatment 1988;3(2):153–65.
7. Strober M, Bowen E. Hospital management of the adolescent with anorexia nervosa. Clinical Psychologist 1986 Spr;39(2):46–8.
8. Deering CG, Niziolek C. Eating disorders: Promoting continuity of care. Journal of Psychosocial Nursing & Mental Health Services 1988;26(11):7–15.
9. Nusbaum JG, Drever E. Inpatient survey of nursing care measures for treatment of patients with anorexia nervosa. Issues in Mental Health Nursing 1990;11:175–84.
10. American Psychiatric Association. Practice guidelines for eating disorders. American Journal of Psychiatry 1993 Feb;150(2): 212–28.
11. See reference 1.
12. Kennedy SH, Garfinkel PE. Patients admitted to hospital with anorexia nervosa and bulimia nervosa: psychopathology, weight gain and attitudes toward treatment. International Journal of Eating Disorders 1989;8(2):181–90.
13. See reference 3.
14. See reference 2.
15. Tinker DE, Ramer JC. Anorexia nervosa: Staff subversion of therapy. Journal of Adolescent Health Care 1983;4:35–9.
16. Conrad N, Sloan S, Jedwabny J. Resolving the control struggle on an eating disorders unit. Perspectives in Psychiatric Care 1992;28(3):13–8.
17. See reference 3.
18. See reference 2.
19. See reference 7.
20. See reference 16.
21. See reference 10.
22. See reference 3.
23. See reference 6.

24. Schlemmer JK, Barnett PA. Management of manipulative behavior of anorexia nervosa patients. Journal of Psychosocial Nursing 1977;15: 35–37, 40–1.
25. See reference 9.
26. Tours SW, Beaumont PJ, Glaun D, Phillips T, et al. Combination of lenient and strict operant conditioning programmes in refeeding patients with anorexia nervosa. British Journal of Psychiatry 1984:144:517–20.
27. Irwin EG. A focused overview of anorexia nervosa and bulimia: Part II. Challenge to the practice of psychiatric nursing. Archives of Psychiatric Nursing 1993 Dec;7(6):347–52.
28. See reference 16.
29. Winnicott DW. Maturational processes and the facilitating environment. New York: International Universities Press, 1965.
30. See reference 4.
31. See reference 8.
32. Stern S, Whitaker CA, Hagemann NJ, Anderson, RB. The hospital's role in family treatment. Family Process 1981;20:395–408.
33. See reference 9.

11. Elderly Psychiatric Patients

Inpatient treatment designed for adults may not be appropriate for the older patient, but contrary to typical psychiatric stereotypes, the elderly respond to active therapeutic approaches. The older patient may need ways to compensate for increasing deficits of various kinds. Elderly patients require a multidisciplinary approach providing attention to physical disabilities as well as social services and rehabilitation [1–2].

Family participation should be mandatory when an elderly patient is admitted. The family can be integrated into the treatment team and make a strong contribution to the patient's rehabilitation. The patient's future social support will have a bearing on the permanence of treatment. Some family members may benefit from instruction in techniques for modifying behavior [1–2].

SPECIFIC TREATMENT ISSUES FOR THE ELDERLY

Elderly patients are dealing with the challenge of retirement, bereavement, social isolation, and declining health. They often have depressive symptoms: suicidal preoccupation, weight and appetite loss, feelings of boredom, inability to concentrate, helplessness, despondency, somatic complaints, and sleep disturbances. Often this depression has deteriorated into a state of emptiness and apathy. Elderly patients often show some organic central nervous dysfunction as well, but they are still able to benefit from treatment. If the dysfunction is severe, their treatment can be made more simplified and less active. Many patients, initially believed to be mentally impaired, have had cognitive abilities restored after their medication was decreased and their depression lifted. There may also be a group of patients diagnosed with late-life paranoid symptoms, whose paranoid ideation may be a defensive response to unacceptable changes in life [1–3].

Group treatment is often superior to individual psychotherapy, since it can meet the patient's need for peer support and can help in problem-solving. The patient can rebuild a social network and restore social skills. There may be many different groups available for the patient, with each designed to fulfill a specific need. Groups may address such areas as community living, reality orientation, psychotherapy, exercise and body movement. These many therapeutic groups revitalize the elderly person and encourage active participation in meaningful interactions with others, a strong contrast to their earlier isolation in the mainstream of life. Individual psychotherapy with the elderly patient is no longer contraindicated, but is usually of the supportive kind, dealing with issues of later life, including loss and bereavement. The patient may also rework issues from earlier life. Emphasis on open communication and the encouragement of the person's autonomy, activity and responsibility will strengthen positive results. Careful planning for discharge can prevent relapses [1–3].

Milieu Staff

If possible, staff should be selected on the basis of their interest in the elderly. The assignment of a primary staff member responsible for the patient's care on a 24-hour basis decreases confusion. Many elderly persons respond well to some form of physical touch. Touching provides comfort for many of the elderly who feel isolated, who have lost a spouse or many friends. It helps to maintain their orientation and is reassuring for many. Yet the staff member must proceed carefully and not infantilize the patient. The staff member should address the patient on a first-name basis only after the patient requests it, not before. Billig and Leibenluft report that the combination of older patients with younger staff or patients often stimulates transference and countertransference problems. It may be difficult for the elderly to have much younger people making decisions in their lives [2–5].

Special Programs

Roskos and colleagues describe a successful therapeutic community program for the elderly that emphasized activity, taking responsibility for one's self and others, a planned review of the past, and careful planning for the future. They conclude that the psychiatric hospital treatment of the elderly can be vital and rewarding and that patients often leave as hopeful people, fully engaged with life [6].

Some would legitimately question the separation of the elderly from other patients. If there is not a special unit, some exceptions should be made in the general milieu rules to allow elderly patients to be less restricted and given frequent pass privileges. Contrary to earlier beliefs, the elderly psychiatric patients do not necessarily require a lengthy stay. They can benefit from short-term treatment if discharge planning and liaison with community resources are in place [7].

References

1. Roskos SR, Lerner S, Kline BE. The elderly patient in a therapeutic community. Comprehensive Psychiatry 1979 Jul/Aug;20(4):359–69.
2. Polinquin IN, Straker M. A clinical psychogeriatric unit: organization and function. Journal of the American Geriatric Society 1977;25(3):132–7.
3. Liptzin B. The geriatric patient and general hospital psychiatry. General Hospital Psychiatry 1987;4:198–202.
4. Whall AI, Conklin C. Why a psychogeriatric unit? Journal of Psychosocial Nursing & Mental Health Services 1985 May;23(5):23–7.
5. Billig N, Leibenluft E. Special considerations in integrating elderly patients into a general hospital psychiatric unit. Hospital & Community Psychiatry 1987 Mar;38(3):277–81.
6. See reference 1.
7. Meier HMR, Besir M, Sylph JA. Psychiatric hospitalization: terminable or interminable? Canadian Journal of Psychiatry 1992 Apr;37(3):157–62.

12. Firesetters

Inpatient treatment of children who set fires is rarely discussed in the literature although residential placement may often be necessary for this serious behavioral problem. Children who set fires often have intense feelings of rage, are impulsive, and have poor self-control. Their firesetting may be an acting out of unexpressed aggression toward their parents. They can often project this anger upon other adults in the treatment center [1].

Kolko and colleagues demonstrate that an educational preventive approach can be effective for young inpatient firesetters. They compared the effectiveness of two approaches, a Fire Safety/Prevention Skills Training Group and a Fire Assessment Awareness program. The awareness program involved meetings with staff nurses to assess and discuss firesetting behaviors. The skills training group was associated with a significant reduction in contact with fire-related toys and matches and less overall involvement with fire than the awareness program. The skills training program for 12 children, ages four to eight, included didactic presentation, modeling, role-playing, self-instruction and reinforcement. The first session discussed how fires help and hurt people and the need for adult supervision with fires. In the second session, children were taught the difference between safe object and objects which should be used only with adult supervision—such as matches, lighters, and sparklers. Children were given a worksheet and asked to place red stickers over forbidden items. Hand-puppets and simulated matchbooks were used in the third session. Children role-played what to do if they found matches. The final session was directed toward personal safety in case of fire and how it felt to be burned [2].

DeSalvatore and Hornstein describe an inpatient program for juvenile firesetters. Although they report that over 75% of the fires that were started by the 52 patients they have treated were started because of anger at parents or friends, the treatment approach they describe directly addresses the firesetting behavior rather than attempting to change their anger. At the same time the treatment does involve a close examination of the family system with the hope of changing the parent-child relationships. The Smokey the Bear program was chosen to appeal to the childhood population. Since children often identify with animals in stories to help them master the world around them, Smokey, the protector of the forest, was chosen with the hope that children could identify with him and help him to do his job [3].

The treatment approach was designed to be carried out by any specially trained member of the mental health team and includes educational components and behavior modification techniques. In contrast to treatments that discuss fire prevention in the abstract, this program allows controlled experimentation with matches and lighters in the staff member's presence. Treatment takes place in a supportive, nonthreatening, nonblaming atmosphere, which encourages children to participate. The children receive many positive reinforcements such as verbal praise, star charts, and snacks [3].

FAMILY INVOLVEMENT.

In the Smokey the Bear program, parents participate actively, completing specific assignments for work at home on weekend visits. They will discuss these assignments later with the therapy staff. This parental involvement establishes a triadic model (parents, child, therapist) of therapy in which changes can be continued by those who have significant relations with the child [3].

Phases of the Smokey the Bear program

Each child has an individual program that can be modified to match the level of functioning and the time needed. The treatment takes place in sessions which last from 30 to 60 minutes, either once or twice weekly. Activities are selected for each individual child [3].

ASSESSMENT

The first phase is assessment. The staff compiles information about the child's family environment and firesetting behaviors. Both the parent and the child complete a questionnaire about firesetting, the child's friendships, school behaviors, and family relationships. The phenomenology of the child's firesetting behavior is charted and is represented by a graph that charts the child's feelings, external stimuli, and firesetting behavior in a time sequence. The child is asked to describe in chronological order what happened before, during and after setting a fire, and then to describe feelings when it happened. The child is also asked to draw several pictures about fire, some showing fire as useful and some as dangerous. These drawings help the child release these feelings in another medium. At the end of the assessment, the staff presents the child with a packet of materials for use in the program, which includes a folder, a junior forest ranger handbook, a Smokey the Bear emblem and bookmarks, a pencil, pen, ruler, a notebook with the emblem and words to a song about Smokey the Bear, all of which were obtained from the U.S. Department of Agriculture and the forestry departments of various states [3].

The Educational Phase

Children learn the potential dangers of fire, fire safety and prevention during this phase. The children begin by analyzing fire as a chemical process that requires three elements: a spark, material to burn, and air. The child then gets to go on "hazard hunts" at home and in the woods to find potential fire hazards. A study of pictures that requires the child to identify hazards and means to correct them is the next activity [3].

Then the staff member teaches the child the safe procedure for lighting trash and campfires. The child practices all these steps outside with staff supervision without actually lighting the fire. This is followed by a rock-gathering activity to teach the child about fire size. The staff and child collect 20 different sizes of rocks and the child arranges them from the smallest pebble to the largest rock. This is a visual demonstration of the fact that small fires can expand to large fires and can be dangerous [3].

The staff teaches fire safety and prevention by role playing, working with parents, and a system of rewards. Detective activities help the child identify different fire hazards and describe safety precautions for them. The children also need to learn about safety with matches and matchbooks. They earn stars as rewards for turning in matchbooks or lighters to an adult. The child and the staff member practice reporting a fire to the fire department and responding to the firefighter's instructions over the phone. The child learns what to do if clothing catches on fire [3].

The Practice Phase

This phase teaches the proper way to strike and use matches. Parents participate in this lesson, which usually takes place either outside or inside, using a metal wastebasket. The staff member begins by discussing the specific functions of matches and explains that they can be dangerous when not used safely. The technique here is to see one, do one, and then teach one. The staff member describes the safe way to strike a match, then does it. The child then strikes a match based on these instructions. Finally, the child teaches the staff member how to strike a match properly [3].

Graduation

A written and practical test evaluate the child's learning. Younger children complete an oral quiz. There is a graduation ceremony where the child receives a membership card, a badge and posters about forest fire prevention, and as part of the ceremony is declared a Junior Forest Ranger [3].

Follow-Up

A follow-up was conducted at 1, 3, 6, and 12 months after discharge. Of the 52 children studied at the various intervals, recidivism was rare. Only two children were reported to have set a fire. The program did not ignore other aspects of the child's treatment, and the residential milieu provided ongoing support. The juvenile firesetter needs encouragement to learn alternative means of expression. Therapeutic activities were selected according to the severity of the child's problems. While some children set fires because of their fascination with it, others have done it for anger and revenge. It is natural for children to experiment with fire, but parents and staff must provide boundaries and limits for the experimentation that can take place. If fire is presented as a forbidden secret it will increase the child's curiosity and the child will try to master its power through experimenting. Positive and creative approaches are necessary to work with this natural curiosity so children can learn about fire in a safe way [3].

An inpatient approach that combines fire safety skills training with behavior management seems to be the most appropriate for severe cases of young firesetters. However, most children who set fires have severe personality deficits that may eventually need addressing. They may be poorly defended against other expressions of aggression and vulnerable to sudden loss of control and regression. They can become easily enraged at the slightest insult from peers or adults and have poor judgment in social situations. Still, a generalized psychiatric approach to remedy these deficits that does not focus on fire safety may not be effective. This is not to say that the staff must finally be able to completely understand the relationship between family dynamics and the child's pathological firesetting to provide comprehensive treatment [4–5].

Bumpass and colleagues report using a "graphing technique" with child firesetters. By this technique, the child becomes aware of the sequence of events that lead to firesetting: the triggering event, the feeling state and the firesetting behavior which follows. This was in outpatient treatment. The Dallas Fire Department, using this technique, decreased recidivism in juvenile firesetters from 32 percent to 2 percent. This model might also be helpful for adults (6–7).

Geller writes about psychiatric patients who set fires. They usually have poor social skills, are not assertive, and have difficulty expressing their feelings. Firesetting becomes a dramatic way to communicate. Rice and Chaplin, in inpatient treatment of ten male firesetters focused on assertion training (behavior rehearsal, modeling, coaching, instruction and feedback). This training was more effective than nondirected group therapy in improving social skills. One year after discharge there were no known acts of firesetting [8–9].

References

1. Sakheim GA, Osborn E, Abrams D. Toward a clearer differentiation of high-risk from low-risk fire-setters. Child Welfare 1991 Jul-Aug;70(4):489–503.
2. Kolko DJ, Watson S, Faust J. Fire safety/prevention skills training to reduce involvement with fire in young psychiatric inpatients: preliminary findings. Behavior Therapy 1991;22:269–84.
3. DeSalvatore G, Hornstein R. Juvenile firesetting: assessment and treatment in psychiatric hospitalization. Child & Youth Care Forum 1991 Apr;20(2):103–14.
4. See reference 1.
5. Cox-Jones C, Lubetsky MJ, Fultz SA, Kolko DJ. Inpatient psychiatric treatment of a young recidivist firesetter. Journal American Academy of Child & Adolescent Psychiatry 1990 Nov;29(6):936–41.
6. Bumpass ER, Fagelman PD, Bris RJ. Intervention with children who set fires. American Journal of Psychotherapy 1983 Jul;37(3):328–45.
7. Bumpass ER, Bris RJ, Preston D. A community-based program for juvenile firesetters. Hospital & Community Psychiatry 1985;36:529–33.
8. Geller JL. Firesetting in the adult psychiatric population. Hospital & Community Psychiatry 1987 May;38(3):501–6.
9. Rice ME, Chaplin TC. Social skills training for hospitalized male arsonists. Journal of Behavior Therapy & Experimental Psychiatry 1979;10:501–8.

13. The Hearing-Impaired Psychiatric Patient

There are few inpatient psychiatric programs that provide treatment for hearing-impaired patients. There are few mental health professionals who are skilled in sign language, the primary mode for communication for most of the hearing-impaired.

Gerstein reports on the development of a psychiatric program for hearing-impaired patients. Several major steps were made before the hospital attempted to serve this population. Workshops with the deaf community helped the staff to develop sensitivity to the lives of the hearing-impaired. Staff members became aware of the conceptual framework of sign language and the differences between it and spoken language. Every effort was made to facilitate communication in the program: the purchase of sophisticated electronic equipment to facilitate hearing, intensive staff training in American Sign Language (the standard visual language for the deaf) and the hiring of skilled interpreters [1].

The plan was to integrate hearing-impaired patients into the ongoing program. Both groups responded well to this integration. Some of the adolescents on the unit became interested in learning finger spelling. Gerstein reports that the staff continued to feel energized working with hearing-impaired patients. The establishment of an advisory board assured that the program maintained ongoing coordination with the hearing-impaired community. Members included representatives from educators of the hearing-impaired, interpreter specialists, deaf activists and mental health professionals [1].

Larson and McAlpine discuss the integration of hearing-impaired patients in a chemical dependency unit. This integration was made possible by the addition of an interpreter to the staff as well as inclusion of patient advocates for the hearing impaired who could advise on communication and social problems. The patients' sign language interpreter joined the program for the daily lectures, individual sessions, recreational therapy, leisure education and the two daily sessions of group therapy. In the evenings when the interpreter was not there, the deaf members interacted by gestures and writing. There were no other staff members or patients who could use American Sign Language in this program. A teletypewriter was available to transfer telephone messages and an employee of the state services for the deaf provided periodic interpretation for initial interviews. A crucial ingredient to the success for the deaf person was the feeling of being welcome and included in social and recreational activities [2].

The paucity of literature on milieu programs for the hearing-impaired indicates that this population has been neglected, both by programs and in literature describing them.

References

1. Gerstein AI. A psychiatric program for deaf patients. Psychiatric Hospital 1988; 19(3):125–8.
2. Larson EW, McAlpine DE. Treating the hearing-impaired in a standard chemical dependence unit. Journal of Studies on Alcohol 1989 Jul;49(4):381–3.

14. The Homosexual Population and Homosexual Behavior

The gay and lesbian population requires special consideration in the treatment setting. While sexual orientation should be irrelevant when it comes to access to care, it can't be irrelevant in planning treatment. Since homosexual behavior itself may also be a normal episodic activity for heterosexuals, the staff also needs to consider appropriate responses to all forms of such expression.

A group living situation heightens adolescents' concerns about sexual identity. Close living arrangements, separation by gender with the absence of the opposite sex, and same-sex roommates increase the likelihood of homosexual behavior. Residential life creates family-like relationships and closeness develops because of the amount of time spent together, the absence of privacy, and the emotional intensity of the living situation. This closeness is often emotionally intense, threatening and yet fulfills many needs. The experience of this closeness, as well as other activities such as horseplay can stimulate fears about sexual identity or homosexual panic. In addition, large numbers of adolescents experimentally engage in sexual experiences with members of the same sex. Homosexual thoughts and fantasies are common in adolescence and beyond [1].

The traditional approach in treatment is for residents struggling with relationship issues to talk about them in individual, group or family therapy. Yet because of homophobia and ignorance, those who openly explore sexual identity issues risk rejection from the peer group or family. Many gay and lesbian adolescents simply withdraw from adolescent experiences. Rejection from same-sex peers can happen once sexual orientation is known, except in extraordinary therapeutic milieus. Gay and lesbian adolescents may be victimized, ostracized or physically abused. A careful choice of roommates for the gay or lesbian adolescent can make a difference. All efforts should be made to assure that there is no victimization, and that they are not isolated or scapegoated [1].

Residential treatment settings are rarely prepared to work with gay or lesbian teenagers, even those who are fairly well adjusted. They will undoubtedly experience homophobia and rejection. The limited confidentiality that occurs when many staff members work with one patient will make the adolescent reluctant to openly explore sexual identity issues. Information disclosed to one staff member will be necessarily shared with others [1].

SEX EDUCATION FOR STAFF AND RESIDENTS

Sex education and healthy, normal interaction with homosexual peers will be the most helpful ways to immunize the treatment center against homophobia. Adolescents concerned about sexual identity issues related to homosexuality will benefit from knowing that:

1. Homosexual feelings are a common part of the human sexual experience.
2. Homosexual activity is relatively common and it does not make someone gay.
3. For those who discover that they are gay or lesbian there is an active community in which to participate [1].

Staff members should receive the same education the residents receive. Simply because they are mature, competent, and experienced does not mean that they are well equipped to understand and respond appropriately to homosexual behavior. AIDS education must also be a part of the curriculum. This basic information should be shared with all, since it may not be easy to determine who needs it most. Staff members are with children and adolescents in situations where all conceivable topics will come up, and all imaginable behaviors, including homosexual ones occur. They should be armed with information so that they can make these key teachable moments productive and affirming for everyone [1].

Sexual Behavior

Patients will be sexually active, so that the treatment center will need policies and procedures for addressing sexual activities. If there are no policies in place, the staff will use their own widely variant judgments on how to handle sexual situations. Treatment centers operate with different guidelines about what sexual activities should be reported. There should be an appropriate concern not to taint sexual behavior with shame and allow each person some appropriate privacy and dignity in sexual expression [1].

At the same time, the sexual behavior of residents often requires a response. The staff member who must respond to same-sex behavior should first think what the response would be for similar heterosexual behavior. Just as in heterosexual behavior, the situation must be assessed to assure that the behavior was not nonconsensual, exploitative, or assaultive [1].

Creating Inclusion and Respect

When staff or patients use derogatory words to refer to homosexuals, their language should be confronted. Permitting this language conveys a message that gays and lesbians need not be treated with respect. The treatment center's policies and the language should reflect the reality that gays and lesbians are equal and respected members of the group and of society. Gay and lesbian clients and families must also be able to sense this respect. References to families or future families of clients should use such words as companion, partners, or significant others, rather than husbands or wives. The administration might also assure that sexual orientation is a protected category in nondiscrimination clauses for employment and services. This inclusion once again clearly reinforces to both staff and patients the treatment center's commitment to treating gays and lesbians respectfully and equally [1].

Affirmation of the Gay and Adolescent Person

The day may come when a gay and lesbian orientation will be treated as a variant of normative sexual behavior. At present, great care must be taken in selecting a responsive treatment setting for the homosexual adolescent. Religious settings that treat homosexual behavior as a sin can't be of help to the adolescent struggling with identity issues. The staff can work to positively affirm the gay or lesbian person. Education can build but not guarantee peer support.

Gay or lesbian adolescents have few opportunities to learn about their own sexuality in the adolescent culture that surrounds them. This socialization can only occur through contact with a local gay and lesbian community. There are many myths about homosexuality that can cause adolescents a great deal of pain and loss of self-esteem that information and help from this group will clarify. The chance for a gay-oriented peer group for an adolescent rejected by peers can be both rewarding and therapeutic. Reading material, both fiction and nonfiction, can provide information and affirmation in a nonthreatening manner [1].

MANAGING HOMOSEXUAL BEHAVIOR

Appropriate interventions should be planned for sexual liaisons among children and adolescents. If they are not responded to properly they may produce anxious and guilty feelings that will affect the adolescents' treatment. A degree of vigilance is also advisable. What might seem to be a positive interaction between children may be a form of exploitation of one by another. There may be boys who have been previously involved in homosexual liaisons in other settings and wish to continue. There are liaisons resulting from attachments intensified by institutional living. There are others who may offer sex for protection or privileges or who become involved in sex out of fear. There may be sexual exploiters who demand sexual favors from weaker peers. If the staff denies the possibility of such behaviors, this can progress to neglect or institutional maltreatment [2]

There will be instances when heterosexual males and females engage in homosexual behaviors that do not in any way necessarily lead to bisexuality or homosexuality. If the staff knows that this can be normal, it will help them not to overreact and be able to assess whether the behavior is a form of exploitation or an expression of attachment. If these encounters do not involve mutuality or consent, they can constitute assault. These episodic homosexual encounters may be consenting liaisons that must be assessed and managed and not immediately labeled [2].

The treatment center staff has three possible approaches to adolescent sexuality: eliminate it, accept it, or cultivate it. If the staff chooses none of these options and ignores it, there can be dangerous and unacceptable consequences. Acceptance involves giving good information and helping children or adolescents understand the meaning of sexual behavior. Cultivation means viewing sexuality as a fully accepted dimension of life. Niles believes that sexuality is a normal aspect of adolescence, that homosexual behavior may be a part of that experience and that we may expect children or adolescents to engage in both heterosexual and homosexual behaviors. No single approach toward homosexual behavior has received unequivocal support, but there are some general guidelines. There should be administrative involvement since the potential for abuse or maltreatment is too serious not to involve the administration [2].

Although therapeutic involvement after such incidents has usually been the domain of the therapist, there is a role for child care workers that is distinct from that of other staff members. It may be the child care worker who first discovers sexual activity and the worker's response will be first therapeutic interaction with the children involved. Child care workers are important in the children's lives and their response either to sexual activity or its reporting by a child is crucial in helping the child understand and grow from it [2].

RESPONSE TO SEXUAL ACTIVITY

There are several steps that follow the discovery of a sexual or homosexual encounter: ending the activity and directing the patients to their rooms or scheduled activity, assessment and follow-up. If there were any rule violations, such as being out of bed during curfew, the staff should inform adolescents about the sanctions for it. However, they should also know that the sanction is not for the sexual activity unless the institution has a public policy of prohibiting sexual activities. Since staff members can't know what the activity means to the children, they should attempt a kind but firm response, conveying neither approval nor disgust. Assessment of the incident should rapidly follow its discovery. Several factors will play a part in the assessment: knowledge of the children, an investigation of possible exploitation or victimization, the "normative" nature of the behavior, and the significance or effect on the children involved [2].

The assessment of what is normal or what is harmful depends upon several factors:

1. The age of the partners. If the age difference is as much as five years staff must investigate whether victimization has occurred.
2. The participants' relationship. For example, is it between a new resident and someone who had been in the setting longer? Could it possibly be an initiation, or testing, or payment for protection?
3. The nature of the sexual behavior itself.
4. Each person should be asked separately to learn how it was initiated, so that it can be learned whether it was consensual, or might result from manipulation, exploitation, or victimization.
5. Each person's own history will play a part so that the staff can determine whether such behaviors have become compulsive or assaultive, or whether one of the partners is extremely vulnerable and might remain a victim. The answers to all of these questions will then bear on the therapeutic follow-up with the staff and the children or adolescents [2].

Successful Programs with Gay and Lesbian Adolescents.

Mallon describes a residential treatment program that has successfully integrated gay, lesbian, and straight adolescents. Although integration is not easy, the benefits clearly outweigh the difficulties. The program not only created a safe and nurturing environment for homosexuals but also went a long way in correcting homophobic attitudes by giving straight and gay peers the chance to interact and get to know each other. Educating the other residents and the staff about gay and lesbian issues and asking them to examine their own responses to homosexuality improved treatment. Well-planned training and a strict antislur policy helped to make it successful. Mallon stresses the importance of recognizing that sexual orientation is only one dimension of the adolescent's personality and that the exclusive focus on the sexual aspects of homosexuality obscures the total person [3].

Mallon describes three common sexual adaptations available for homosexual adolescents: 1) repression of desire; 2) suppression of homosexual impulses with concurrent attempts to be heterosexual or asexual, and 3) disclosing and deciding to be what they are. Each of these adaptations can cause difficulties in treatment. The repressed adolescents often act out. The suppressed adolescents often have great difficulties with identity formation, feel inadequate and unacceptable. Those who disclose find themselves rejected by peers [3].

PROACTIVE PREPARATION

Increased sexual activity often occurs during slow unsupervised times, when new residents arrive or when groups of isolated and lonely children seemed to cling together. There may also be more unpredictable or transferential occurrences in response to the presence of extremely charismatic or attractive staff members or when staff members became engaged or pregnant. If children or adolescents have the chance to discuss and feel included in such unit happenings, and are not just outsiders then they may be less likely to seek sexual expression [4].

Sexual orientation is the preferred term when referring to homosexuality. Staff and peers should realize that homosexuality is not a choice to be corrected but an orientation to be respected, just as we respect all human differences. The homosexual population has not been well served in inpatient treatment. The pain of social stigmatization causes them to be more vulnerable than their peers to chronic depression, substance abuse, rejection by families and suicidal ideation. The development of programs for this population is an equity issue, not a sexual issue. Caring for the child or adolescent is the real issue at hand [4].

References

1. McMillen C. Sexual identity issues related to homosexuality in the residential treatment of adolescents. Residential Treatment for Children & Youth 1991;9(2):5–21.
2. Niles WJ. Managing episodic homosexual behavior of adolescents in residential settings. Child Care Quarterly 1986 Spr;15(1):15–26.
3. Mallon GP. Serving the needs of gay and lesbian youth in residential treatment centers. Residential Treatment for Children and Youth 1992;10(2):47–61.
4. Johnson WH. Childhood sexuality: The last of the great taboos? SIECUS Report 1977;V:1–15.

15. The Multicultural Population

The most exciting difference in all institutions in the last decade has been the emergence of a multicultural population. Assimilation for this population is no longer the answer. The milieu staff must learn to provide culturally sensitive and culturally responsive treatment for this varied group. Cultural sensitivity can enable us to understand and respect the values and behaviors of all ethnic groups. We must reevaluate clinical practices for each population and learn what might be considered normal and abnormal in each society. We need to improve diagnosis and classification and understand belief systems and communication patterns in order to continue with treatment [1].

We can no longer assume that the theoretical and treatment principles of psychiatry are international. Attempts to change the patient to fit the institution's structure may be impractical, dehumanizing, and produce negative results. Inpatient evaluations frequently ignore the principal foundations for identity—the person's ethnicity and culture. We must become familiar with the person's sociocultural milieu to assess not only psychopathology but also resources and coping behavior. This education may need to continue on a patient-by-patient basis. There are several ways to build cultural sensitivity: the intensive study of a culture, consultation with cultural anthropologists, spending time in other cultures, and consulting with peers from many ethnic groups. Once ethnic minorities are represented in the clinical and administrative staff, the task will become easier. Recruitment and training of a diverse clinical and research staff should be a priority. A culturally diverse staff will, of course, bring adjustment problems of its own, but it will be best equipped to deal with psychopathology that might be mistaken for cultural differences [1–6].

Not only must the staff be culturally sensitive, but the treatment center itself must become culturally responsive. This will mean being careful not to overwhelm the patient with culturally unfamiliar treatment. It will mean providing literature, magazines, and television programs that respect ethnic diversity, as well as food and changes in decor. Staff members cannot become culturally responsive without examining their own cultural biases and countertransference—confronting them honestly with an openness to new experience. Past experiences reveal that racial and ethnic bias has affected treatment. Stereotypes and unfamiliarity have played a role in misdiagnosis and treatment planning for many African-American patients. Bond and colleagues, in a study of race and violence in a psychiatric setting, find that although there was no difference in the number of violent acts between white and nonwhite patients, the white hospital staff physically restrained nonwhite patients nearly 4 times as often as they restrained whites. Increasing interracial contact reduced this difference. There have been significant differences reported between African-Americans and whites in the assessment of the psychiatric ward atmosphere, with African-Americans reporting a much more negative perception. White patients have been found to remain longer in inpatient treatment, while more black patients left against medical advice. Some of this bias is also related to stereotyping. We must be careful when we describe certain characteristics as prominent in Native Americans and remember that there are at least 400 different American Indian tribes in the United States alone. We cannot confidently speak of a Latino or Hispanic culture when such a group encompasses persons from Mexico, Cuba, Puerto Rico, El Salvador and the Philippines. There is no truly distinct "Asian" culture. We shouldn't make the mistake of viewing all members of a particular ethnic background as so similar that they need the same form of therapy [6–13].

We must also consider the interaction of ethnicity with acculturation. Ethnic identity refers to the person's commitment to living within a native cultural tradition. Even if the person is bilingual, we should not necessarily presume that ethnic identity is not fully preserved. The individual member of an ethnic group must first be seen as a person and it is this sharing of human bonds that transcends ethnic and racial differences [13].

This discussion of the multicultural population is cautionary rather than comprehensive and focuses more on the mistakes that can be made and the questions to be considered rather than providing thorough descriptions of each cultural group.

DIAGNOSTIC ISSUES FOR MULTICULTURAL POPULATIONS

Placement in what seems to be a foreign environment can create a serious distortion of reality that should not be mistaken for pathology. Morrisette describes the distortions experienced by Native American youth in residential treatment. When these adolescents learned that Native American values were not accepted they were left without a foundation for their lives [14].

INTERVIEWING AND INTERACTING WITH PATIENTS FROM OTHER CULTURES

When the patient is required to speak in another language, the consequences become immediately uncertain. Whenever possible, a native speaker should conduct the admissions interview, since even English-speaking foreigners revert to their native language when they become ill. If the interviewer has learned the patient's language, it will still be of little value if the person's cultural values are not known. The interviewer should formulate probing questions with great discretion. In some cultures, even small details become closely guarded secrets. Questions that allow the person to withhold some information while still answering will help to build rapport. Questions that bring forth information and the selection of alternative answers rather than a simple yes or no answer will help keep communication open [15–16].

We must understand and respect varying speech patterns. Native Americans speak more softly and pause much longer before responding. They find a virtue in silence, and express emotions in a more subtle manner. They may prefer few words over many. These language behaviors may make them seem uninvolved or passive-aggressive. Japanese Americans respect periods of silence [15–17].

Languages differ in the use of metaphor, and we can make mistakes when taking words too literally. Clients may speak of hot stomachs or sad eyes, or of ancestral spirits, all of which reflect the culture's metaphorical construction of experience. Haitians, for example, often speak idiomatically and in proverbs. Emotional expression also varies with ethnic groups. Japanese Americans may not easily share their feelings. They may display a form of ritual self-denigration that should not be interpreted as low self-esteem or depression. Emotions are usually understated [17–18].

Eye contact varies among many ethnic groups. While they will periodically make visual contact, Japanese may view staring or an intense visual expression of interest as a sign of contempt. African-Americans or Asians may often look down or away in respect for authority, and this behavior should not make others suspect distrust or evasion. Native American children may be reluctant to look an adult in the face [17–19].

Mind body relationships

Ethnic groups vary in their conception of the relation of mind and body. Hispanics may feel that mind and body are inseparable. Asian Americans often express their emotional distress in somatic complaints [19].

Delusions and hallucinations

Clinicians may interpret the religious beliefs or the world views of the patient as a delusion or mistake delusional material for a cultural belief. Paranoid symptoms, from basic mistrust to ideas of references and hallucinations may be a normal reaction to placement away from a familiar milieu or an adaptive response to adjusting to a perceived hostile environment. The trance or altered state of consciousness that is achieved in many ethnic cultures should not be misinterpreted as a dissociative or hysterical state [20].

Religious Beliefs

Spiritual practices play a central role in the lives of many ethnic groups and these beliefs should be carefully examined before they are interpreted as delusional. Many Asians believe in the influence of their ancestors on current events. Some Puerto Ricans believe that spirits surround the material world and can reincarnate themselves in people and objects. Spirit possession is also a folk belief in some Caribbean cultures. Even when the spirits are not corporal entities, communication can take place with them. Spirit possession is not necessarily bad, for those possessed by spirits often play important social roles and are held in high esteem. Communication with the dead is a culturally accepted means of grieving and mourning in many Latino cultures. Many ethnic groups also believe in evil spirits or forces. Arredondo writes that alcoholism in Hispanic culture is often attributed to evil forces that take the form of a curse by a vengeful person, or it can be interpreted as a punishment from God or as a test of a family's faith. Alcoholism treatment must be based on the family's own interpretation of its cause. Religious beliefs and spiritism will affect the way the family interprets the cause of mental illness. Schwartz asserts that the treatment community must relate to the patient's own view of the cause in order for healing to take place. Many ethnic groups recognize both natural and supernatural causes. Schwartz warns against cultural imperialism—imposing psychiatric theory upon the belief systems of others. Reeves notes that since the best of western scientific thought cannot explain the cause of illnesses such as schizophrenia, we should be able to respect and understand the Hispanic's attraction to folk beliefs [20–23].

The ethnic family may want to include native healers in the treatment process. Folk healers should be consulted in the overall treatment plan, and they may eventually become a part of the hospital's treatment network. The healer's views must be respected as we respect those of any other professional. The staff should be willing to respond to the family's desire for a healing ceremony. This will strengthen the treatment alliance and can lead to an improvement in symptoms. Arredondo suggests that the staff explore alternatives for the treatment of alcoholism in Mexican Americans, who may choose to consult the *curandero* or folk healer before seeking American treatment, with the hope of having a hex removed. *Curanderos* also prescribe an aversive form of therapy. A toasted seed is added to food or drink, which causes the drinking person to vomit. *Curanderos* are often willing to work with chemical dependency staff [20–23].

Many programs have been successful by integrating cultural symbols, metaphors, and rituals into the daily life of the treatment community. Programs that help Native Americans reconnect with their culture can build on a spiritual foundation. Rituals, such as the sweat lodge, allow emotional release in a safe environment. Tribal traditions have always included ritual and prayer in the healing process [24].

The idea of harmony is significant in many cultures and may be used to explain a diagnosis. Native Americans interpret illness as a lack of harmony with nature. Conventional treatment may need to be supplemented by native rituals to restore disrupted harmony. Behaviors that disrupt the harmony of family or community functioning may be interpreted as brought about by witchcraft and special ceremonies may be used to address this disharmony [25].

The Cambodian culture also emphasizes harmony and equilibrium. There is a basic theme in the Khmer culture of a need for equilibrium, calling for a balance in food intake, emotional state, interpersonal relations, leisure time and spiritual life. There is also a moral balance, with good deeds balancing out transgressions on the path to reincarnation. Culturally approved behaviors such as generosity and a nondirect approach to conflict help to achieve equilibrium. Cambodian beliefs may conflict with the American belief in openness or confrontation. Internal disequilibrium is expressed in such culture-bound syndromes as wind illness, which may result from the suppression of anger or grief. Diseqilibrium may also be caused by *koucherang,* or thinking too much, a culture-bound syndrome characterized by depression, suicidal behavior, or intrusive thoughts. The Khmer adolescent who is diagnosed with *koucherang,* may be counseled by the culture to fight sad thoughts through laughter or keeping busy. Frye and McGill advise that the Cambodian family can best accept a psychiatric diagnosis framed within a context of harmony and equilibrium, or with an additional chemical or biological perspective. They believe that cognitive therapy can effectively address the symptoms of *koucherang,* which are similar to those of anxiety, depression or post-traumatic stress disorder. The exploration and modification of cognitive patterns can attempt to restore balance and harmony with the self, family, and community [26].

Family Structures

A cardinal rule for work with ethnic groups is respect for the family and its differences. Each family will differ, depending on its identification with its own ethnic origins or with the dominant cultural group. The staff must remain curious about any behavior that seems unusual and be eager to learn. The staff will quickly learn who makes the decisions for the family. In a Native American family, members of the extended family, which may include the matriarch of the clan, may need to approve of a child's hospitalization. Relatives will see any attempt to rush this process as disrespect and disempowerment of the family hierarchy. In Hispanic families, the staff must show respect for the father as the decision-maker. More than two family generations may participate in family therapy for Hispanic and Native American clients. Healing usually requires the full participation of the Hispanic family, which respects the importance of the family members' interdependence. African-American children may have had multiple caretakers, and this may represent a security net, not inconsistent childrearing. The support from the extended family will play a significant role in treatment planning for African-American, Hispanic, and Native American families. The staff should also welcome the minister of the African-American church as a collaborator in the support system. The client's role in a cohesive community can become a source of growth and self-esteem [27].

The mental health staff member who lectures ethnic families about co-dependence or separation-individuation or adolescent autonomy should be ready to be laughed out of the room. Families will more easily accept therapies that emphasize family dependence rather than independence and autonomy. The focus should be on restoring the patients' harmony with significant people in their lives. Many ethnic groups give priority to the group or the collective identity over the person. The maintenance of a strong family takes precedence over individual priorities in traditional Japanese culture. The Native American adolescent is never considered independent in personal relationships, and takes appropriate responsibility for family support [27–28].

The instilled beliefs of family alcoholic treatment should be tossed out when working with Hispanic or Native American families. The Hispanic family name must be protected. The male has the right to drink as long as he provides for and protects his wife. If the alcoholic male can no longer provide for the family, he will continue to protect his family name by limiting outside intervention. The concept of codependence is a value-laden "Anglo" cultural narrative with little applicability to the Hispanic patient and any changes recommended based on this interpretation are in serious conflict with the Hispanic value system. Arredondo describes techniques for substance abuse programs with Hispanic families. *Machismo* can be reframed as being brave, honest, and a family provider. The family is recognized as a strong support to draw upon. The family may still learn to see alcoholism as a family illness and participate in family education, therapy and Al-Anon. The extended family is also included and makes treatment decisions [28–29].

There are other techniques that should not be used with ethnic groups. Touching, for example, has various meanings in different cultures. Japanese patients may find it uncomfortable, preferring a more formal or symbolic expression of concern. Patients from other minority groups will expect or even require smiling or a handshake. Many ethnic groups will interpret confrontation techniques as rejection. If it is necessary for clarification, the staff member might indicate that there are two conflicting pieces of information and ask for help in understanding the disparity. Confrontation violates codes of Asian conduct. Confrontation with Hispanics is a serious challenge to *machismo*. Even the use of traditional group and individual psychotherapy may not be of value in working with many ethnic groups. Hispanic males will resist self-disclosure in groups. Revealing their own pain and fears will make them feel too vulnerable, presenting an image that contrasts too strongly with the Latino version of male strength. Expressive therapies that allow feelings to be expressed through metaphor will finally be more effective [29–30].

Special Programs for Ethnic Groups

Programs tailored for a particular ethnic group have met with some success, and will also contribute toward providing insights into program elements that can be integrated into a program serving several ethnic groups.

NATIVE AMERICAN PROGRAMS

Kline and Roberts describe an early alcoholism treatment program that was not completely successful. It was apparently not possible to attract Native American staff to work in the program. Individual therapy proved to be more helpful than group therapy, since apparently the participants felt that their comments were worthless, that they were powerless, and that no one would listen to what they said. A willingness to take an active role in the group usually resulted in ostracism. Weibel-Orlando finds that treatment techniques designed for the dominant society ignore the social and cultural background of Native Americans. She suggests that programs that include indigenous curing practices will have greater success [31–32].

The Native American Church (NAC) provides indigenous strategies for healing. Weibel-Orlando notes that of the more than 50 Indian substance abuse interventions she has observed since 1978 the ones that appeared to be the most viable and which attracted the most enthusiastic clients shared certain traits:

1. Clients initiated the program.
2. Leaders had charismatic qualities and served as role models. In some instances the leader was a shaman who had won a battle against alcohol. In other instances a tribal leader near to self-destruction had returned to long term sobriety and balance.
3. They all involved the recovering clients in ongoing therapy and interaction with the group, both as clients and healers.
4. The community formed an alternative society to the drinking culture.

The notion of a healing community is a powerful one. The healed become healers themselves [32].

Manson and colleagues find that many traditional Indian and Alaskan native healing practices are gradually being incorporated into contemporary approaches to mental health treatment of Indian patients. Three traditional therapeutic strategies have received considerable attention: the four circles, the talking circle and the sweat lodge. The talking circle is a form of group therapy. The group members sit in a circle, and no one can leave once it begins. Handshaking establishes a physical connection that continues around the circle. Once the handshake is completed, the leader begins to share his innermost feelings with everyone. Each participant is then free to speak without fear of rejection or contradiction, but no one replies directly to the remarks shared by any one person. There are no interruptions and one may speak for long as he wants. The talking circle closes with a joining of hands and a brief prayer. The group chooses whether what was discussed will remain confidential or shared with each other. The knowledge that other group therapies have not been effective makes this particular form of greater value [33].

Anderson describes a six-week family chemical dependency program for native peoples in British Columbia that is based on a quiet, gentle and respectful approach. The complete family population meets together three to five times a week for a half day—a group process where clients work slowly to share their lives, although they have come from a community that has usually communicated little about emotions. Here they learn to trust, accept and give support. The group uses a charismatic Catholic healing exercise, the Healing of Memories, which takes an entire day in the 4th week of treatment. This includes a guided meditation that culminates in a powerful experience of forgiving and healing. Group members sit or lie quietly with eyes closed, visualizing various scenarios of healing and forgiving. The energy released by the forgiving process helps them to heal. Those who attend later set up circles for treatment in their home communities [34].

Not only Native American techniques but also Native American cultural concepts will be the most effective way to help the adolescent group. Contact with tribal elders and strong members of the culture will help Native American chemically dependent adolescents relearn those cultural values that will protect them from drug abuse.

LATINO TREATMENT PROGRAMS

Dolgin describes an Hispanic treatment program with staff of Hispanic heritage. The program emphasized the use of linguistic and cultural elements as well as customs and beliefs characteristic of Hispanic culture. The treatment team created a familiar and comfortable environment reflecting Hispanic culture. Staff and residents celebrated traditional Hispanic holidays with special emphasis on food and activities [35].

Since folk beliefs were an important aspect of the patients' reality, therapists used them as a context for providing interpretations. It was important to differentiate delusions from culturally specific syndromes such as *susto* (fright), *mal ojo* (evil eye) and *mal puesto,* a hex cast upon someone. Family involvement was a strong part of the program [35].

Culture intensive psychotherapeutic approaches included *macho* groups for male patients led by male cotherapists. Many of their problems involved relationships with females, which could be discussed in a safe atmosphere without threats to masculinity. There were also female groups, where female patients could discuss subjects that were taboo in mixed groups. Cultural identity groups examined culture-specific elements relative to their relationship to the dominant society. Patients attempted to look at themselves and their environments from a realistic perspective. Their suggestions were incorporated into the treatment regime. The program strengthened the identity and improved self-confidence while increasing the capacity to assess stressful situations in a multicultural society [35].

Zepeda describes a Hispanic substance abuse program established so that residents could express ideas and feelings in their primary language. The goal of the 30-day program is total abstinence using the 12-step tradition. The unit treats not only the person but also the entire family. Weekly family days address family dysfunctions. The family comes to understand the use of denial and learns not to blame the patient for all family problems. The patriarchal Hispanic structure places a strong emphasis on family unity and the program has designed different dyads and techniques to address these needs. Zepeda believes that the Hispanic community has tolerated alcoholism for many centuries and the Hispanic family often enables it. The program focuses on practical economic and social matters rather than theoretical or analytical issues. Assertiveness training is very useful tool for Hispanics who often identify assertiveness with aggressiveness. These methods have been useful in defocusing their sense of powerlessness [36].

African-American Treatment Programs

Smith and colleagues describe a successful African-American extended family program for a chemically dependent population. The church-sponsored program adapts the 12-step principles to the African-American community in the inner city. African history classes are an added component. Those who join the program become members of an African-American extended family. Day support groups begin with the singing of a selected spiritual, and the meeting is structured around the meaning of the song. The program makes an analogy between substance abuse and slavery. Each support group becomes as a "generation" of addicts born into recovery. Each generation celebrates in a ritual graduation. The church regularly devotes Sunday services to the graduating generation to acknowledge their new knowledge and accomplishments. They speak before the congregation and are ritually given birth again, passing through a "placenta" of previous generations. These rituals help to enhance the members' self-esteem and provide support [37].

Smith and colleagues describe the problems that some African-American experience in conventional 12-step programs that not only seem exclusively white and middle class but also provide some difficult messages for their community. A community that has felt powerless too long will naturally resist an admission of powerlessness. Smith and colleagues add that Native Americans also find this difficult because it disagrees with tribal mores of self-reliance and stoicism. In this African-American program the use of the word "surrender" is described in terms of joining a winning team and essentially gaining power rather than losing it, by calling on the higher power and having the support of the African-American fellowship [37].

Inpatient treatment programs must progress from cultural awareness to cultural competency. Cultural competency includes cultural sensitivity, knowledge, and skill. Cultural sensitivity will include examining one's individual bias and prejudices and avoiding cultural imposition on others, imposing one's own beliefs, values or patterns of behavior on others. Cultural knowledge is the educational foundation for knowing other cultures. Cultural skill will involve conducting a cultural assessment in order to formulate culturally relevant interventions. This means not only knowing about the cultural group, but also assessing the individual's values, beliefs and practices, as well as the person's perception of the illness. This cultural assessment develops appropriate interventions [38].

Cultural competency will require understanding and appreciation of cultural differences as a background for developing focused interventions, communication and support. Informed multicultural treatment will be developed from the combined literature of psychiatry, anthropology, sociology and public health. An understanding of what is culturally normative behavior will influence both diagnosis and treatment planning. All components of treatment should be examined in order to learn which can be shared and which should be culturally specific. Cultural competence will finally assure that all barriers to treatment will be removed. Laosa writes of cultural democracy—the belief that there are many valid ways to choose what, how, and when to do things. Since culture represents the person's real world, if cultural values are ignored, the person will feel alienated. Mental health should not require the abandonment of life style and cultural background [39–40].

References

1. Westermeyer J. Clinical considerations in cross-cultural diagnosis. Hospital & Community Psychiatry 1987 Feb;38(2):160–5.
2. Schwartz D. Caribbean folk beliefs and western psychiatry. Journal of Psychosocial Nursing & Mental Health Services 1987 Nov;23(11):26–30.
3. Laureano M, Poliandro E. Understanding cultural values of Latino male alcoholics and their families: a cultural sensitive model. Journal of Chemical Dependency Treatment 1991;4(1):137–65.
4. Campinha-Bacote J. Culturological assessment: an important factor in psychiatric consultation-liaison nursing. Archives of Psychiatric Nursing 1988;2(4):244–50.
5. Zweben JE. Editor's introduction: Culturally relevant substance abuse treatment. Journal of Psychoactive Drugs 1993 Jan-Mar;25(1):1–4.
6. Spurlock J. Assessment and therapeutic intervention of black children. Journal American Academy of Child Psychiatry 1985;24(2):168–74.
7. Worthington C. An examination of factors influencing the diagnosis and treatment of black patients in the mental health system. Archives of Psychiatric Nursing 1992;6(3):195–204.
8. Allon R. Sex, race, social class and process reactive schizophrenia ratings. Journal of Nervous & Mental Disease 1971;153:343–59.
9. Bond CF, DiCandia CG, McKinnon JB. Responses to violence in a psychiatric setting: the role of patients' race. Personality & Social Psychology Bulletin 1988;14(3):448–58.
10. Flaherty JA, Naidu J, Lawton R, Pathak D. Racial differences in perception of ward atmosphere. American Journal of Psychiatry 1981 Oct;131(10):815–7.
11. Flaherty JA, Meagher R. Measuring racial bias in inpatient treatment. American Journal of Psychiatry 1980 Jun;137(6);679–82.
12. Beauvais F. An integrated model for prevention and treatment of drug abuse among American Indian youth. Journal of Addictive Diseases 1992;11(3):63–80.
13. Givler TL. Working therapeutically with parents of Hispanic and American Indian children and adolescents in the hospital. In: Hendren RL, Berlin IN, eds. Psychiatric

inpatient care of children and adolescents: A multicultural approach. New York: John Wiley, 128–42.
14. Morrisette PJ. The therapeutic dilemma with Canadian native youth in residential care. Child & Adolescent Social Work 1991; 8(2):89–99.
15. Collins JL, Mathura CB, Risher DL. Training psychiatric staff to treat a multicultural patient population. Hospital & Community Psychiatry 1984 Apr;35(4):372–6.
16. Leveck PG. The role of culture in mental health and illness. In: Cook JS, Fontaine KL, eds. Essentials of mental health nursing. Menlo Park, CA: Addison-Wesley, 1986, 158–61.
17. Marsella AJ. Counseling and psychotherapy with Japanese Americans: Cross-cultural considerations. American Journal of Orthopsychiatry 1993 April;63(2):200–8.
18. Gustafson MB. Western voodoo: Providing mental health care to Haitian refugees. Journal of Psychosocial Nursing & Mental Health Services 1989 Dec;27(12):22–5.
19. Cravener P. Establishing therapeutic alliance across cultural barriers. Journal of Psychosocial Nursing & Mental Health Services 1992 Dec;30(12):10–4.
20. See reference 1.
21. Arredondo R, Weddige RL, Justice CL, Fitz J. Alcoholism in Mexican-Americans: Intervention and treatment. Hospital & Community Psychiatry 1987 Feb;38(2):180–3.
22. See reference 2.
23. Reeves K. Hispanic utilization of a mental health clinic. Journal of Psychosocial Nursing & Mental Health Services 1986 Feb;24(2):23–6.
24. Rowell RM, Kusterer H. Care of HIV-infected Native American substance abusers. Journal of Chemical Dependency Treatment 1991;4(2):91–103.
25. Keltner BR. Native American children and adolescents: cultural distinctiveness and mental health needs. Journal of Child & Adolescent Psychiatric Nursing 1993 Oct;6(4):18–23.
26. Frye BA, McGill D. Cambodian refugee adolescents: cultural factors and mental health nursing. Journal of Child & Adolescent Psychiatric Nursing 1993 Oct-Dec;6(4):24.
27. Berlin IN, Hendren RL. Effective treatment planning. In: Hendren R, Berlin IN, eds. Psychiatric inpatient care of children and adolescents: A multicultural approach. New York: John Wiley, 67–87.
28. Inclan J, Hernandez M. Cross-cultural perspectives and codependence. American Journal of Orthopsychiatry 1992;62(2):245–55.
29. See reference 21.
30. DeLeon G, Melnick G, Shoket D, Jainchill N. Is the therapeutic comunity culturally relevant? Journal of Psychoactive Drugs 1993 Mar;25(2):77–86.
31. Kline JA, Roberts AC. A residential alcoholism treatment program for American Indians. Quarterly Journal of Studies on Alcohol 1973;34:860–8.
32. Weibel-Orlando J. Hooked on healing: anthropologists, alcohol, and intervention. Human Organization 1989;48(2):148–55.
33. Manson SM, Walker RD, Kivlahan DR. Psychiatric assessment and treatment of American Indians and Alaska natives. Hospital & Community Psychiatry 1987 Feb;38(2):165–73.
34. Anderson EN. A healing place: ethnographic notes on a treatment center. Alcoholism Treatment Quarterly 1992;9(3/4):1–21.

35. Dolgin DL, Salazar A, Cruz S. The Hispanic treatment program: Principles of effective psychotherapy. Journal of Contemporary Psychotherapy 1987;17(4):285–99.
36. Zepeda R. Hispanic Program: Careunit Hospital of Los Angeles. Journal of Substance Abuse Treatment 1986;3(2):135–7.
37. Smith DE, Buxton ME, Bilal R, Seymour RB. Cultural points of resistance to the 12-step recovery process. Journal of Psychoactive Drugs 1993 Jan-Mar;25(1):97–108.
38. Campinha-Bacote J. Transcultural psychiatric nursing: diagnostic and treatment issues. Journal of Psychiatric Nursing & Mental Health Services 1994;32(8):41–6.
39. Cultural competence: An interview with Warren Hewitt. Journal of Psychoactive Drugs 1993 Jan-Mar;25(1):5–7.
40. Laosa LM. Child care and the culturally different child. Child Care Quarterly 1974 Win;3(4):214–24.

16. Multiple Personality Disorder (Dissociative Identity Disorder)

Multiple personality disorder (MPD) develops as a protection against repeated traumatic experiences. The person who suffers repeated trauma and does not have the benefit of disclosure or comforting may use a form of self-hypnosis and split off feelings and memories from awareness. These dissociated experiences and feelings become the nucleus for the formation of other personalities or alters. Experiences, thoughts, and feelings are consequently not integrated within a single personality. It is important to remember, however, that each personality continues to represent a layer of the whole person and must be treated with full seriousness and respect. The staff must not challenge these essential dissociative defenses [1–2].

Persons with multiple personality disorder are usually treated in an outpatient setting, but may require hospitalization when they feel suicidal or out of control, or when they need structure and safety during certain stages of treatment. The initial treatment stages are concerned with establishing the diagnosis, gaining access to the most available personalities, gathering the history and mapping the personality system. Hospitalization may be required, usually in the later stages, when the person becomes aware of early traumatic experiences. Kluft describes this stage as "metabolism of the trauma." The various personalities become aware of the trauma. The defenses can finally be challenged. The patient is extremely vulnerable, overwhelmed by these painful experiences with no strategies for coping. The recall of memories recreates the painful experience in the present. This process, called abreaction, may involve screaming, episodes of intense anger and out-of-control behaviors. The last stage of treatment is devoted to fusion and integration [3].

Staff skepticism about the diagnosis can present serious problems. Persons will multiple personality disorder usually feel isolated and "freakish" since they have seldom met others who share their disorder. This is all the more traumatic when the staff members find it so unbelievable that they feel the person is "putting on an act." This is complicated by the fact that the patient may be in treatment many years before the actual diagnosis of multiple personality disorder is made. Steinmeyer writes, however, that neither understanding nor acceptance of the MPD diagnosis will guarantee adequate patient management. Since extensive staff debates about the validity and meaning of the diagnosis seem only to destroy staff morale, Steinmeyer finds it more productive to concentrate instead on designing interventions that will manage behavioral difficulties and insure safety. The staff member's inexperience with the MPD patient may lead to a fascination that merely reinforces pathology rather than encouraging normal adaptation. Staff members may feel called upon to protect these patients from further "abuse" and this special treatment will prevent therapeutic progress or normal interaction in the milieu [4].

Staff members should understand the goals for the patient, which usually correspond to the stages of treatment. Regardless of the stage of treatment, the primary function of the milieu is to provide a supportive and safe environment. The person with multiple personality disorder may not have previously been able to build trusting relationships or disclose feelings and reactions to traumatic events. Indeed, the person with multiple personality disorder may create situations where the staff will appear untrustworthy. The staff can be made powerless by the patient whose behavior recreates the punitive and chaotic environment where the disorder first emerged. Anderson and Ross suggest ways for the staff to work toward a trusting relationship. The patient should be given an orientation to the unit, its expectations and rules, but with some flexibility to negotiate some aspects of treatment. Mutual honesty is vital. The staff is advised to carefully avoid double bind situations [4–5].

Experiences in the hospital may bring about painful memories or trigger flashbacks or nightmares and the staff must see the patient through them, providing reassurance that the hospital will be safe. The inpatient milieu can provide the necessary external controls when the process of discovering other personalities begins. The therapist helps the patient become conscious of the other personalities or alters, many of whom will release catastrophic feelings and memories to full awareness. Abreaction cannot necessarily be restricted to the therapy hour. During these times the staff comforts the patient, gives reassurance that the traumatic experience occurred in the past, not in the present, and that the patient is safe now and can't be hurt. Steinmeyer recommends that the primary staff member stay with the patient, record the materials the patient presents, and finally reorient the patient to the present and safe environment. In these circumstances, the primary staff member may often need to request the healthy alter's assistance to take control of the patient's body [4–5].

All staff members must be trained what not to do. The staff is not to press into consciousness the presence of other personalities. This is done only in therapy. If this happens in the milieu it will create even stronger defenses. The patient may actually develop new alters, try to elope, or even attempt suicide. Sakheim and colleagues urge the staff to protect the patient who feels compelled to discuss traumatic material with staff and other patients. They caution that the patient's relationship with others is not sufficiently strong or longlasting enough to support the disclosure of this difficult material. After such disclosures, the patient may feel even more isolated, vulnerable or abandoned. The staff should not ignore these disclosures but should advise the patient to discuss them with the primary therapist. The staff's role, then, should not be to uncover but to provide containment and support. The treatment team and the patient must together determine if the patient can maintain control over behavior in the face of such powerful emotions. If the patient cannot be helped to develop internal controls, then external ones must be used. A behavior contract can be helpful, but it should focus on how the patient wishes to be treated in certain situations. For example, it might stipulate that child alters must never be touched without their permission. Steinmeyer reports that staff members who work closely with MPD patients are at risk for becoming enmeshed in tense, demanding relationships and must be prepared to set limits around personal boundaries—the time to be spent with the patient and the limits on inappropriate behavior. However, limits that are too strict will make the patient feel rejected. These patients may find the standard hospital routine to be coercive, uncaring, and the effect may be one of retraumatization. They may find, for example, that their own privacy has been severely compromised [4–7].

RESPONSE TO OTHER PERSONALITIES

The emergence of new personalities (the alters) presents problems the treatment staff has never encountered before. The staff must form a treatment alliance, not just with the host personality but eventually with each separate personality. Milieu treatment will need to be provided for each of the personalities, and each will present its own problems in adjustments and relationships. There will be questions about how much responsibility and autonomy to give the person whose ego states are often changing. For example, Davidson and colleagues write about whether they should give a patient car privileges when they feared that the child alter might suddenly appear at the wheel. There is the interesting question of whether to consistently address the "host" personality even when another personality predominates. Since dissociation is necessary for the patient, the alter should be treated with kindness and respected as another part of the patient's self. However, Anderson and Ross believe that in many situations, the alter can be carefully reminded that she is part of the host personality. What should happen, for example, if one personality must accept the consequences for a behavior she does not remember? Anderson and Ross believe that the patient must be treated like everyone else in the milieu. The consequences stay in effect and the patient is told that the behavior occurred when another personality was out. When one personality complains about another, the staff member should try to help each understand the other. This will provide a step toward the goal of integration [4–8].

The treatment team should be equipped to understand all of the personalities. This can be accomplished by mapping them so that they will be recognized when they appear. When it is deemed appropriate, the patient should be fully included in the mapping process. Although the presentation of alters is often frightening, Anderson and Ross note that the reason for hospitalization is to make it possible for them to appear and abreaction to occur. The staff should assure alters that they are safe, that it is safe to feel and talk about everything, and that they will not be hurt. Anderson and Ross then ask the logical question. If staff members don't discourage the appearance of alters, are they bringing about further dissociation? They believe that the process must resemble other forms of psychotherapy, where the client is assisted in revealing all aspects of the self to appear and be explored [4–8].

THE MPD PATIENTS AND OTHER PATIENTS IN THE MILIEU

Another protection that must be offered the patient is protection from embarrassment. When child alters appear, it is wise to keep the patient away from others. Kluft describes some of the reactions of other patients, reporting that patients with multiple personality disorder often stir up feelings and conflicts that other patients try to suppress. Ross believes that MPD patients can be managed on a general adult unit without severe disruption of the milieu and that many patients simply do not display their disorder to others and would rather that they not know about it. Many patients seriously resent the amount of staff time that is taken up by MPD patients in the milieu [4–9].

The Organization of the Milieu

Steinmeyer stresses the need for clear communication among the primary therapist, treatment team, and nurses. In the program she describes, the primary therapist meets with the treatment team before the patient's admission to discuss what is known about the individual alters and their relation to the patient's ego system. The treatment team presents a protocol outlining strategies and limits that will be set. The next meeting should include the patient and can be devoted to a discussion of both the patient's and team's expectations for treatment [10].

Structure, staff communication and cohesion can protect the integrity of the milieu. Steinmeyer suggests a communication notebook where the staff and primary therapist can record their own questions, issues, and recommendations for each patient, a place for materials not usually placed in the medical record. This will allow the development of specific interventions [10].

Steinmeyer recommends the assignment of primary nurses to the patient for both the day and evening shifts, but with rotating assignments arranged so that no staff member works with a given patient for more than three days. A staff member with less experience works with each primary nurse and interacts with the patient in daily 2:1 sessions. This way of organizing solved the problem of the intense pathological staff/patient bonding that had prevailed before. Dispersing the relationships over a number of staff relieved the patients from the feelings of panic and abandonment they suffered in the absence of their primary nurse. Treatment team meetings could then be devoted to productive therapeutic issues rather than conflicts about the unavailability of staff members. Staff members felt relieved from having the exclusive responsibility for the MPD patient and were much more comfortable when it was shared. Steinmeyer writes that this integration of staff members in an organized structure around the patient provided a helpful metaphor for the concept of integrated ego functions that the patient must finally achieve [10].

Steinmeyer feels that MPD patients can benefit from heterogeneous groupings in group psychotherapy, assertiveness training, gender groups, and all other milieu activities. Although they should not be expected to discuss the more dramatic presentations of their illness, Steinmeyer writes that the alters who could function in groups were able to develop more adaptive and socially appropriate behaviors through these normal milieu interactions. Early emphasis on milieu participation then seemed consistent rather than coercive, as it had been when presented later in the patients' stay [10].

Kelly, who writes about the treatment of MPD in partial hospitalization, recommends an individual treatment coordinator who can organize all aspects of the person's "chaotic world," to insure a safe environment that will contain the patient, provide treatment, and teach self-care. The treatment coordinator works with the patient to identify problems, formulate short and longer term goals, and determines the resources to be used [11].

Dissociation, of course, is a major problem and will require documentation of the patient's symptoms, such as anxiety, panic attacks, flashbacks, voices urging self-harm, rage, psychotic thinking or phobias. The patient and coordinator may choose two or three goals which may address the problems of dissociation and begin to attain mastery over their complex internal world [11].

THE REACTION OF THE STAFF

Staff members may find themselves overwhelmed and frightened by MPD patients, particularly in response to the dramatic and changing self-presentations. These patients threaten the competence of the milieu. Sakheim and colleagues warn that the staff will encounter its most intense countertransference with them. Staff members often feel tricked and manipulated. Lego describes some of these feelings: skepticism, strong reactions to their frightening histories, embarrassment, fear of anger. She describes anxiety about identifying with the patient, a fear that part of the staff member's own self is crudely exposed, with its rage, sexual feelings, or childish longings. Because no one knows what personality might suddenly appear, there is a feeling of loss of control. The staff can resent the helplessness it experiences with these patients or feel angry at the psychiatrist who admitted them [12–15].

Anderson and Ross recommend support meetings for staff to talk over countertransference feelings. This is particularly important because of the splitting which sometimes seems inevitable. It may occur because of doubts about the diagnosis and differing views about the patient. Educational sessions with the psychiatrist will also help, as well as a good orientation and written unit guidelines. It might be more honest to realize that the patient does not really split the staff. The staff splits itself by letting opposing points of view determine professional behavior. Kluft describes this complex process as group projective identification. The staff makes certain assumptions about the patient and exerts such unconscious pressure that the patient will demonstrate those behaviors which create difficulty in the treatment setting. This splitting can flourish if there are any breakdowns in communication. Consistency must be developed through effective planning of care and staff members may often have to be willing to sacrifice their own personal opinions [14–15].

Boundaries

Kelly describes MPD as a disorder of broken boundaries. The milieu staff must be able to set firm limits and boundaries in order to contain maladaptive behavior. The patient must be helped to learn to anticipate and delay action, tolerate anxiety, and achieve a stronger sense of autonomy. The milieu staff must set appropriate boundaries for it will need protection in working with these difficult patients [16].

Treatment Protocols and Patient Contracts

Many writers recommend a treatment protocol which will clearly outline expectations, acknowledge the patient's strengths, and help to create a trusting relationship with a staff that will understand the patient's specific problems. Given the fragmentation of multiple personality disorder, straightforward written communication in contract form can often add clarity. In the contract the patient might agree to

1. Inform the staff of any self-destructive impulses, actions, plans.
2. Explore and develop strategies for self-soothing.
3. Select places in the treatment center that feel safe.
4. Select staff members who can help the patient feel comfortable and safe.
5. Use structure appropriately.

Contracts should include the patient's own suggestions. Copies should be given to the treatment team, therapists, and all who are involved in the patient's care [16].

Techniques for helping MPD patients

The patients' interpersonal relationships often reflect their broken boundaries. They have little trust in others, and yet are dependent and traumatized by separation. They may require individual social skills training to learn how to listen and respond, ask for help, be assertive, negotiate, and learn how to resolve conflicts. Kelly suggests that the milieu staff encourage patients to keep a journal, which could serve as a "self-paced healing tool." Not only will it help the patient release emotion, it will record the shifts in the patient's world, helping the patient to reflect, not merely react [16].

Patients can learn to help themselves by developing self-soothing techniques. These might include exploring deep-breathing exercises, relaxation tapes, exercise, guided imagery, crying, walking, singing, music, hot baths, hot tea, being with supportive friends. They may even try having internal dialogues with alters for problem solving and decision making. Partial hospitalization or long-term treatment should be designed to develop autonomy. The person should become increasingly responsible for a daily routine, and should be encouraged to use calendars, lists, organizers, even post-it notes, if these can be of help [17].

Treating Children with Multiple Personality Disorder

Hornstein and Tyson discuss the inpatient treatment of children with MPD, and give a significant role to the primary nurse. The beginning tasks are to establish a secure and nurturing environment and a therapeutic alliance. Improvement of ego functions and management of behavior problems may need to be accomplished before working with alters. Early in treatment the staff must identify and prioritize the behaviors that require intensive intervention. Limits on destructive behaviors may be set by redirecting the child or by brief time-outs. Specific coping behaviors should be introduced to replace dysfunctional ones and positive reinforcement should be designed for more functional behaviors. Seclusion or physical restraint should not be used unless there is a danger of physical damage to the child [18].

THE THERAPEUTIC ALLIANCE WITH THE CHILD

The therapeutic alliance cannot easily be achieved without full acceptance of the child's inner experience of having separate personalities. The inpatient staff should learn to treat these experiences in a matter-of-fact way. Empathy will help the staff member to know the individual experience of the alters and their own reactions to staff. This manner of treatment will allow the child to comfortably reveal these personalities without anxiety. Hornstein and Tyson believe that, strangely enough, full acceptance of these alters may decrease the child's use of dissociation. The child should simply not be pushed to accept an identity as only one person with one name. Reassurance of safety is important. Staff should intervene to be sure that the children do not misperceive or misinterpret their environment. This will decrease dissociative episodes [18].

Each child should have therapeutic sessions with the primary nurse, with the final goal of developing mastery over switching. To achieve this, the child begins to identify the thoughts and feelings that are a part of each personality. At the same time, the child is encouraged to call upon alters for help in difficult situations, and is asked if there is someone inside who can help or soothe. The strengths of each alter and its individual importance should be discussed with the child. The final goal is integration of this comforting capacity into the child's full self. All of the child's alters are acknowledged and assured of safety. As with adults, there are consequences given even for the behavior of another personality [18].

The person with multiple personality disorder needs to understand the diagnosis and to learn why dissociation exists. The final goal of patient education is to learn new ways to cope with the stress associated with confronting painful experiences. The hospital environment provides a safe place to practice behaviors and coping skills without needing to dissociate, The proliferation of literature on multiple personality disorder is an indication that the number of patients has significantly increased or that it is being more frequently diagnosed. In any case, clinicians are understanding it better and an informed milieu staff is better prepared to integrate the person into treatment. Steinmeyer advises that it may be more helpful to consider multiple personality disorder not as a single illness, but rather as an illness with multiple ego states, each of which may represent a personality disorder. There may be an alter which displays borderline personality characteristics and another with anorexic behavior. Management of the symptoms and dynamics of each alter may finally be required [19].

References

1. Sakheim DK, Hess EP, Chivas A. General principles for short-term inpatient work with multiple personality-disorder. Psychotherapy 1986;25:117–24.
2. Lego S. Multiple personality disorder: an interpersonal approach to etiology, treatment, and nursing care. Archives of Psychiatric Nursing 1988; 2(4):231–5.
3. Kluft RP. Hospital treatment of multiple personality disorder: an overview. Psychiatric Clinics of North America 1991;14(3):695–719.
4. Steinmeyer SM. Some hard-learned lessons in milieu management of multiple personality disorder. Psychiatric Hospital 1991 Win;22(1):1–4.
5. Anderson G, Ross CA. Strategies for working with a patient who has multiple personality disorder. Archives of Psychiatric Nursing 1988;2(4):236–43.
6. See reference 1.
7. See reference 3.
8. Davidson J, Allen JG, Smith WH. Complexities in the hospital treatment of a patient with multiple personality disorder. Bulletin Menninger Clinic 1987;51(7):561–8.
9. Ross CA. Inpatient treatment of multiple personality disorder. Canadian Journal of Psychiatry 1987;32:779–81.

10. See reference 4.
11. Kelly KA. Multiple personality disorders: treatment coordination in a partial hospitalization setting. Bulletin Menninger Clinic 1993 Sum;57(3):390–8.
12. See reference 1.
13. See reference 2.
14. See reference 3.
15. See reference 5.
16. See reference 11.
17. Turkus JA. Psychotherapy and case management of multiple personality disorders: Synthesis for continuity of care. Psychiatric Clinics of North America 1991;14:649–60.
18. Hornstein NL, Tyson S. Inpatient treatment of children with multiple personality/dissociative disorders and their families. Psychiatric Clinics of North America 1991;14(3): 631–48.
19. See reference 4.

17. Obsessive-Compulsive Disorders

Persons with obsessive-compulsive disorders are usually treated in outpatient settings. Those who are not able to develop self-management of their symptoms or who experience disabling symptoms may require an inpatient program. Behavioral methods are the predominant nonpharmacological treatment, According to the learning theory model of avoidance conditioning, every occurrence of compulsive responses reinforces abnormal behaviors. Response prevention therefore becomes a goal. This means that strict control over the person's behavior is mandatory in inpatient treatment. The staff's attempt to maintain this control can lead to severe conflicts and even escalation of the patient's symptoms. A good, supportive therapeutic relationship and a high degree of staff coordination is extremely important. Treatment of this intensity cannot be accomplished on a general psychiatry unit, and usually requires a special behavior therapy program [1].

Inpatient behavioral programs work toward placing behavioral therapy and self-management into the hands of the patient. In the program Megens and Vandereycken describe, exposure *in vivo* rather than response prevention is the predominant therapeutic principle. Patients are provided with confrontations of the situations they fear. Following this exposure, they are asked not to carry out compulsive rituals—a self-imposed response prevention [1].

The patient receives a detailed description of the program and an explanation of its rationales before admission. Those who are admitted must be accepting of the program, play an active role, and have a strong motivation to change. The behavioral therapist does not force participation in fearful situations. Rather, participation is voluntary. Following the confrontation, the patient is given encouragement but not external supervision to control the rituals. The goal is to help the patient develop the ability to overcome fears and thus control the rituals associated with them. Any external supervision could undermine the patient's actual participation in treatment [1].

Thornicroft and colleagues describe an inpatient behavioral psychotherapy program for obsessive-compulsive patients which stresses the development of both self and family treatment. Family members live in apartments on the ward with the patient for short periods of time and learn to be cotherapists. From the beginning of the program patients learn that behavioral treatment cannot be imposed on them and that they will become their own therapists. They keep a schedule of self-treatment tasks and document them in records that will be reviewed regularly. They learn coping strategies that will help them deal with problems after discharge to decrease the risk of relapse. Patients go on home leaves several times during the program in order to practice self-treatment skills in a natural environment, phoning the unit daily to report on their progress [2].

Each patient has two therapists, one of whom is a key worker, who participates in the assessment and negotiates the planning and implementation of homework practice with the patient as well as the evaluation of progress toward goals. A few patients are asked to sign a contract, particularly those who have problems with alcohol or violence. When patients are noncompliant they are asked to go home on a week's leave to decide whether to continue treatment. Since family members, in their attempt to help the patient, often reinforce the rituals, they are taught how to not participate in rituals and how to withhold reassurance about them. When the patient seeks reassurance to continue with rituals, family members are taught through role play to say in a neutral way: "Hospital says no answer"—a type of broken record response. During hospitalization they are asked to monitor the patient's self-exposure tasks and to practice withholding reassurance [2].

Thornicroft and colleagues report that although few patients were totally cured by behavioral psychotherapy their handicap became less disabling and they and their families were able to lead normal lives. Before inpatient treatment their disabilities had been as severe as that for persons with chronic schizophrenia, with a diminished ability to work or carry out household tasks [2].

Drummond describes a successful program for patients with chronic and resistant obsessive-compulsive disorder using exposure and response prevention. The individual treatment plan was based on an analysis of why previous treatment had failed. If a patient fails to make progress when the plan is implemented, the behavioral psychotherapy team reviews the hypothesis and revises the plan. In addition to the behavioral therapy regime, specific interventions were designed for each patient. The therapist also participated with the patient in exposure treatment. This was necessary for highly anxious patients and to allow for direct observation of any problems. When patients later gain confidence they are encouraged to take more responsibility for their treatment, to use self-exposure and to monitor and record their progress in self-exposure homework diaries [3].

These programs all required specialized training. Calvocoressi and colleagues present treatment guidelines for work with patients with obsessive-compulsive disorder on a general psychiatric unit. These guidelines are for staff members without special training in behavioral methods. Patients with obsessive-compulsive disorder my require hospitalization because of disabling symptoms. They may also have concurrent psychiatric disorders which can't be treated in specialized behavioral units. The treatment team evaluates the patient's ability to participate in behavioral treatment. They are told that the staff will help them establish normal functioning. They will be expected to participate in mealtimes, scheduled meetings and take their medication. Patients who initially have difficulties complying will negotiate contracts outlining the conditions they believe they can fulfill. Family members are requested to support the treatment contract. If patients can't comply, the staff will help [4].

Patients with obsessive-compulsive disorders often display both strong control and dependency needs and can be extremely disruptive to the hospital milieu. Other patients are angered by the attention they get from the staff. While some patients can comply with treatment, others who have consistently used their obsessive-compulsive symptoms to control interpersonal relationships arouse conflicts among patients and staff. Their compulsions can interfere with the use of bathrooms and disrupt mealtimes and meetings. Calvocoressi and colleagues recommend locking bathrooms for patients who can't stop compulsive handwashing. While some fellow patients become angry, others may turn toward helping the patients complete their rituals. They can be angry toward the staff for letting these patients upset the unit routine. However, the group tension can also be turned toward changing the patient's behavior. They finally become aware of the its upsetting effects and changing it becomes more imperative than it had been at home. The social pressure that has been generated can help them change. If these patients are willing to share their treatment plan with the community, they can actually get others to help them comply with the unit norms. Patients also need to learn how their needs for dependency or control can be met in more adaptive ways in interactions with others. Relaxation techniques can also help them control the anxiety caused by the changes imposed by the hospital program [4].

Calvocoressi and colleagues describe a community meeting where patients complained about their limited access to the bathroom because of a male patient's compulsive behaviors. They criticized the staff for not controlling him and were confused about how such a helpless person could control an entire unit. The staff asked the group if they would help him to control his illness by feedback and constant reminders. This particular patient was concerned about others and was willing to try to change. Staff members may find themselves responding as if they were patients with borderline personality disorders, feeling protective at times and at other times, harsh and angry. Staff conflicts will center around whether or not these patients can voluntarily control their behaviors. Those who advocate control will recommend strict behavioral contracts while others will find this punitive. These staff conflicts mirror the patient's own internal conflicts related to control and dependency needs [4].

Staff conflicts can be managed in the same way as is usually done for borderline personality disorders. The staff must be educated about the patient's intrapsychic issues and how they are reenacted in the milieu. This will help staff members to understand and control their own reactions as well as work productively in a group. Despite the staff members' interest in intrapsychic issues, they should be instructed to respond primarily to the patient's overt behaviors. If the staff turns to speculation about whether these behaviors can be voluntarily controlled, this will only delay interventions in critical situations [4].

Since hospitalization on a behavioral unit is not always possible, staff members even without specialized behavioral training can help patients with obsessive-compulsive disorders stabilize their functioning and decrease their symptoms. These patients can be helped by the external support and control the staff provides as well as by the social pressure or influence of the community. A well-structured program can limit the opportunity to engage in rituals [4].

References

1. Megens J, Vandereycken W. Hospitalization of obsessive-compulsive patients. Comprehensive Psychiatry 1988 Jan/Mar;30(2):161–9.
2. Thornicroft G, Colson L, Marks E. An in-patient behavioural psychotherapy unit; description and audit. British Journal of Psychiatry 1991;158:362–7.
3. Drummond L. The treatment of severe, chronic, resistant obsessive compulsive disorder. British Journal of Psychiatry 1993;263:223–9.
4. Calvocoressi L, McDougle CJ, Wasylink S, Goodman WK, et al. Inpatient treatment of severe obsessive-compulsive disorder. Hospital & Community Psychiatry 1993 Dec;44(12):1150–4.

18. Patients with Paranoid Disorders

The person with paranoid traits is usually extremely vulnerable. The vulnerability is often masked by a facade of self-sufficiency, a tendency to blame others, and concerns over being powerless. The person with paranoid traits has difficulty with authority figures, difficulty fitting into a social structure, and usually feels like an outsider. Thought processes are characterized by suspiciousness, delusions and possible grandiosity [1–2].

The staff soon discovers that its usual repertoire of caring behaviors is not effective with the person with paranoid traits. Warmth, friendliness, and efforts to get close should never be excessive. The staff should approach the person straightforwardly using clear and simple language, avoiding overly friendly or patronizing behavior. The staff should not touch the patient or approach too quickly. The person with paranoid features should not be surprised. There should be great respect for the need for territorial space. These patients must be absolutely sure that medication is not poisonous. Education about medication will be needed, including why it is prescribed, and assurance that it won't remove the patient's own control [2].

Despite barriers, it is the staff who must take the initiative in providing treatment since the patient will not ask for help and does not wish to appear inadequate. Staff members must realize that they are going to be angry and at times will probably want to punish the patient. By arousing anger, the patient is actually forcing the staff to confirm a view of the world as hostile and punitive. Staff members will have much to learn about the patient and will need a forum for discussing emotional reactions. They must learn that it is normal to have intense reactions to paranoid patients—fear, anxiety, frustration, and hopelessness. Although withdrawing from the patient seems natural, the staff should determine not to let it happen. Staff members must always be completely honest with these patients, who lack basic trust and have a very low tolerance for ambiguity. Any attempts to gain their compliance by tricking them or using half-truths can be seriously damaging. The patient should work with the same small number of staff each day so that there will be an opportunity to build trusting relationships. However, it is the patient who will need to lead the way in making them, since one characteristic of the disorder is a fear of intimacy [2–4].

Milieu Activities

In contrast with usual milieu procedures, persons with paranoid features should not be pushed to interact with other patients. They may enjoy quiet activities with staff members they have come to trust or be pleasantly diverted by solitary activities. Requiring them to socialize with other patients can make them feel panic or aggression. When the person becomes more comfortable on the unit, there may be opportunities to gradually introduce other staff and patients [4].

Violence

Paranoid patients can be hostile and threatening and the staff is justifiably frightened. The patient must be told that violence is not acceptable under any circumstances and should be informed of the consequences of violence and the hospital's procedure for handling outbreaks. Timely interventions can often prevent it. Williston Di Bella indicates that paranoid patients' violence does not appear "out of the blue." Mounting tension or excessive angry brooding usually precede violent actions. If an episode does occur, it should be discussed with the patient. In addition, staff members should meet to relieve their own feelings about it, and plan ways to prevent its happening again. Patients on the unit should also be encouraged to discuss the incident to seek reassurance [5].

PROJECTION AND DELUSIONS

The person with paranoid features feels at the center of others' interest. Feeling one's self as the center also means feeling one's self as the target. This helps to explain the feelings of vulnerability. It will be the therapist's role to work with the patient's projections. Staff members' challenging of the person's projections will only stimulate opposition. The staff should not tell the patient that treatment is to correct delusions. No matter how intense the delusional feelings the patient has toward others, the staff must strive to build a working relationship [6].

Working successfully requires respect for the patient's fragile and threatened autonomy. Any decision that is made in the hospital should be discussed with the hope that the patient can make or be consulted on most treatment decisions. These patients will not be cured by simply living in a beneficent milieu. The staff's task will be to provide a therapeutic and non-threatening environment and through experience develop controls and ways to handle feelings in working with them.

References

1. Meissner WW. Paranoid Personality Disorders. In: American Psychiatric Association Task Force on Treatments of Psychiatric Disorders. Treatments of psychiatric disorders. v. 3. Washington, DC: American Psychiatric Press, 1989, 2705–12.
2. Williston Di Bella GA. Educating staff to manage threatening paranoid patients. American Journal of Psychiatry 1979 Mar;136(3):333–5.
3. Roth M. Delusional (Paranoid) Disorders. In: American Psychiatric Association Task Force on Treatments of Psychiatric Disorders. Treatments of psychiatric disorders. v. 2. Washington, DC: American Psychiatric Press, 1989, 1609–48.
4. Justic M. Nursing care for the hospitalized patient with psychotic symptoms. In: Wells, LA, ed. A handbook of psychiatric nursing. St Louis: Warren H. Green, 1989, 245–87.
5. See reference 2.
6. Sparr LF, Boehnlein JK, Cooney TG. The medical management of the paranoid patient. General Hospital Psychiatry 1986 Jan:8(1);49–55.

19. Post-Traumatic Stress Disorder

Establishing a therapeutic alliance with patients with Post-Traumatic Stress Disorder is a major hurdle in treatment. The milieu staff and therapists must be able to not only provide an explanation for the patient's distress but also instill a sense of hope. Most of the literature on inpatient treatment of Post-Traumatic Stress

Disorder is devoted to programs for veterans, but some of the same principles will apply for all forms of trauma [1].

Those who work with patients with post-traumatic stress as a result of traumatic war experiences indicate that debriefing, no matter how distant from the event itself, is essential. The ultimate goal of treatment with veterans is to help them resume the transition to adulthood and normal life that the war interrupted. A program that serves veterans can remove some of the stigma they may feel as mental patients by simply calling it a veteran's program rather than a post-traumatic stress unit. The building of mutual support and group solidarity is essential to a program for this population. It may help if the unit can be explicitly designed as a therapeutic community that uses not only peer support but peer pressure. Self-help principles are effective [2].

Program Models

Berman and colleagues describe three treatment phases in a therapeutic community program for male Vietnam veterans with Post-Traumatic Stress Disorder. The program includes 65 therapy groups serving a patient population in crisis, who are anxious, depressed and often psychotic. The goal of the first phase is to resolve the crisis, develop trust in the treatment staff, and ventilate feelings. The content of this phase will be devoted to a review of the veterans' life situations before military service and the changes that took place during the war. The replaying of their lives in combat is central, and together the veterans go through the painful acts that have ignited their own intrusive thoughts, nightmares and flashbacks. Anger, rage and feelings of disillusion are the predominant emotions during this phase. They will find themselves blaming the Vietnam War for everything that went wrong in their lives. The group and the leader do not discourage this during this phase of treatment. The veterans are also given the strength to "clean up" the lives they left before hospitalization, e.g., make an arrangement to pay unpaid rent, resolve child-support, call employers to negotiate a return to work [2].

With completion of the first phase, the veteran has a more objective view of himself, both before and during the Vietnam war, and understands more about the social context within which the war occurred. In order to maintain group cohesion, every attempt is made to move the veterans together into the second phase. In this phase the veteran is out of crisis and more settled into the program. The thrust of this phase is to help the veterans take more responsibility for their actions, both before, during and after the war. The veteran's blaming of the war for all difficulties is not responded to in the same way, not because the blaming isn't valid but because it isn't productive. Each person is helped to recognize and develop his own strengths to master the challenges of life and to triumph over earlier problems, whether they began in childhood or during the war. This phase ends when the veterans can develop solutions and make plans for reintegration into the community [2].

The third phase, that of psychosocial rehabilitation, is devoted to making this possible. Each veteran devises a plan that includes employment or education, a social support system, plans for housing and income. The veterans begin work in the community but return to the medical center at night. They work toward final independence, living and working in the community [2].

Perconte describes a day hospital program for veterans with the treatment goals of reducing anxiety and compulsive behaviors and resolving issues of blame and guilt to restore self esteem. Social skills training and improving family communication reduced the veterans' social anxiety and increased their participation in the community. Treatment began with the discussion of problems. The veterans were later able to release the blocked emotions of guilt, fear and sorrow and reexperience the impact of the war events. The next stage was a sharing of these experiences and feelings with family members. The veteran who could start to make changes was able to begin to participate in community and social activities and formulate both short term career and family goals. The program goals were implemented primarily through the various therapy groups. Veterans attended groups for up to 12 hours per week [3].

References

1. McFarlane AC. The treatment of stress disorder. British Journal of Medical Psychology 1989 Mar;62(2):81–90.
2. Berman S, Price S, Gusman F. An inpatient program for Vietnam combat veterans in a Veteran's Administration Hospital. Hospital & Community Psychiatry 1982 Nov;33(11):919–22.
3. Perconte S. Partial hospitalization treatment of Post-traumatic Stress Disorder. International Journal of Partial Hospitalization 1986 Dec;3(4):21–30.

20. Psychosomatic Disorders

The primary goal of treatment for the psychosomatic patient is an improved sense of physical well-being sufficient to allow a surrender of the sick role. This will not be possible without developing improved coping skills and social functioning. Specific goals are formulated for each patient and then broken down into short-term objectives which can be reviewed at weekly rounds. Abbey and Lipowski recommend that the psychosomatic patient be assigned a primary nurse who will coordinate the treatment plan [1].

The Milieu Program

The foundation for the treatment program for psychosomatic patients is the therapeutic milieu and the formation of a milieu culture which rewards activity and discourages illness behaviors. When patients begin to focus on symptoms, they should be redirected toward thinking of rehabilitation. The family must be included in many of the therapeutic aspects of the program [1–2].

GROUP TREATMENT

The development of coping strategies is central, and groups can play a significant role. Abbey and Lipowski describe several groups in the psychosomatic medicine unit. Patients can review their short term goals and successes in a goal-setting group which meets three times a week. There is a stress-management group with a life skills approach that meets twice a week. Members have homework assignments and review results in the following session. A family relations group concentrates on the patient's relationships in the family and its response to the patient's illness. This group can generate discussion by selecting a specific theme such as the family life cycle, or the expression in anger in families. A daily exercise group helps to reactivate these patients and make physical activity a source of pleasure. Inpatient treatment can prepare patients for outpatient psychotherapy by helping to develop a problem-solving orientation [1–2].

References

1. Abbey SE, Lipowski ZJ. Comprehensive management of persistent somatization: an innovative inpatient program. Psychotherapy & Psychosomatics; 1987;48:110–5.
2. von Rad M, Sellschopp A. The integrated psychosomatic inpatient unit. Psychotherapy & Psychosomatics 1987;48:101–9.

21. Schizophrenic Disorders

Milieu therapy is potentially harmful for persons with schizophrenia. Drake and Sederer describe the most obvious form of mistreatment of schizophrenia as prolonged, unnecessary hospitalization. They allow that intensive and stimulating milieu treatment may help some patients, but unfortunately it is not possible to know which ones. Intensive milieu treatment usually results in negative treatment outcome: regression, treatment noncompliance, premature discharge and even greater alienation from others. Milieu treatment as usually defined is simply not helpful. This does not mean, however, that persons with schizophrenia need understimulating, unstructured environments. Guidelines for beneficial interactions are still necessary [1–2].

There may be a population of persons with schizophrenia who are never hospitalized. Hospitalization may occur only during a crisis. The literature makes a distinction between the acute and chronic schizophrenic patient, and the term "chronic patient" often seems another way to say "schizophrenic." Coursey reports that we no longer discuss psychotherapy for the person with schizophrenia but instead concentrate upon psychiatric rehabilitation, vocational rehabilitation, family support and education [3].

A background in the biological nature of the illness is helpful in designing treatment. Persons with schizophrenia have impaired information processing. Their ability to filter events that occur at the same time is impaired. They cannot necessarily generalize learning. They therefore need special help in adjusting to new settings. Eaton advises that admission to the hospital may be more disruptive and disabling than any other experience associated with a schizophrenic illness. Verbal instructions and interventions require multiple repetitions. New behaviors require frequent practice [4–5].

Any form of active treatment must be balanced by the knowledge that the person with schizophrenia has to be able to modulate stimulus levels. An overstimulating environment is destructive. Patients will need to socially withdraw and doing so is beneficial. A milieu with multiple meetings, group therapies, and treatment through exploration of feelings or confrontation can be harmful. Families now learn to maintain a low-stimulus home environment for the family member with schizophrenia. Research suggests that the schizophrenic person who returns to a family with high "expressed emotion" relapses more frequently. The family with high expressed emotion is likely to more critical, more hostile, or emotionally overinvolved. Although these findings remain controversial and do not go unchallenged, empirical studies conducted with families have implications for all group living arrangements for persons with schizophrenia. It may seem that we are left with a better understanding of what not to do, rather than what to do [6–7].

The Role of the Staff in Treating the Person with Schizophrenia

What is important then in the positive treatment of schizophrenia? The creation of trust is the most essential and the most difficult task. Brown advises that the patient should be given one staff person per shift as a primary contact to give consistency in the new environment. The staff can serve as crucial "primary objects" who will eventually serve as models for identification and present new patterns for interaction. Developing a trusting alliance that still respects the person's need for distance is the most crucial step in treatment. Huszonek counsels that the difficulties in making contact with the patient will not really be solved by saying the right things and that saying too much will be intrusive and frightening. The best way to begin to increase a sense of trust is to relate to the patient as a real person. The quality of the relationship bond may initially depend on whether the person sees the staff member as helpful. The staff works for empathic understanding. Pao writes that following a schizophrenic episode, the person loses self-cohesion and is like a toddler taking the first steps—but unlike the toddler, will not keep trying [8–12].

If a treatment alliance develops, both staff and patient can share responsibility for working toward treatment goals. These goals should be modest and clearly defined. The staff member must become a dependable part of the patient's support system and interactions should be both supportive and educational. A final goal is to enable the person to become an agent of personal change, rather than being a passive recipient of treatment. Staff can encourage patients to participate in the program and to take more risks. The patient's ability to make choices and be in charge will help develop the self-cohesiveness needed after discharge. In an article reviewing her own treatment as a patient, Leete contrasts the nonparticipatory treatment she received in the hospital with her participation in a residential treatment center. In the residential treatment center, she no longer encountered authoritarian postures, so power struggles were eliminated. The treatment team considered her a partner in her own treatment and encouraged her input. The mutual fear that she and the staff experienced in the hospital was replaced by mutual acceptance in residential treatment. This does not mean, of course, that every person with schizophrenia is capable of such participation [13].

Many patients will be unmotivated and not cooperative during treatment, but resistance, withdrawal and passivity are not enduring characteristics of schizophrenic disorders. Patients with schizophrenia can be goal-directed, have an active will, and try to cope with their illness as best they can. Carr's exploration of the ability of persons to cope with schizophrenia demonstrates that they are not passive victims of the illness. Carr finds that for many the experience of schizophrenia resembles a learning process in which patients can actively attempt to master their illness and not allow it to dominate them [14–16].

Gunderson states that the staff and therapists who work with patients with schizophrenia need a shared philosophical orientation, clear leadership and distribution of responsibility. There must be a recognition of the patient's deficits and individual needs. Gunderson reports that it is the very busy staff with high morale and involvement that will work well with schizophrenic patients—not the staff that has time on its hands and doesn't feel occupied. Having several patients in the unit functioning at a high level will help social participation and provide role models. The program should also provide expectations and rewards for social interaction and participation [17].

The Treatment Team

The treatment team's support is of great importance in the care of the schizophrenic adult patient. The severity of the illness can leave staff members feeling as helpless and hopeless as the patient. The insights that the team can produce by sharing perceptions build an integrated team perspective and empathic understanding that can prevent countertransference reactions. Levy describes the countertransference that occurs when the staff member with strong wishes for caring and nurturing is rebuffed by the patient with schizophrenia. When staff members are deprived of exercising this important function they feel guilty and often will reject the patient. Being able to nurture the patient's embryonic pattern of attachment while allowing the distance the patient needs becomes a major challenge. Kahn and White advise the treatment team to be alert for negative group dynamics which are extremely contagious for the patient with schizophrenia. A reading of the ward atmosphere and its impact upon the patient should be considered at staff meetings [18–20].

The Concept of the Holding Environment

Despite its roots in psychoanalysis, the concept of the holding environment can also be applied to the treatment of persons with schizophrenia. Kahn and White describe five elements of the holding environment for the schizophrenic patient: safety, structure, support, socialization, and self-understanding. After the most crucial needs are met for safety and structure, there may be an opportunity to provide socialization and self-understanding [20].

Safety is provided by planned interventions such as suicide precautions or time-outs. Structure is accomplished by careful orientation of the patient, appropriate patient guidelines, a schedule of activities and a plan for managing noncompliance when it occurs. Scott writes about the hospital's role as a holding environment in an illuminating way. He describes the boundaries of the person's self as disrupted so that personal thoughts begin to be experienced as originating from outside. He sees the hospital as a container that can establish definite boundaries for the person. The hospital provides the structure that becomes the container for the psychosis. The functions of the patient's ego pass temporarily into the guardianship of the staff. Scott describes the world of the schizophrenic person as having the following features: loss of ego boundaries, loss of control, loss of constancy in the experience of self, and the need for containment which does not invade the boundaries that remain [20–21].

Scott believes that the relationship with the staff can provide an identification, a process by which the patient's ego functions can be reintegrated and then returned. The patient's capacity to maintain an image of the caretaker even when absent can build a relation to the outer world. The containment function of the hospital can be used to restore the patient's ego which has lost its internal control and boundaries. Leete, describing her own schizophrenia, reports that her identity began to fragment and blend with the environment. She felt merged with the wind [21–22].

Hallucinations and Delusions

Schizophrenia usually involves hallucinations during some phase of the illness. Lally, providing the patient's perspective, writes that it is usually hallucinations which mark the person's own recognition of mental illness. When these hallucinations are experienced as real and originating from outside, there is a splitting of the real from the unreal. The person can no longer always distinguish inner thoughts from outer reality. Although hallucinations are usually controlled by psychotropic medication, the milieu staff should explore ways to help the patient who has them. Field's description of the stages of hallucination is helpful. The person creates a perception. An inner thought becomes a voice speaking. The person then believes the voice is coming from the outside world. The third stage in the process occurs when the person does not realize it is an inner or created perception [23–24].

When hallucinations occur in the milieu, Field suggests that the staff member lead the person to a private surrounding and gently inquire about hearing voices. If the person confirms this, the staff member suggests a way to try to get rid of it. And that is to say: "Go away and leave me alone." Field suggests that this be done loudly and distinctly several times. This gives the person a sense of control. When there is no privacy, the hallucinating person can be advised to sing softly as a control. Puskar and colleagues describe the care of medication-free psychotic patients in a schizophrenia research unit. The patient's trust in the primary nurse is crucial. Patients are encouraged to speak about their internal experience. Nurses are encouraged to interrupt and distract them from hallucinations by one-to-one contact, music, or activities [24–25].

The person with schizophrenia is also subject to delusions, fixed false beliefs that are maintained despite contrary evidence. Schizophrenic delusions often appear without any reason. Staff members may feel helpless and impatient in the face of delusions, but they should not attempt to overcome them with logic, take a humorous approach to them, or pretend that the delusions are true. These actions will only distance and confuse the patient. Although neuroleptics can usually control hallucinations and delusions, many patients have devised coping strategies such as distraction and self-verbalization [26]. (For more information about hallucinations and delusions, consult Chapter VII.)

Treatment Methods

ACUTE TREATMENT IN AN INTENSIVE CARE UNIT

Cohen and Khan describe acute treatment of schizophrenia in a locked intensive care unit, with an average stay of 12 days. Each patient is given a single room and interpersonal contact is kept at a minimum for the first 48 hours. The patient is secluded with staff rounds every 15 minutes. Psychopharmacotherapy is the treatment of choice. Results demonstrated dramatic clinical improvement during the first two days of treatment. Cohen and Khan describe this treatment as having an antipsychotic effect. The Brief Psychiatric Rating Scale demonstrated a reduction in psychotic symptoms such as conceptual disorganization, suspiciousness, hallucinations, and unusual thought content, when compared to the control group. Cohen and Khan advise that in acute treatment the first two days be devoted to treatment that provides minimal stimulation and interaction, focusing on reality orientation [27].

Graduated Therapy with the Schizophrenic Patient

Patients with schizophrenia come to the inpatient setting in various phases of the illness and with varying abilities. Kahn and White propose a sequential therapy beginning with an orientation to the treatment program and developing goals. This is followed by education, helping the patient learn about the illness, its causes and treatment, and ways of coping. The final step is understanding. Whereas the earlier steps are processes that can be done for the patient, the final step, understanding, is more difficult and dependent upon the patient's own ability. The patient must be able to integrate the experience of the psychotic episode into a present identity and be able to carry the lessons of the hospital into the context of the real world. Each of these steps of treatment offer elements matched to the patient's progress. Each requires a greater tolerance of stress and a higher organization of thinking [28].

Kahn and White advise that as patients are able they can join the less demanding activities available in occupational, art, music, and recreational therapies. Corrigan and colleagues find, for example, that patients who participated in direct recreational activity decreased the frequency of their bizarre and inappropriate behaviors and increased their prosocial behaviors. Recreational activities in general seem to replace bizarre behaviors since they are not compatible with sustained activity. Activities that are enjoyable also help the patient sustain attention [28–29].

Later patients may be ready to be placed in supportive group therapy. Since one of the most frightening aspects of the psychotic episode is alienation from others, group therapy can provide peer support and be the first step toward social reintegration. Patients have described the following therapeutic results from group therapy: the restoration of hope, the ability to share common experiences of the crisis situation, and self-understanding. The group can help the patient gain some mastery over the crisis situation and regain connections with people [28–29].

The Rehabilitation Model

The rehabilitation model introduces a new value system in treatment, a realization that persons with chronic schizophrenia are not merely "schizophrenics." The staff must make empathic contact with the real person and help the person to accept the chronic illness but find the highest level of functioning. Smith and colleagues describe the principles of rehabilitation psychiatry in the treatment of a woman with paranoid schizophrenia, that focuses on the patient's strengths and motivation rather than on symptoms and disabilities. The treatment must take into account the schizophrenic patient's vulnerability to stress. Wasylenki writes that the one feature that schizophrenic patients have in common is not really the presence of the illness but rather the presence of the vulnerability. The patient's ability to cope breaks down under stress and in the absence of social support. Treatment must prepare the patient for establishing social support and restore the ability to cope, but it must also teach those in the person's milieu how to maintain a less stressful environment [30–31].

The goal of rehabilitation is to help the person with schizophrenia to acquire the physical, emotional, social and intellectual skills in order to live and work in the community with the least amount of support. The goal is accomplished not only by teaching specific skills but also by increasing the environmental resources necessary for support. Bradshaw compares the effects of coping skills training and a problem-solving approach on patients with schizophrenia. Group coping skills training included cognitive restructuring, relaxation techniques, and social skills training. Although all of these methods had been used before, they had not been combined in a comprehensive approach to develop stress management. Problem solving group treatment was arranged in four steps: problem identification, designing possible solutions, implementing them, and monitoring the results. Members of the group share ideas and support each other in solving problems of living. Of this small sample, patients in the coping skills group were significantly closer to their goals. Their rehospitalization rate for the first year was 7%, much lower than the reported national average of 35–50% for schizophrenic patients [32–34].

Glynn and Mueser report that nursing staff and well-trained paraprofessionals have been able to remediate bizarre symptoms, self-care and social deficits of severely impaired schizophrenic patients by the use of behavioral assessment and therapy. Liberman and colleagues describe behavioral rehabilitation. Behavioral rehabilitation differs from other psychosocial approaches to schizophrenia in that it requires a behavior analyst or therapist. Positive reinforcement must be given consistently and frequently for appropriate social behavior. Glynn and Mueser describe social learning for patients with schizophrenia that concentrates upon integrated procedures for skill acquisition and education. This is best accomplished in a token economy structure with consistent pacing and generalization training. It was Paul and Lentz who made the definitive argument for social learning and a token economy in a comparative study of three forms of treatment, custodial, milieu therapy, and social learning. This study was comprehensive in its comparisons as well as in its rigorous methodology, virtually demonstrating that social learning is the most effective and lasting treatment for the population with chronic schizophrenia. After the program of social learning, patients who had been hospitalized for an average of 17 years achieved higher rates of release and longer community stays [35–37].

The program was based on learning principles of associative learning, problem-solving, reinforcement, modeling and shaping. Patients spent 85% of their working hours in structured activities. It was also accomplished primarily by a nonprofessional staff (80%), but a staff that had carefully learned behavioral techniques. Although the results of this program demonstrated without question the superiority of behavior techniques, they have not been shown to produce fundamental or lasting changes in the illness [35–37].

The development of social skills can defend the person against various stressors. Social competence is the best single predictor for remaining in the community after discharge. There are several training models available for the individual patient: attention-focusing procedures, problem solving models, and social skills training. Social skills training (SST), when behavioral techniques are used, shapes the person's behavior by reinforcing appropriate verbal skills, such as conversational responses, assertive responses, voice volume, and nonverbal responses such as eye contact and appropriate smiling. Job interview skills are also important. SST has proved to be a helpful technique for building social competence. It is a well-structured educational technique that uses modeling, role playing and social reinforcement. The training breaks down complex social repertoires into smaller elements, such as maintaining eye contact and providing social responses. Patients practice each element and then learn to combine them. Follow-ups at 6 or 12 months indicate maintenance of training. Benton and Schroeader's meta-analysis of research on social skills training for persons with schizophrenic disorders indicate that SST signficantly improves social behavior and self-perception and reduces social anxiety. Dobson and colleagues found that both social skills training and social milieu treatment improve schizophrenic symptoms but that SST is more effective for improving what are called the negative symptoms of schizophrenia: lack of affect and social deficits. The results of this nine-week training program began to decline after six months, which led the authors to consider the need for longer training [35–40].

Inpatient Treatment of Schizophrenia in Children and Adolescents

Parker believes that for the schizophrenic child or adolescent, nothing is more important than skill development. He describes the need to control the psychotic process so normal developmental skills may be acquired. After the patient is stabilized most of the treatment is devoted toward improving adaptive functioning and creating a support network outside of the treatment center to protect the child or adolescent's progress. Attending to stress and the proper degree of stimulation is also necessary with children and adolescents. Either too little or too much stimulation can stop the progress of treatment. Bizarre behaviors on the part of the patient will signal that a stress threshold has been reached [41].

Treatment team meetings are important because the staff will have a great need to exchange results of planned interventions, ideas and strategies. The team can ascertain which staff member might be most successful in building a personal relationship. Parker's guidelines for the goal oriented treatment meeting begin with the clear identification of the problem, statement of the desired outcome, exploration of solutions with anticipated results. The team should then select the solution, put it into action and evaluate the results [41].

WORKING WITH THE FAMILY

Work with the family should begin at admission. The staff should obtain the family's permission for the use of psychotropic medication. All families will need support and education and a great deal of planning to prepare for the patient's life after discharge. Families should learn about early symptoms of relapse, and become familiar with the literature about expressed emotion. Findings about expressed emotion must be approached carefully, since the research has used an oversimplified unidirectional model of the family 's effect on symptoms, not the total social context which must also include the patient's effect on the family [42].

Descriptions of Special Programs

Descriptions of successful programs for the treatment of schizophrenia are now rare in the literature. Since there are no definitive answers for schizophrenia, descriptions of such programs instill hope. Few current empirical or controlled studies are available, so descriptions of programs usually provide only helpful ideas, not tested techniques. Although there are good descriptions of behavioral programs, the programs discussed in this section are programs which do not necessarily require special training or technology.

Soteria was a program for a small group of schizophrenic persons located in a house staffed primarily by non-professionals. Length of stay was three to six months. There was a guiding philosophy that there were significant benefits in treating psychosis without medication. Outcome for the Soteria graduates was compared with that of medicated schizophrenic patients from a community mental health center (mean stay, 25 days). Results after one year showed no differences in the two groups in symptoms, social functioning, or rate of relapse. Follow-up after two years revealed that a greater number of Soteria patients were able to live away from families and work at a higher level occupation [43–44].

The staff's goal at Soteria was to provide a warm, supportive, nonintrusive social environment, to share responsibilities and decisions with the residents, but not to cure them. Mosher described this as a "phenomenological" approach to schizophrenia—being able to share the person's experience as much as possible without judging or invalidating it. It was hoped that the person could feel not only accepted but understood and that somehow the psychotic experience could be integrated into present life. The beneficial results led Mosher to believe that it is possible to design an interpersonally based therapeutic milieu that is as effective as neuroleptics in reducing acute psychotic symptoms in newly diagnosed persons with schizophrenia. This positive long-term outcome may have been helped by the growth of the unplanned and informal Soteria network that provided friends, support, recreation, and even housing for former residents and staff [43–44].

Gunderson describes some shared characteristics of these small effective programs: high patient-staff ratio, 20 beds or less, as well as youthful staff members working in a program known to be nonconventional. These programs have an orientation that interpreted schizophrenic signs and symptoms of schizophrenia as meaningful expressions of the person's experience. Gunderson also describes a distribution of responsibility among all staff members. Staff and patients were greatly involved in the community and both assumed social responsibilities. Some but not all of these characteristics could be transferred to other treatment settings [45].

Brey writes about PREP (the Psychosocial Rehabilitation Entry Project), a 32-bed inpatient unit, where all persons share responsibility for unit life. The community elects officers and holds daily meetings to discuss community problems. The resident group also makes work assignments and plans activities. Residents are expected to keep their rooms clean; fellow residents inspect rooms and make notes on residents who are not performing tasks. The staff's role and influence are minimal. They attend meetings but are there only to observe and advise when consulted. Their observations of adaptive and maladaptive behaviors are communicated, not in meetings, but in notes to the group. Each small group meets daily without the staff to discuss these communications, with all members encouraged to give their opinion. Then the entire group takes action and communicates to the staff. The staff then provides the residents with feedback on their problem solving. The staff's communicating in writing reduces its influence on the group's ability to solve its problems and helps strengthen the peer support system. When a note describes a resident's behavior, it is the group that must learn how to work with it and how to gain the resident's cooperation. PREP also includes a privilege system and work program so that individual progress can be achieved and recognized. Discharge can be accomplished after the resident is ready to complete a plan for outpatient therapy, housing, and sources of financial support. PREP provides a small group treatment modality closer to real life situations. This small group approach could also be used in halfway houses and in day treatment and could be modified for other forms of inpatient treatment [46].

A study by Vaglum and colleagues finds that even after 40 years, not enough is known about beneficial milieu therapy for schizophrenic persons. A beneficial milieu for schizophrenic disorders usually requires a low level of anger and aggression, and a high level of order and organization, support, and practical orientation. Some of the unit characteristics which can be detrimental are a large number of patients, a high percentage of psychotic patients, and high staff turnover. They warn against group therapy that is confronting or community groups that often become antitherapeutic "pseudo-groups " [47].

We have learned a great deal (but not yet enough} about the treatment of the patient with schizophrenia in the last two decades. Previous discussions of earlier treatment such as the "total push" method now give us retroactive shudders. Drake and Sederer enumerate the basic principles for successful psychosocial treatment as we now know them. Treatment should focus on adaptation and growth rather than psychopathology. Family and other social support systems should be integrated into therapy. The development of an alliance between the patient and the staff member is crucial. Drake and Sederer caution that unless selection criteria for intensive treatment is clear, the treatment should begin with less intensive treatment. Kahn and White believe that treatment should build slowly on the patient's gains and be tailored to the phase of the illness. Interventions should be simple, focused and highly structured. Patients should know that relapses might be expected but that they are not a permanent defeat. Eckman and colleagues report that there is some evidence that patients retain the benefits of treatment for at least six months. The staff's level of expressed emotion and criticism should always be considered; Snyder and colleagues discovered that the effect of staff caretakers' expressed emotion on their residents was similar to those of family members on adult children. The more critical the staff, the poorer the quality of the residents' lives and the greater the increase of their hostility and suspiciousness. Patients should know that relapses might be expected but that they are not a permanent defeat. There is some evidence that patients retain the benefits of brief treatment for at least six months. The illness will probably require multiple treatments carried out in an integrated fashion over a long period of time. Even persons who are severely impaired can learn new behaviors which will help them maintain an adequate quality of life [48–51].

References

1. Drake RE, Sederer LI. The adverse effects of intensive treatment of chronic schizophrenia. Comprehensive Psychiatry 1986;27:312–26.
2. Glynn S, Mueser KT. Social learning for chronic mental inpatients. Schizophrenia Bulletin 1986;12(4):640–8.
3. Coursey RD. Psychotherapy with persons suffering from schizophrenia: The need for a new agenda. Schizophrenia Bulletin 1989;15(3):349–53.
4. Eaton WM. Long-term course of hospitalization for schizophrenia: Part I. Risk for rehospitalization. Schizophrenia Bulletin 1992;18(2):217–28.
5. Kahn EM, White EM. Adapting milieu approaches to acute inpatient care for schizophrenic patients. Hospital & Community Psychiatry 1989 Jun;40(6):609–14.

6. Vaughn CE, Snyder KS, Jones S, et al. Family factors in schizophrenic relapse. Archives of General Psychiatry 1987;42:1169–77.
7. Lefley HP. Expressed emotion: conceptual, clinical and social policy issues. Hospital & Community Psychiatry 1992 Jun;43(6):591–8.
8. Brown LJ. A short-term hospital program preparing borderline and schizophrenic patients for intensive psychotherapy. Psychiatry 1981;44:327–36.
9. Selzer MA. Preparing the chronic schizophrenic for exploratory psychotherapy: the role of hospitalization. Psychiatry 1983;46(4):303–11.
10. Huszonek JJ. Establishing therapeutic contact with schizophrenics: a supervisory approach. American Journal of Psychotherapy 1987 Apr;41(2):185–93.
11. Axelrod S, Palgi E. Developing an alliance with schizophrenic patients in day hospital treatment. Bulletin Menninger Clinic 1990;54:340–52.
12. Pao PN. Schizophrenic disorders: Theory and treatment from a psychodynamic point of view. New York: International Universities Press, 1979, 405.
13. Leete E. The treatment of schizophrenia: a patient's perspective. Hospital & Community Psychiatry 1987 May;38(5):486–91.
14. Bellack AS, Mueser KT. Psychosocial treatment for schizophrenia. Schizophrenia Bulletin 1993;19(2):317–26.
15. Strauss JS. Subjective experience of schizophrenia. Toward a new dynamic psychiatry-II. Schizophrenia Bulletin 1989;15:179–87.
16. Carr V. Patients' techniques for coping with schizophrenia: an exploratory study. British Journal of Medical Psychology 1968;41(4):339–62.
17. Gunderson JG. A reevaluation of milieu therapy for nonchronic schizophrenic patients. Schizophrenia Bulletin 1980;6(1): 64–9.
18. Levy ST. Aspects of countertransference in the treatment of schizophrenia. Journal National Association of Private Psychiatric Hospitals 1979;10:60–7.
19. See reference 9.
20. See reference 5.
21. Scott RD. A conceptual model of a hospital as an aid to the everyday handling of psychotic patients. Psychiatry 1962;25:208–18.
22. See reference 13.
23. Field WE. Hearing voices. Journal of Psychosocial Nursing & Mental Health Services 1985 Jan;23(1):8–14.
24. Lally S. "Does being in her mean there's something wrong with me?" Schizophrenia Bulletin 1989;15(2):253–65.
25. Puskar KR, McAdam D, Burkhart-Morgan CE, Isadore RB, et al. Psychiatric nursing management of medication-free psychotic patients. Archives of Psychiatric Nursing 1990;4(2):78–86.
26. Rosenthal TT, McGuinness TM. Dealing with delusional patients: discovering the distorted truth. Issues in Mental Health Nursing 1986;8:143–54.
27. Cohen S, Khan A. Antipsychotic effect of milieu in the acute treatment of schizophrenia. General Hospital Psychiatry 1990;12:248–51.
28. See reference 5.
29. Corrigan PW, Storzbach DM. Behavioral interventions for alleviating psychotic symptoms. Hospital & Community Psychiatry 1993 Apr;44(4):341–7.

30. Smith TE, Woo-Ming AM, Lang E, DeFelice L, et al. Treatment planning: Rehabilitation psychiatry in the inpatient treatment of a woman with paranoid schizophrenia. Hospital & Community Psychiatry 1994 Dec;45(12):1179–81.
31. Wasylenki DA. Psychotherapy of schizophrenia revisited. Hospital & Community Psychiatry 1992 Feb;43(2):123–27.
32. Anthony WA, Liberman RP. The practice of psychiatric rehabilitation: historical, conceptual and research base. Schizophrenia Bulletin 1986;12(4):542–59.
33. Liberman RP. Handbook of psychiatric rehabilitation. New York: Macmillan, 1992.
34. Bradshaw WH. Coping-skills training versus a problem-solving approach with schizophrenic patients. Hospital & Community Psychiatry 1993 Nov;44(11):1102–7.
35. See reference 2.
36. Liberman RP, Glynn SM, Phipps CC. Rehabilitation in schizophrenic disorders. In: American Psychiatric Association Task Force on Treatments of Psychiatric Disorders. Treatments of psychiatric disorders. v. 1. Washington, DC: American Psychiatric Press, 1989, 1567–83.
37. Paul GL, Lentz, RJ. Psychosocial treatment of chronic mental patients. Cambridge: Harvard University Press, 1977.
38. Wallace CJ, Nelson CJ, Liberman RP, Aitchison RA, et al. A review and critique of social skills training with schizophrenic patients. Schizophrenia Bulletin 1980;6:42–43.
39. Benton MK, Schroeader HE. Social skills training with schizophrenics: a meta-analytic evaluation. Journal of Consulting & Clinical Psychology 1990;58:741–7.
40. Dobson DJG, McCougall G, Busheikin J, Aldous J. Effects of social skills training and social milieu treatment on symptoms of schizophrenia. Psychiatric Services 1995 Apr;46(4):376–80.
41. Parker DR. Treatment of schizophrenic children and adolescents. In: Lyman, Robert D, Prentice-Dunn S, Gabel S, eds. Residential and inpatient treatment of children and adolescents. New York: Plenum Press, 1989, 259–64.
42. See reference 14.
43. Mosher LR. Soteria: A therapeutic community for psychotic persons. International Journal of Therapeutic Communities 1991;12(1): 53–67.
44. Mosher LR, Menn AK. Dinosaur or astronaut? One-year follow-up data from the Soteria Project. American Journal of Psychiatry 1976 Aug;133(8):919–21.
45. See reference 17.
46. Brey KH. The mental hospital revisited: a program. Schizophrenia Bulletin 1981;7(3):522–6.
47. Vaglum P, Friis S, Karterud S. Why are the results of milieu therapy for schizophrenic patients contradictory? An analysis based on four empirical studies. Yale Journal of Biology & Medicine 1985;58:349–61.
48. See reference 1.
49. See reference 5.
50. Eckman TA, Wirshing WC, Marder SR, Liberman RP, et al. Technology for training schizophrenics in illness self-management: A controlled trial. American Journal of Psychiatry 1992 Nov;149(11):1549–55.
50. Snyder KS, Wallace CJ, Moe K, Liberman RP. Expressed emotion by residential care operators and residents' symptoms and quality of life. Hospital & Community Psychiatry 1994 Nov;45(11):1141–3.

22. Victims of Sexual Abuse

Although there are few specific inpatient programs for victims of sexual abuse, a large number of patients in psychiatric treatment settings have sexual abuse histories. Milieu treatment planning should always consider this history of sexual abuse. Survivors of sexual abuse may recreate abusive acts as a way to master the earlier trauma that they have not been able to process. In inpatient treatment the reenactment may take the form of power struggles with staff and peers and attempts to elicit punitive and negative reactions from them. Zahn and Schug write that the earlier relationship between the sexual abuse victim and victimizers was one of power. The victim of sexual abuse has internalized the feelings of powerlessness. In reenacting the trauma, the victim may shift between being victim and victimizer. Both self-abuse and aggressive behaviors result. The sexual abuse survivor may also join with peers who have had similar histories in order to symbolically play out such roles as victims, perpetrator or witness [1–2].

Staff Reactions to Patient with Sexual Abuse Histories

Staff members need a working knowledge of the effect of sexual abuse on children to understand the fears, fantasies, and feelings they may experience in working with them. Kohan and colleagues studied whether certain behaviors were more frequent in children with sexual abuse histories and whether the clinical staff have difficulties in managing these children. Common staff reactions included denial, disgust, restrictions, and punishment. Staff members expressed greater discomfort, particularly fear and anxiety. They often felt angry and uncomfortable with the children's symptomatic behavior, which often included exhibitionism, seductiveness, sex play with others and masturbation. The sexual behavior was hard to understand, and they didn't know how to respond. Staff members didn't know what to do when the children touched them. Although sympathetic, they were simply upset by sexual behavior and frightened of the children's explosive acting out [3–4].

The enormous pain of these survivors and the damage that has been done makes the staff feel helpless and inadequate. The survivor may have learned to sexualize all relationships, leaving the staff member to wonder how to establish a relationship that is appropriate and nonsexual. Rather than directly addressing the child's inappropriate behavior, the staff may avoid the child. These children can elicit feelings of anger and hurt. Staff members often demonstrate many unhelpful responses to the child with a history of sexual abuse. They can unconsciously express disgust and find restrictions and punishment a convenient therapeutic device. They may be puzzled as to what is therapeutic. Not knowing what to do seriously affects the building of therapeutic relationships and communication. This is complicated by the children's own distrust since their earlier trust in persons in their lives was betrayed. Staff members who overcome the relationship barriers may feel that they have rescued the child and their overprotectiveness may then create new barriers in working with the child's parents [4].

MILIEU MANAGEMENT

Some but not all children with a history of sexual abuse continue to act out sexually, and they will need close supervision to prevent it. Many aspects of the environment may need to be rearranged to protect the larger group until the child gains control over sexual behaviors. Staff members must be vigilant about inappropriate pairings of children. Some survivors will be flirtatious, seductive, or exhibitionistic. Those who work in the milieu must be able to understand and contain this behavior, however difficult it is to empathize or understand the child who produces it. These children make the staff angry because they seem to do so little to respond to any attempt to protect them. The staff will require additional training to learn how to handle these overt sexual behaviors. When they don't know how to do this, they are vulnerable to feeling anxious and ineffective, and this lack of self-confidence can lead to many inappropriate actions [4].

These children may seem developmentally arrested because of the sexual abuse, and may benefit from milieu systems that reward them for performance. Others may have become precocious, with adult-pleasing behaviors. Uninformed staff members may inadvertently reinforce this behavior. They may not realize how important it is for these children to interact with peers at an age-appropriate level and build peer support, rather than being thrust into the world of adults and adult sexuality. Some sexual abuse victims will use manipulation and evasion, skills that once helped them to survive their victimization [5].

The anger of sexually abused persons can often be directed inward in a self-destructive manner. They will often require 1:1 staffing to help decrease stimulation and to protect them from self-mutilating or suicidal behaviors. Their acting out has a panic-inducing, exhausting quality because it is not understood. An appropriate environment and an understanding milieu can eventually diminish this need for acting out. The milieu can ultimately give these children the feeling that they are now in a setting that makes sense to them and which, in turn, can understand them [5].

CHARACTERISTICS OF SEXUALLY ABUSED CHILDREN

These children often have low-self esteem. They have little competence in handling feelings or relationships or knowing what's expected of them. Any new relationship may have the potential for further victimization. Making peer relationships or dating will not be easy for them. Their relationships may be inappropriate or destructive. Yet some patients with this history are overcompliant and easy to please. Because they aren't able to share their feelings, they cannot always receive the benefits of a therapeutic relationship. They are likely to be depressed, feel alone and rejected, and believe that no one would understand what they have endured. They feel that their peers will not believe that they have been abused or blame them for it. They often feel that they are to blame for it as well. They can feel damaged, dirty, and guilty. Sexual abuse and its conspiracy of silence only increases their shame. When the child can come to address it with others in the milieu a serious block to building self-esteem is removed. Both boys and girls will be comforted when they learn that this kind of abuse has happened to others and their sense of confusion and anger can be shared. Abused boys need healthy role models for identification and male staff members can be important in teaching about healthy affection and male-female sexual relationships. As treatment progresses, young boys will need trusted staff members who can discuss questions of sexual orientation [5].

Strategies of Treatment

The specific treatment process for survivors of sexual abuse will include improving communication so that they can identify and express the complex feelings that are the result of the trauma. They need help to understand what happened to develop a perspective upon it that neither exaggerates nor minimizes the experience. Bennett believes that sexually abused children will need to find ways to express their rage toward the perpetrator, either by using drawings, writing letters, or making a pretend phone call to the abuser. Helping the child to express anger safely may be an important part of the treatment [5].

Reeves finds that young sexually abused children have not been able to develop a sense of self and that the "roots of selfhood have withered." Those in the milieu must provide a substitute parental caring, with all its immediacy and intensity, as well as the objectivity of the analytic encounter. He describes interpretation through action, with informed responses having to do the same work as insightful interpretations [6].

Expanding the Range of Behaviors

Since all of these problems aren't easily eliminated, Oles recommends that treatment attempt to extend the person's range of behaviors and develop effective behavior rather than trying to directly solve problems. This would help to increase rather than limit the child's behavioral repertoire. The milieu staff can teach the child how to use social support. Social support can decrease feelings of isolation and powerlessness. It can decrease vulnerability and alleviate some of their self-destructive impulses [7].

Conceptualizing the Patient's Difficulties as Post-Traumatic Stress Disorder

Oles finds it helpful to view these patients as suffering from Post-Traumatic Stress Disorder (PTSD). Their traumatic life experiences may be continually reexperienced with symptomatic behaviors until they can successfully integrate the trauma into their life experience. Since these persons are young, their own cognition and defenses are still developing. As these change, they are bound to re-work the trauma, with new understanding and interpretations and more mature defenses. PTSD provides a concept to integrate the work. Abused adolescents can understand that they will be vulnerable to stress, since that is a normal reaction to abuse. This will help them understand what is happening to them. Adolescents also can easily understand that they will be vulnerable to crisis because the trauma of abuse has made them suspicious of others and thus not open to their help. Viewing their problems this way keeps them from feeling guilty and frees them to find new ways to cope. Oles suggests framing the patient's identity as that of a survivor. The word survivor is a hopeful one, describing victims who have worked through the abuse in their lives and then moved on. This helps to take away the feelings of powerlessness [7].

Understanding these behaviors as PTSD is not only beneficial for the patient but will help the staff to know that the patient may not have fully recovered. The staff then understand how the patient may replicate previous destructive relationships in the hopes of gaining some mastery and having it end differently than in childhood. The staff must be alert to potential abusive relationships where the patient can become either perpetrator or a victim. These patients are vulnerable to exploitation and domination by both peers and adults because of their desperate need for security and nurturance. They may have also learned to use their sexuality to influence or manipulate relationships, although this is more prevalent in abusers [7–8].

Gaining support

Sexual abuse victims need to know how to get support from others. The milieu staff can show them that getting support is a good way to start solving problems, modeling ways to make interpersonal connections and get peer support. Sharing feelings and getting help from others will prevent the interpersonal situations that brought about abuse. Support groups will allow disclosure and acceptance and increase the person's feeling of being believed. The group provides a forum for modeling, rehearsing and mastering skills that can help enlist support from the environment. These patients can satisfy their dependency needs in the peer group without the intensity of individual therapy and this will help them to depend on peers rather than adults. It can provide a corrective emotional experience that directly challenges the fear of betrayal. This repeated sharing of painful emotions can provide cognitive and emotional mastery over the abusive events. A group which emphasizes support seeking skills forms the nucleus of a support network after discharge. The formation of the support group in the treatment center is a concrete expression of the program's commitment to openness and mutual support [7–8].

Social Skills training

Social skills training will also help sexually abused persons to expand their repertoire. They will need to understand how they can use these skills to help prevent them from repeating their mistakes. They should learn how to read situations and people clearly, know how to get information and feedback, and how to influence situations. Bennett writes that sexually abused boys often have poor social skills and that assertiveness training will be valuable. These boys must have the opportunity to say no during their hospitalization, for overcompliance can be considered countertherapeutic for the abused child [7–9].

The Adult Survivor of Sexual Abuse

Adult survivors of sexual abuse are often admitted to inpatient treatment because of mood or anxiety disorders, suicidal ideation, or incidents of self-mutilation. The inpatient experience may serve as a place for soothing and respite in a safe therapeutic environment. Despite confidentiality, it can also convert the patient's private information into public information [10].

The well-functioning unit with rules and structure may create terror in the sexual abuse survivor who fears control or manipulation by strangers. The staff must be prepared for intense emotional outbursts. While such outbursts may seem regressive, for these patients they may represent a working through of traumatic memories. Such distinctions will be difficult to make. Managing these episodes can be difficult because every effort should be made to respect the person's interpersonal and physical boundaries. Nor is trust easily earned. In the midst of such turmoil, Dominiak advises that a familiar, calming, and soft voice may help the patient. Milieu staff members will find that their relationships with the sexual abuse survivor are emotionally exhausting, but they should not feel compelled to act as therapists. Their own fresh outlook and practical relationship orientation will benefit the patient. Staff education on techniques of stress management, modulating affect and self-soothing can help members work with the patient to develop ways of controlling these experiences of crisis. Victims of sexual abuse will need a staff that is comfortable addressing issues of self-esteem, and body image and gender. Working with both adolescent and adult patients who have been sexually abused can bring about feelings of disbelief, blaming, repulsion, pity and overprotection. The staff will be continually challenged to offer support and containment that will not repeat the patient's earlier experience of victimization [10].

References

1. Reeves C. The role of milieu therapy in the treatment of sexually abused children. Child & Youth Care Forum 1993 Apr;22(2):111–24.
2. Zahn BS, Schug SE. The survivor's project: a multimodal therapy program for adolescents in residential treatment who have survived child sexual abuse. Residential Treatment for Children & Youth 1993;11(2):65–88.

3. Charles G, Coleman H, Matheson J. Staff reactions to young people who have been sexually abused. Residential Treatment for Children & Youth 1993;11(2):9–21.
4. Kohan MJ, Pothier P, Norbeck JS. Hospitalized children with history of sexual abuse: incidence and care issues. American Journal of Orthopsychiatry 1987;57(2):258–64.
5. Bennett C. Sexually abused boys: Awareness, assessment, and intervention. Journal of Child & Adolescent Psychiatric Nursing 1993 Apr-June;6(2):29–35.
6. See reference 1.
7. Oles TP. Complementing the therapist: Child care work with sexually abused youth. Journal of Child & Youth Care 1991;5(1):43–50.
8. Stanisz MM. A support group for inpatient abused adolescents. Journal of Child & Adolescent Psychiatric Nursing 1991;3(1):14–7.
9. See reference 4.
10. Dominiak GM. Inpatient psychiatric care for victims of sexual abuse. In: Shapiro S, Dominiak GM, eds. Sexual trauma and psychopathology: Clinical intervention with adult survivors. New York: Lexington, 1992, 161–74.

23. Sexual Offenders

Most sexual offenders committed their first offenses during early adolescence. If treatment is to be effective, it will require specific programs which will allow interventions at an early stage. The conventional treatment approach in psychotherapy that encourages the patient to set the therapeutic agenda, stresses confidentiality or places the therapist in an advocate role careful not to impose values on the patient will not work with the sexual offender. Treatment programs must directly address the person's deviant sexual desires and fantasies and try to teach self-control methods so that the offense will not occur again. The thought processes that have brought about sexual offenses and assaultive behaviors must be explored, with the goal of modifying errors of thought and cognitive distortions. The personality deficits that contributed to the person's assault must be explored and treated [1–2] .

CONFIDENTIALITY IN THE TREATMENT PROGRAM

The traditional standards of confidentiality between residents and staff members and various parts of the treatment can't be applied in treatment programs for sexual offenders. This openness among all members is necessary to overcome the denial and secrecy with which aberrant sexual behavior patterns develop [1–2].

BEHAVIORAL GUIDELINES

Certain behavioral guidelines apply to all residents in order to maintain a safe environment, such as no physical assaultiveness and no sexual contact. Some residents need more guidance in order to meet these standards and it is expected that peers as well as staff will identify warning signs until residents can gain more personal control. If both staff and peers set community boundaries, the staff has more time and energy to provide a whole atmosphere of caring [1–2].

Assessment

Assessment of the offender should help to identify the specific personality deficits that relate to the sexual deviance. The staff will need to know if the person has difficulties with social interactions, whether control of anger is a problem, or if there are developmental disorders or substance abuse problems. Beyond this assessment, more needs to be known about the person's own sexuality, sexual arousal, and sexual needs. Offenders may lack basic knowledge of human sexuality [1–2].

A first step is to help the offenders overcome denial and begin to take responsibility for their behavior. Challenging the cognitive distortions that have led them to committing abuse will be of value. They often have serious social deficits and poor coping skills, so work in socializing them in the milieu and practicing social skills with others is helpful. They must be able to develop empathy with others and begin to understand the plight of the victim. A more intensive therapy will explore the person's own history of trauma and victimization and its relationship to present behavior. The program should integrate the family into treatment and both the offender and family need to be aware that there are many risks that the offense will recur again. The support of family and spouse in helping the person meet treatment goals is vital [1–2].

Treatment and the Group Process

The group process usually becomes the primary therapeutic modality in inpatient treatment. The therapist and more experienced group members confront the person's denial of sexual abuse, point out cognitive distortions and wait for the person to accept responsibility. The offenders will initially deny, minimize or give excuses before admitting that they had actually made a choice to commit the sexual offense. Patients discuss their life histories, their own sexuality and aggression in the group, searching for what their lives hold in common and what is unique. The group and the person need to clarify the experiences in which the youth was the perpetrator and when the victim. Many programs explore the offender's own victimization in an attempt to understand later behaviors. Unresolved childhood trauma may have prevented normal attachments and the development of a sense of internalized accountability. If these traumatic experiences can be explored and resolved, the person can move beyond them and be directed toward a normal path of development. Some programs stay away from this approach, since it allows the offender to continue using rationalization and blame. Members should be called upon to examine the sexual assault cycle: their feelings, thoughts, and behaviors before, during and after offenses. They can then practice making interventions to interrupt the cycle in treatment [1–2].

ACCOUNTABILITY

One part of taking responsibility will involve recognition of the harm that has been done and awareness of the damage that sexual abuse brings about. The treatment program can address this in a number of ways, including literature, videotapes, role play, through letters from victims and face-to-face discussion with them. This presentation of the victim's perspective can help develop empathy. Victim reconciliation and reparation are recommended if it can be done. Victim-sensitive therapy should always have reparation to the victim as one of its goals. The orientation to another rather than to the self underlies all the work with the offender. Accountability can be learned from both giving and receiving it. A consistent approach to limit setting will help the residents learn to count on staff for teaching personal accountability. Limits and consequences may vary depending on the resident's individual needs and time in the program. These differences should be carefully explained to the group so the residents can join with the staff in supporting them [1–2].

BEHAVIOR THERAPY

Treatment of the sex offender can be based on social learning principles, using behavior modification to counter what is perceived as learning deviant sexual behavior and reinforcing normative sexual patterns. Behavior therapy may be used to reduce abnormal sexual arousal. By applying the foundations of learning theory, abnormal behavior is extinguished and replaced with socially desirable responses. Behavior therapies generally include social skills acquisition, modeling, role playing therapy, and assertiveness training. Many offenders take aversive conditioning training to decrease their sexual interest in children: pairing shocks with pictures of nude and seminude children. The offender must be helped to determine the kind of external or internal psychological events which precedes or triggers sexually assaultive behavior and learn how to resist and control these compulsions [1–3]

RESOCIALIZATION OF THE SEX OFFENDER

Specific treatment of the offense is absolutely necessary, but resocialization of the person into the human community may also be a key to treatment. Many offenders will need to reexamine their own concept of masculinity and learn to develop relationships that are not involved with intimidation or coercion. The offender will need to learn to express vulnerability in relationships. Many sex offenders really have limited knowledge of the opposite sex and don't respond appropriately. They can seriously misinterpret friendliness from women as a sexual invitation. Increasing social competence through individual and group counseling can help correct social and sexual adjustment problems [4].

Later in treatment, it becomes important for the adolescent not to view his role as a sexual offender as his only identity. While the treatment staff will never minimize the seriousness of these offenses, work also need to be done to provide these adolescents with the opportunity to redefine themselves [4].

Bremeer writes about a successful program with adolescent sexual offenders that works to develop meaningful prosocial child-adult attachment, since this may be the only way that true socialization occurs. These "resocializing" attachments can form only if the community sets clear boundaries, maintains them and is willing to define negotiable areas relevant to any given current population. In the center that Bremeer describes, each staff member, regardless of job description, individually contributes to the growth and development of the residents. Residents are encouraged to develop ways of expressing nonsexual affection with each other and staff. Staff and residents always have the right to check out the meaning of a gesture. The program is devoted to building relationships. Family involvement with the program is also central [5].

Adolescents in this program reported that experiencing a caring relationship and/or identifying and expressing their inner emotional selves was what helped them to change. Other factors reported in follow-up were: gaining a sense of security, learning the meaning of or how to have relationships, and the ability to express feelings and understand and identify with the feelings of others. Bremeer feels that these young men were saying that the key to maintaining a nonabusive lifestyle was the way that they were treated in the program, not the content in and of itself. All program elements described above may exist but won't be effective unless the staff and residents can develop a therapeutic, resocializing relationship [5].

Relapse Prevention

Relapse prevention techniques focus on identifying one's individual pattern of offense and relapse and developing appropriate interventions. Nelson and colleagues describe a cognitive-behavior model to help the sex offender gain control over sexually aggressive behavior. The model identifies the decisions that are made prior to the offense, situations that pose high risks, and the cognitive and emotional precipitants in the offense pattern. Relapse prevention treatment is particularly useful when the patient has a network of social support, family and friends, employers, probation officers and fellow group members who have a thorough knowledge of the pattern and can reinforce appropriate interventions [6].

Although the successful program elements may be clear, they will have stronger effects on some than on others. The sexual offender's deviance is a complex combination of physiological affective, cognitive, social and cultural factors. The type of technique that works for a single person varies widely. For some the social interaction of the group is most curative. For many, behavioral reconditioning techniques redirect their sexuality. Regardless of techniques used specifically to address the sexual behaviors, attention to building attachments and resocialization should gain in importance in the final treatment [7].

Despite the fact that some treatment programs can demonstrate clinically significant improvements in offenders' mental health and personality measures, child molesters are at serious risk of further offenses for many years. Hanson and colleagues studied 197 child molesters from a successful treatment program, and found that 42% had been reconvicted for a sexual offense. Sixty-three per cent of this group were followed for 20 years [8].

References

1. Bremeer JF. Serious juvenile sex offenders: treatment and long-term follow up. Psychiatric Annals 1992;22(6):326–30.
2. Schwartz MF. Sexual compulsivity as Post-Traumatic Stress Disorder: treatment perspectives. Psychiatric Annals 1992;22(6):333–8.
3. Saunders EB, Awad GA. Assessment, management and treatment planning for male adolescent sexual offenders. American Journal of Orthopsychiatry 1988 Oct;58(4):571–9.
4. Scavo R, Buchanan BD. Group therapy for male sex offenders: a model for residential treatment. Residential Treatment for Children & Youth 1989;7(2):59–74.
5. See reference 1.
6. Nelson C, Miner M, Marques J, Russell K, et al. Relapse prevention: A cognitive-behavioral model for treatment of the rapist and child molester. Journal of Social Work & Human Sexuality 1989;7:125–43.
7. See reference 2.
8. Hanson RK, Steffy RA, Gauthier R. Long-term recidivism of child molesters. Journal of Consulting & Clinical Psychology 1993;61(4):648–52.

24. Substance Abuse Disorders

The inpatient treatment of chemical dependence is designed to immediately end drug abuse, begin rehabilitation, and prepare the person for outpatient treatment. This is primarily accomplished by establishing a staff of both recovering addicts and specialists as well as a peer group community that uses techniques similar to outpatient self-help groups. Patient homogeneity is usually necessary in treatment for drug addiction, and those being treated for substance abuse should not be combined with other psychiatric patients [1–2].

Establishing rules for the Unit

If drug units are to operate effectively, rules should be established and each new patient should receive a copy of them. There may be some rules, which when violated, are serious enough to warrant discharge: e.g., drug use or physical violence. Patients are usually expected to submit random urines for drug analysis and comply with various medical precautions. All drug unit staff members in recovery may also be expected to submit urine samples for analysis. There also may need to be a way to screen all visitors for drug addiction. This may require being searched for drugs before a visit or submitting to urine samples. If the program is to be effective, access must be closed to addicted family members or friends who may bring drugs into the unit. The treatment program should have a level system with graduated privileges. The daily schedule should be busy with many periods of activity. This will help to relieve the boredom that can lead to drug craving or subversive behavior and also provides a model for outpatient treatment where expanses of free time should be avoided [1–2].

Admission of Patients

Gallant describes the value of group intake sessions that help to alleviate the individual patient's feelings of alienation and isolation. When three or four patients are admitted at the same time, they do not feel lonely or as threatened by professionals or authority figures. Those admitted together are told that successful treatment will depend on their participating in the group. The patient with the most severe problem is then asked to discuss personal problems of addiction. Group cohesion develops as the other patients identify with the person and also realize that they have something to offer the group. In the program that Gallant describes, the therapist unites the group in a common anxiety situation by describing the physical damage that results from advanced stages of substance abuse. These group sessions proceed more rapidly and more efficiently than individual evaluations and allow little time to elapse between the patient's admission and the beginning of treatment [1–2].

Patients can also be accompanied by other patients at their individual psychological evaluation, where they are asked to bring one or two others whom they trust. Their presence helps to defeat the substance abuser's neurotic defenses, particularly the skilled use of denial because it creates a forum where several substance abusers may discuss their common problems [1–2].

Patient Evaluation and Treatment Goals

The program Gallant describes also asks that patients assist in their own self-evaluations and help staff formulate treatment plans. They become even more involved in their treatment by reading their charts at least once a week and voicing any difference in opinion. To fulfill treatment goals patients must evaluate their own strengths and weaknesses, and be willing to accept the role denial plays not only in alcohol and drug abuse but in their emotional problems. The final goal is to learn to enjoy life without alcohol and drugs. They must also contract for a year of follow-up outpatient treatment in their home clinic. This treatment program uses such techniques as individual and group therapy, assertiveness training, and behavior modification for phobias and anxiety. Marital and family therapy, pastoral counseling and occupational and recreational therapy are also available [1–2].

STAFF

The innovative treatment program that Gallant describes outlines treatment goals for staff members as well as for patients. The four staff treatment goals are to care about patients as individual persons, to listen to them even while disagreeing with their rationale or perceptions, to be completely honest and admit to mistakes, and to convince patients of the staff's ability to diagnose and treat psychiatric disorders and substance abuse. Each staff member learns to function in variety of roles, including serving as group therapist. The staff versatility plus the free services provided by Alcoholics Anonymous and Narcotics Anonymous accounts for much of the program's cost-effectiveness. At discharge patients receive the phone numbers of six key staff members, including the medical director, with permission to call them at home during times of crisis rather than waiting for their next appointment. The patient's family can also call the staff, although no confidential material can be discussed. The staff members' willingness to be called at home illustrates the depth of their commitment [1–2].

EDUCATION

Substance abuse programs should also help patients understand addiction and ways to recover. Addicts learn that they must avoid all addictive substances including marijuana and alcohol. The patient may need to find new peer groups in order to avoid those who use substances. Previous settings that stimulate the urge to use drugs are linked to relapse and must be viewed as dangerous. Patients learn that the inability to control drug use is permanent [1–2].

CREATING THE GROUP PROCESS

Peer groups can be formed if drug patients with similar psychosocial and addictive backgrounds can be grouped together. When possible, they might be grouped according to substance of use, such as heroin, cocaine, or alcohol. A strong peer group may turn out to be the most important element of inpatient substance abuse treatment. Twelve to 16 patients appear to be the optimal number of patients in a viable inpatient peer group. If the unit is larger than that, patients can be divided into smaller groups. Dramatic changes can often be produced by a cohesive group of peers. The staff's effort to develop the peer group often involves facing initial cynicism, rebelliousness, and manipulation. The patients must come face to face with their own responsibility not only for recovery but also for their behavior and attitudes. They learn to attend all meetings, be honest and help each other by caring confrontation. Much of the work is done in group meetings can be run by recovering staff members with professional training [2].

Galanter and colleagues describe a day program for cocaine abusers which combined peer-led self help groups with professional psychiatric service. Thirty-nine per cent of the these patients, a group of serious abusers, had a successful outcome. The groups are managed by patients who had been in the program for several months, with consultation with a counselor who was a recovering addict. Group communication was honest but supportive. There were also seven staff-led groups each week, as well as the "home group," which included the primary therapists and patients in their caseload. The peer-led meetings included a daily session which reviewed each patient and selected the day's theme. There were two groups on relapse prevention, one on stress management and 12-step instructional groups. The 12-step group provided the transition to community reintegration. Two AA groups and Cocaine Anonymous were available in the hospital and three 12-step groups in the community were selected for off-site attendance [3].

Other groups included a self-disclosure group, three-hour encounters, interactional sessions to address patient's relationships with each other, and a community meeting which encouraged patient management of the program's administration. While the peer-led model is a successful treatment in nonmedical facilities, combining it with psychiatric professional services in a hospital setting provided maximal social influence without sacrificing medical and psychiatric services [3].

Peers in adolescent drug treatment become the primary agents of change. The relationship with peers is of greater significance to adolescents than those with the administration or staff. Peers are less threatening and usually immune from the negative transference adolescents often have toward adults. Peers who have made progress in treatment can serve as models of self-control. Ex-addict staff members present other positive aspects for role modeling. They seem organized and decisive and seem to have the answers. Confused adolescents are easily impressed by someone who shows a strong sense of identity and can give them direction and purpose. Sometimes peers are tougher with each other than the staff would be, but coercive peer authority may produce only token adherence to rules and superficial behavior change. The adolescent's personality difficulties and basic conflicts will then stay hidden rather than be resolved [4].

Numerous daily groups are the most important aspect of patient rehabilitation These may be open-ended groups or groups devoted toward a particular patient or treatment issue. Drug groups should have a similar philosophy as outpatient self-help groups such as Cocaine Anonymous, Narcotics or Alcoholics Anonymous. These groups have a strong belief system than can provide patients with a sense of meaning, purpose and direction for their lives. It tells them what to believe and how to behave. Everyone in the program is positive about what is right and what is wrong, which gives them a strong direction and purpose. This can be irresistible to someone who is lost and floundering [4].

MILIEU COUNTERTRANSFERENCE

Substance abusers with severe character pathology can evoke intense staff countertransference. Instead of trying to analyze it or avoid the person, it will be more helpful to simply maintain a limit-setting stance rather than therapeutic abdication in order to counteract dangerous and manipulative behavior [5].

Experience and research have indicated that the two most important elements for continued therapeutic progress for an adolescent treatment program are identification with a positive peer group and commitment to continuing helpful physical activity. Progress in treatment for older patients is based on the development of internal motivation for recovery, honest self-disclosure and commitment to outpatient treatment. In some cases hospitalization is the only intervention powerful enough to end the active cycle of addiction [6].

References

1. Gallant DM. Gold Award: Individualized treatment for substance abusers. Hospital & Community Psychiatry 1984 Nov;35(11):1141–4.
2. Davis CA, Gold MS, Estroff TW. Inpatient treatment of addiction. In: American Psychiatric Association Task Force on Treatments of Psychiatric Disorders. Treatments of psychiatric disorders. v. 2. Washington, DC: American Psychiatric Press, 1989, 1359–78.
3. Galanter M, Egelko S, De Leon G, Rohrs C. A general hospital day program combining peer-led and professional treatment of cocaine abusers. Hospital & Community Psychiatry 1993 Jul;44(7):644–9.
4. Rachmann AW, Heller ME. Peer group psychotherapy with adolescents drug abusers. International Journal of Group Psychotherapy 1976;26(3):373–84.
5. Imhof J, Hirsch R, Terenzi E. Countertransferential and attitudinal considerations in the treatment of drug abuse and addiction. International Journal of the Addictions 1983;18(4):491–520.
6. Brock TF. A model adolescent hospital-based program. In: Lawson GW, Lawson AW, eds. Adolescent substance abuse: etiology, treatment and prevention. Gaithersburg, MD: Aspen,1992,105–119.

25. Substance Abuse Treatment in the Therapeutic Community

Therapeutic communities provide the most comprehensive form of drug abuse treatment. This section will focus primarily on the comprehensive therapeutic community model in long-term treatment, particularly the treatment model that has been successful at therapeutic communities, such as Phoenix House or Daytop Village. Clients with a wide variety of emotional disorders, including serious character disorders, can be successfully treated in a therapeutic community that assimilates the person into a community that shares expectations and values. The primary therapist or teacher is the therapeutic community itself: peers and staff who are role models of successful change and serve as guides in the recovery process. The community provides a 24-hour learning experience in which individual changes in attitudes, behaviors, and emotions can be observed and mutually reinforced [1].

A Belief System

The therapeutic community offers a systematic approach which is guided by shared beliefs about substance abuse, recovery and right living. Therapeutic communities usually share a belief about personality change. It may have various names, but it is often referred to by members of these programs as the Concept, a belief system with a statement of philosophy that members recite, mottoes, and its own language. The belief system gives the members meaning and direction. Everyone in the program feels positive about these beliefs that can change the lives of substance abusers who are lost and floundering. Repetition of the belief is important. The concept of recovery and the right ways to live are continuously repeated in various aspects of the program [1–3].

In most therapeutic communities, it is believed that the problem is not just the use of drugs. Drug abuse is indicative of arrested personality development or chronic deficits in social and educational skills, and involves all areas of functioning. Thinking may be unrealistic. The person may lack a system of values. The community usually shares a concept of what constitutes the healthy person and shares such values as a belief in work, honesty, personal accountability, concern and responsibility for others [1–3].

The Craving for Drugs

The physiological withdrawal from drugs is given little sympathetic attention in the therapeutic communities that DeLeon and colleagues describe. The person is simply encouraged to tolerate it until it gets better. The community must also address the resident's psychological craving for drugs, and may use various behavioral techniques: ignoring (extinction), distraction (interruption, or blocking) or response competition. The residents may be allowed to talk about their desire for drugs, but this is then either ignored (extinction), blocked (told not to think about them), or they are told to try new behaviors and new thoughts (running or exercise). Since drug users seem to have very little tolerance for discomfort, the therapeutic community gives tolerance training. This involves raising the person's tolerance level and developing alternative behaviors for reducing or avoiding discomfort through positive or less self-defeating responses. The person develops awareness of the chain of cognitive and behavioral events which reflect poor tolerance. A primary technique for increasing tolerance is to delay expected outcomes or rewards so that the person can come to deal with uncertainty, frustration, or disappointment [1–3].

SOCIAL LEARNING

Changes in the person can occur only in the social context. What is learned is identified with the people involved in the learning process, peers and staff, as credible role models. Key staff, who are recovered addicts are visible role models who illustrate the possibility of personal change. Without new social connections, new ways of coping are threatened by isolation and its potential for relapse. The therapeutic community structure builds the individual's identification with the community of others and relationships of mutual responsibility. The principal aim of the therapeutic community is a total change in the way the person lives. This will mean radically altering the patterns of feeling, thinking and behaving that lead to drug use. The community will promote abstinence and the elimination of antisocial activity, and the resident is helped to develop prosocial attitudes and prepare for useful work in society. The residents are taught to develop awareness of their own feelings, learn to express them and also to manage them so they will no longer lead to drug use or self-defeating behaviors [1–3].

One interesting technique is called "acting as if." Residents are asked to behave as if they are the person they should be rather than the persons they have been. That is, they act as if the problem is resolved. This helps change both current beliefs and perception of the problem and may finally result in actual behavior change. The cognitive and emotional changes that occur from "acting as if" can make the behavior permanent. The changed self-image and the feelings that accompany it often follow rather than precede the permanent change in behavior. This is based on the belief that a socially responsible role comes from acting it out. This technique does not overlook the necessity for insight to change behavior. DeLeon and colleagues state that insight is insufficient without felt experience and somehow "acting as if" can accomplish it [1–3].

MUTUAL SELF-HELP

The broad goal of recovery in the therapeutic community can be achieved only through mutual self-help. Treatment of the whole person requires a 24-hour observation of behavior as well as credible and constant feedback to make changes. All persons in the therapeutic community serve as both trainees and trainers. The core elements in the mutual self-help process are

> *Confrontation and responsible concern:* Community members confront each other about their attitudes and behavior, but with caring and concern, as a way of taking responsibility for others.

Feedback: Feedback can be both positive and negative and is usually about changes in attitudes and behavior.

Support: Support is given to keep trying and to stay in the program and is also given indirectly by identifying with others in the change process [1–3].

Role Models

The addict's lack of stable identity can best be overcome by providing role models, the residents who have progressed in the program. Role models help to train others and new residents change their behaviors by imitating and identifying with them. Their success in the program gives others hope. They can make contrasts between their present and earlier behaviors. The role model's own behaviors and attitudes are reinforced when they teach others. Role models instill motivation and provide hope for change [1–3].

Therapeutic Community Structure

The therapeutic community structure helps to provide a stable environment for those who have come from the chaotic world of addiction. A demanding schedule helps to combat boredom, negative peer groups, and preoccupation with drugs. Activities usually include classes, seminars, training, and work. Morning meetings bring everyone together to begin the day with optimism. These meetings may include singing, readings, and recitation of the therapeutic community philosophy. Although individual differences are recognized, all residents usually follow the same activity schedule [1–3].

Privileges and Sanctions

Privileges are rewards that reinforce achievement. They are awarded for behavior, attitude change, job performance and overall clinical progress. Privileges can be lost by negative attitudes or inappropriate behavior, but can be earned back when improvement is shown. They are not just given but are earned and earning them requires an investment of time and energy and attempts to change. The privilege system is related to clinical progress and time in the program. It may begin with phone privileges and progress to frequent weekend passes. Sanctions are used to preserve safety and health and teach healthy interactions. In the therapeutic community everyone usually has the duty to see that rules are enforced [1–3].

Group Activities

DeLeon and Rosenthal describe four forms of group activities in the therapeutic community: encounters, tutorials, probes, and marathons. Encounters use confrontations to change attitudes and behaviors. They are used to manage individual and interpersonal difficulties as well as provide an emotional catharsis. Experienced members participate in a more advanced form of encounter where the group vigorously and repeatedly attacks antisocial, self-defeating, and immature behaviors. The targeted member's only defense is honesty. Probes are directed toward psychological insight. Marathons are longer group sessions used to help the person resolve life experiences. Tutorials are used for teaching and training. Both positive and negative pressure to change influence recovery; the pressure of the group continuously strengthens motivation [1–3].

WORK ASSIGNMENTS

Work assignments, usually arranged in a hierarchy, provide both education and therapy. The residents move through a series of jobs that acquaint them with every part of the community. It is essentially an arrangement for upward mobility. Job assignments begin with the most menial tasks but can lead to management levels. Residents can come as patients and leave as staff. Job mobility is an effective therapeutic tool, providing a measure of the resident's growth and further incentives for change. Mobility is based not only on work performance but also on how well the resident has assimilated the community's teaching. Each job level represents a broadly defined behavioral repertoire that indicates competence at that level. DeLeon notes that progression in work assignments resembles mobility in the real world, but in the therapeutic community the resident can fail safely and be able to try again [1–3].

The Therapeutic Community Staff

The therapeutic community's staff is in a position of authority, monitoring the residents' behavior, supervising the groups, making and supervising work assignments. The staff makes decisions on the resident's treatment plan, status, promotion, and discharge. Staff members are expected to train, guide and correct, rather than punish or control. Supporting, correcting and protecting are their primary functions. They will give reasons for their decisions and explain the meanings of consequences. Because of their own experience with recovery, they have strong credibility. [1–3].

The family atmosphere created in the therapeutic community leaves little room for professional distance. Personal lives are not immune from scrutiny. Even staff members are expected to keep few secrets about their lives or feelings. In adolescent substance abuse treatment, the residents often develop strong dependence on the staff. This intimacy with residents is actually much more demanding than relationships with peers [4].

Therapeutic Communities for Adolescents

Although the model described was designed for adult drug abusers, it has been modified for adolescents. There can be many variations on therapeutic community principles for adolescent substance abusers. One of the advantages of the therapeutic community for this age group is the possibility of building peer relationships within a community that provide feedback and confrontation. The staff and peers will point out the adolescents' difficulties in relating to others and the group process can teach them how to improve interpersonal relationships. They will be able to make friendships that will support them in abstinence [4].

CRITIQUES OF THE THERAPEUTIC COMMUNITY

Drug treatment programs have a high drop-out rate and the motivation and work required in the therapeutic community may quickly drive away the less-motivated. This is unfortunate since there is a strong relationship between time spent in the program and successful outcome. Cohen reports that 3/4 of residents may leave before graduating from the program. Sexuality is a problem in the therapeutic community since it is difficult to develop close relationships and at the same time prevent sexual acting out [4–5].

The belief system sustains motivation and helps the person who feels lost in life, but it may also be inflexible and rigid. The belief system defines what is healthy and insists that everyone match this. There is a danger of coercion in producing conformity to the belief system. The individual person's own growth in discovering a philosophy and a way to live is thwarted. There may be a real concern about preserving democracy and freedom in these programs [4–5].

Discussion

The therapeutic community has many features that are worth emulating. None of its features have been tested independently but as a comprehensive program it produces successful outcomes. Many therapeutic communities have an admission policy that eliminates those with low motivation, so that admission becomes an achievement in itself. These communities often have a strong leader who takes authority and makes decisions. Rehabilitation remains the personal responsibility of the resident who will also benefit from the mutual assistance of the community. There is a therapeutic community quotation that says that the person alone can do it, but can't do it alone. Structure and discipline and constant observation are powerful treatment forces. The resident learns through positive and negative reinforcement and is given the opportunity for rising in the hierarchy, and taking on work assignments with more responsibility and privileges [5].

Treatment in an ideal therapeutic community focuses upon the whole person. Drug dependence involves all aspects of the person: psychological, educational, biomedical, emotional, and spiritual. Many therapeutic activities are needed: behavioral management, attention to the psychological and emotional life, nurturing of the intellectual, spiritual and ethical life, as well as work and vocation [6].

The community functions as an extended family that absorbs the new person and provides a new beginning. The person is separated from what was probably a toxic society, and introduced to new values of responsibility, honesty and nonviolence. The therapeutic community differs from other substance abuse programs in that drug abstinence is only the beginning. It focuses instead on the behaviors that brought about and maintain substance abuse. The resocialization process helps the person develop trust in the self and others, and know how to seek help and support while still assuming personal responsibility. From active involvement in such a community, the person can escape from the isolation and self-absorption of chemical dependency into interdependence and true concern for others [7].

References

1. DeLeon G. The therapeutic community and behavioral science. International Journal of the Addictions 1990–91;25:1537–57
2. DeLeon G. Psychopathology and substance abuse: what is being learned in therapeutic communities. Journal of Psychoactive Drugs 1989;21(2):177–88.
3. DeLeon G, Rosenthal MS. Treatment in Residential Therapeutic Communities. In: American Psychiatric Association Task Force on Treatments of Psychiatric Disorders. Treatments of mental disorders. v. 2. Washington, DC: American Psychiatric Association, 1989, 1379–96.
4. Rachmann AW, Heller ME. Peer group psychotherapy with adolescent drug abusers. International Journal of Group Psychotherapy 1976;26(3):373–84.
5. Cohen S. Therapeutic communities for substance abusers. Drug Abuse & Alcoholism Newsletter 1982 Feb;11(2):unpaged.
6. Deitch DA, Solit R. Training drug abuse treatment personnel in therapeutic community ideologies. Psychotherapy 1993 Sum;30(2):305–16.
7. Hulbert RJ. In the spotlight: The Iowa therapeutic community model of chemical dependency treatment. Journal of Substance Abuse Treatment 1992;9:389–93.

26. Tourette's Syndrome

Persons with Tourette's Syndrome are usually not hospitalized. However, the behavioral and social problems that develop in association with the syndrome may require special attention in inpatient treatment. Persons with Tourette's Syndrome are often impulsive and hyperactive, often have obsessions and compulsions, and may be aggressive. They have motor, phonic, or verbal tics which have no purpose. The motor tics may include grimacing, jaw snapping, eye blinking or winking, and general restlessness. They experience rapid, repetitive and involuntary muscular movements and involuntarily utter sounds or words. Tourette's can often be controlled by medication [1].

The inpatient with Tourette's will require structure, behavior management, and education. The person must be carefully educated about the illness and be able to distinguish somehow what is the illness and what is the self. If the initial onset of some of the symptoms can be identified, there may be better ways to establish control. Education will be of help in developing more effective coping [1].

STRUCTURE

Structure will organize the patient's day and time. A specific time schedule for daily activities with steps for settling down in the evening will provide a way to progressively decrease stimulation, with the bedtime schedule including quiet time, a bath, reading, radio time, medication. Structure may include interventions such as establishing contracts for behavior and hygiene that will establish a mutual agreement for the desired behaviors and consequences for non-compliance. The patient can be helped to improve behavior and reach treatment goals with the help of a point plan, which allows the purchase of treats and privileges with points accumulated for behavior. Time-outs may be established to allow the patient to gain control and reduce overstimulation. A sign-in with the staff every hour or half hour will assure contact, and allows the staff to monitor behavior and safety. There will be times when the staff member needs to stay with the patient to prevent aggressive, impulsive or self-destructive behaviors [1].

Patients will benefit from interactions with peers in the milieu and there will be hope that in this environment, acceptance will come once some of the unusual behaviors that characterize the illness are understood. Tourette's is a chronic illness and the patient's response to treatment will be slow [1].

References

1. Rosner TA, Pollice SA. Tourette's syndrome. Journal of Psychosocial Nursing & Mental Health Services 1991 Jan;29(1):4–9.

27. The Young Adult Patient

The young adult patient is now often referred to as the young adult chronic patient and is described as part of a rapidly growing population in the United States. Some distinctions should be made, however, between the literature that addresses the problems of the young adult chronic patient and the programs that are designed for this population that do not presume chronicity. Most of the literature on the young adult chronic population describe patients who are psychotic, substance abusers or have severe character disorders.

The young adult is called upon to complete many life tasks: consolidating identity development, achieving intimacy with others who may become life partners, and selecting a vocation. A hospital program for this population must recognize all of these tasks and, in addition to addressing the emotional issues, help the person embark in these directions. Tashjian described the treatment of young adults as reparative and preparative. The reparative work is usually done in individual psychotherapy and in family therapy addressed to helping the young adult become independent. Hoffman and Mastrianni describe a program that uses an association with a nearby college to help young adult patients reach age-appropriate developmental levels and make the transition from the hospital to an educational setting [1–2].

Many writers feel that young adults are not well served in units designed for adolescents. While adolescents seem primarily concerned with challenging limits and authority, young adults are more concerned with self-definition, autonomy and life direction. They respond better to a more flexible structure, since a rigid discipline would deny them the opportunity to experiment, synthesize and work through to consolidated identity. The program should provide a broader playing field for experimentation. The young clinical staff can provide models for identification and patient-staff relationships can provide a growth-promoting structure. The staff's emotional investment should remain stable despite the wide fluctuations in the functioning of these patients [3].

Patient meetings or group therapy can serve as a foundation for the treatment. Young adults can benefit from these experiences in socialization, can learn that they share common problems, and can overcome their own feelings of isolation. Other groups may also address such issues as independent living, socialization, and leisure. Independent living groups can help the patient learn to obtain information about getting housing or how to budget. Leisure groups can help patients become aware of resources for leisure and help them develop their ability to use free time [3].

In order to manage the self-destructive behavior of many of young adult patients, the program may be designed around a level system. This can provide a predictable environment for patients who lack inner controls. The issues of living together can be discussed in daily community meetings and group discussion about each person's status and therapeutic passes can contribute to their progress through the program. Snyder found that although a level system at first seemed more suitable for use with adolescents, the young adult patients felt a sense of accomplishment and success working through the levels. This seemed to increase their independence and self-assurance [3].

Psychotherapeutic treatment goals will vary with the patient but many will need to learn to stop their self-defeating and self-destructive behaviors and increase their ability to tolerate anxiety and postpone gratification. Developmental goals will be shared with other patients in the program. They will need to accept increased responsibility and become self-reliant and develop a secure sense of self and autonomy [3].

Many young adults will need treatment for substance abuse. If this cannot be accomplished within the treatment center, relationships should be maintained with substance abuse programs and referrals made to Alcoholics and Narcotics Anonymous groups.

LIFE-SKILLS TRAINING

If any of the above goals are to be maintained, patients will require life skills training. The goals of this training would be to help the patient explore vocational interests and aptitudes, learn how to apply for jobs, find housing and learn how to live independently. These goals can only begin to be met in the hospital and further training through adult education and enrollment in vocational schools may be necessary. Such basic skills as balancing a checkbook, preparing and practicing for a job interview, shopping and cooking may be all that can be accomplished in a short-term program. Students should also be encouraged to study for and take the G.E.D. if they have not graduated from high school [3].

THE DIFFICULT YOUNG ADULT PATIENT

Gallop turns attention to the difficult, chronic young adult patient with severe ego deficits in impulse control, affect modulation and reality testing. These patients may abuse drugs, present as angry, verbally and physically abusive. They are demanding and overdependent on the hospital but are nevertheless noncompliant with treatment. They require an active and caring milieu which can offer containment. Such short-term units will have specific treatment objectives and time limits. They will need to know their discharge date and be reminded of it regularly. The hospitalization helps to design a plan which will use community resources to meet remaining treatment needs [4–5].

There must be baseline boundaries for behavior, a predictable structure and clear expectations for patients stated with clearly defined consequences when the patient is admitted. If these are not set immediately, clinical responses may be arbitrary or the staff will be accused of being brutal and sadistic. Gallop believes that individual treatment should still have consistent broad-based rules to guarantee a safe environment. Patients should understand that self-destructive acts can result in discharge or transfer to a locked facility [4–5].

Hospitalization usually occurs during the acute phase of treatment, and the patient should plan how it will be used. The treatment should address the healthy nonregressed part of the young adult. Treatment for these patients requires careful discharge planning for the next step and an examination of the social supports which will be available in their future environment. These patients may be readmitted to the unit many times in their careers and they can be reminded of its future availability to help counteract their feelings of abandonment [4–5].

References

1. Tashjian LD. Treatment programs for the young adult. Journal National Association Private Psychiatric Hospitals 1979;10(3):17–19.
2. Hoffman FL, Mastrianni X. The hospitalized young adult: new directions in psychiatric treatment. American Journal of Orthopsychiatry 1992;61(2):297–302.

3. Snyder S. Comprehensive inpatient treatment for the young adult patient. Occupational Therapy in Mental Health 1985;5(2):47–58.
4. Gallop R. Difficult young adult chronic patients: Re-evaluating short-term clinical management. Journal of Psychosocial Nursing & Mental Health Services 1986 Mar;24(3):29–32.
5. Lehman A, Zastowny T, Kane C, DiMartino E. Intensive inpatient treatment of young adult chronic patients. Psychiatric Quarterly 1986–87 Fall;58(3):167–9.

CHAPTER

VII

Problems in the Psychiatric Milieu

Many problems in the inpatient milieu present interesting intellectual challenges—problems such as manipulation or splitting. Others demonstrate that even in the structure of the psychiatric hospital, human interaction cannot be controlled. A review of the literature about problems over the decades reveals that although the literature records substantial progress, many problems still remain. The problem of violence has accumulated the most extensive body of literature. A few writers, Felthous, Morrison, and Katz and Kirkland have applied cultural, behavioral and organizational analysis to the problem and suggest new, more hopeful solutions. The literature on self-wounding and self-cutting has led the way to increased understanding in the last decade. There is greater freedom to discuss problems such as sexuality or institutional abuse. There are times when the answers to problems are not techniques that the milieu staff alone can carry out—anger control training, for example. However, it will still be comforting to know that there are answers and that both patients and the milieu staff could receive specific training to solve some longstanding problems.

1. AIDS: Protecting Psychiatric Patients from HIV Infection

This section discusses problems that may occur for staff and patients in the face of the difficulties posed by HIV infection. It does not provide medical information but merely discusses the precautionary measures that should be taken. For information about the milieu treatment of patients with AIDS, the reader should consult the section in Chapter VI on milieu techniques for specific populations.

HIV infection is higher in psychiatric inpatients than in the general population. AIDS education should be integrated into milieu programs, particularly for treatment centers that serve adolescents, substance abusers, and chronic psychiatric patients. These sessions should be modified to meet the educational and intellectual levels of all patients, and given frequently, whether or not there are known HIV-infected patients in the hospital [1–2].

Training can include a variety of activities, such as viewing videotapes with subsequent discussions, guest speakers on safer sex practices that reduce risk, and special groups conducted by staff members. Card and colleagues find interactive video an effective educational process for teaching about AIDS. The videos could be viewed in private, with multiple choice questions following the presentation. The program reinforced correct responses and provided further information for incorrect responses until correct answers were given. Goldstein and Yuen describe some special techniques used in a treatment center for substance abuse. Female residents received special sessions informing them of their own ability to control the outcome of their own future sexual encounters. The medical staff distributed condoms in weekend kits with illustrated written instructions and were available to answer personal questions on condoms or sex education. Condom distribution may be a questionable practice in some treatment centers, since it gives the message of condoning sexual behavior, even when it is against the rules. But the rules must be balanced against the threat of HIV infection [3–5].

Patients are often seriously misinformed and fearful of contracting AIDS, so another goal of an education program is to counsel patients that there is no risk from getting AIDS by participating in regular daily activities with HIV-positive persons. The staff should be aware that the fear of AIDS can become a part of the individual's psychopathology or delusional system and proceed with care [6].

PATIENTS WITH CHRONIC MENTAL ILLNESS

Persons with severe mental illness may remain unconcerned about the risks of AIDS transmission and continue risky sexual activities. Graham and Cates, while recognizing that educational efforts will not be guaranteed effective, suggest a videotape format for this population, followed by questions and discussion. The videos should provide simple, straightforward information. They report that viewers identified positively with videos that showed persons in potentially at-risk situations. Videos opened up topics for discussion. For example, the authors reported that no discussion of oral sex had occurred until it was mentioned on the videotape. Effective programs for these chronic patients are simple, concrete, and nonjudgmental. Because they may have short attention spans and high anxiety, they respond best to brief programs, no longer than 20 or 30 minutes. The videotapes should lead in to questions from the viewers and staff members should be prepared to respond to pathological or eccentric responses. In addition to providing education, the staff should assess the patients' own risk status and ability to implement the health practices they have learned [7–8].

Kalichman and colleagues describe a group prevention program consisting of 4 weekly sessions, 90 minutes each. The first session, on videotape, reviewed information about HIV transmission and risky behaviors. A group discussion followed, which covered AIDS myths and testing. Group members were asked to analyze what triggered their own risky behaviors, such as substance abuse, coercion by others, or depression. The second session helped members to develop skills to reduce risks and included condom demonstrations. The third session helped group members learn to resist a partner's coercion to engage in unprotected sex. The final session reviewed materials and skills learned [9].

Staff

It should never be presumed that all staff members have received appropriate education about AIDS. Staff education should include formal training, updates and refresher courses, to build a permanent foundation for AIDS education. Staff fears of contagion usually diminish with education, time, and experience. Inservice sessions are necessary but staff members also need psychological support to enable them to work successfully with AIDS patients. Support groups that will allow them to voice their many emotional reactions in working with patients will be of great help. Individual supervision should explore these topics and the staff member's countertransference in working with these patients. Nonjudgmental acceptance of staff feelings will establish an atmosphere of trust and comfort. If staff members don't feel comfortable in expressing their feelings of terror or hostility they won't be able to understand their origin and work through them [10].

The Duty to Warn

If it is suspected that AIDS patients are having unprotected sex with persons outside the hospital, the staff will face a very difficult situation. All attempts should be made to persuade patients of the need to inform sexual partners of their condition. Professional associations now suggest that in a situation where the patient will not inform such persons, the clinician may need to violate the patient's confidentiality to protect another person. Guidelines from the American Psychiatric Asociation indicate that if the psychiatrist has received reliable information that a patient infected with HIV is engaging in behaviors that place persons at risk, the psychiatrist should seek the patient's agreement to stop and to inform the other persons. If there is evidence that the patient has not done this, it is ethically permissible for the psychiatrist to notify identifiable persons at risk or arrange for public health authorities to do so. If there are unidentifiable persons at risk, it is also ethically permissible to notify public health authorities. In some therapeutic communities for substance abuse, special information nights for sexual partners are arranged to provide information on prevention and discuss how the HIV infection is transmitted. This provides general information and does not specifically reveal the health status of a specific patient [11–12].

PROTECTING PATIENTS AND STAFF

Psychiatric patients who enter the treatment center are not screened for HIV, so that any patient who has sexual relations in the hospital may be at risk. Patients who are in a state of sexual hyperarousal, such as those in a manic state, may require continuous surveillance. Given the extreme risk to patients, Davies advises a change in British law to permit HIV screening in the psychiatric hospital. Volavka and colleagues report that their findings on the seroprevalance rate among high-risk patients was sufficient to suggest that an HIV antibody screening test is warranted for consenting, newly admitted psychiatric patients. They feel that newly emerging treatments for HIV infections make such a treatment program morally imperative [13–14].

All patients and staff must be considered potentially at risk for transmitting or receiving HIV infection. Basic standards of care include: implementing and monitoring infection control procedures, education and supportive services for patients, families, and staff, and appropriate management in the treatment center of emotional, cognitive and behavioral disturbances to reduce risk for both patients and staff. If a patient engages or threatens to engage in behavior placing others at risk for HIV infection, appropriate steps must be taken to control this behavior, including isolation or restraint. Adequate supervision must insure that all patients, regardless of HIV status, are not able to engage in behavior that could transmit HIV [15].

HOSPITAL RESOURCES

The staff should be trained in universal precautions for handling blood and body fluids, and gloves and other protective barriers should be available. Assaultive patients need to be handled in ways that minimize the risk of HIV infection. Assaultive or hypersexual patients may require 1:1 supervision. The hospital staff should be consciously aware of all new research findings in order to provide resources more effectively in organizing HIV care.

References

1. Volavka J, Convit A, O'Donnell J, Douyon R, et al. Assessment of risk behaviors of HIV infection among psychiatric inpatients. Hospital & Community Psychiatry 1992 May;43(5): 482–5.
2. Forstein M, Baer J. HIV infection. In: Sederer LI, ed. Inpatient psychiatry: Diagnosis and treatment. 3rd ed. Baltimore: Williams and Wilkins, 1991,189–211.

3. Card CAL, Jacobsberg LB, Mofatt M, Fixman B, et al. Using interactive video to supplement HIV counseling. Hospital & Community Psychiatry 1993 Apr;44(4):383–5.
4. Goldstein ML, Yuen FM. Coping with AIDS: An approach to training and education in a therapeutic community—The Samaritan Village Program. Journal of Substance Abuse Treatment 1988;5(1):45–50.
5. Cournos F, Hempfield M, Horwath E, Schrage H. HIV infection in state hospitals: Case reports and long-term management strategies. Hospital & Community Psychiatry 1990 Feb;41(2):163–6.
6. See reference 2.
7. Graham LL, Cates JA. How to reduce the risk of HIV infection for the seriously mentally ill. Journal of Psychosocial Nursing & Mental Health Services 1992 Jun;30(6):9–13.
8. Steiner J, Lussier R, Rosenblatt W. Knowledge about and risk factors for AIDS in a day hospital population. Hospital & Community Psychiatry 1992 Jul;43(7):734–7.
9. Kalichman SC, Sikemma KJ, Kelly JA, Bulton M. Use of a brief behavior skills intervention to prevent HIV infection among chronic mentally ill adults. Psychiatric Services 1995 Mar; 46(3):275–80.
10. Hoffman BF, Arthurs K, Lunn S, Meyers L, et al. AIDS: Clinical and ethical issues on a psychiatric unit. Canadian Journal of Psychiatry 1989 Dec;34(12):847–51.
11. American Psychiatric Association. Commission on AIDS. AIDS Policy: Position Statement on Confidentiality, Disclosure, and Protection of Others. American Journal of Psychiatry 1993 May;150(5):852.
12. Carroll JFX. Working with drug dependent residents with AIDS/ARC in a therapeutic community. Alcoholism Treatment Quarterly 1988;5(3/4):163–89.
13. Davies DR. HIV and the psychiatric hospital. (Letter). British Journal of Psychiatry 1987;150:881–2.
14. See reference 1.
15. Silverman DC. Psychosocial impact of HIV-related caregiving on health providers: A review and recommendations for the field of psychiatry. American Journal of Psychiatry 1993 May;150(5):852.

2. Anger and Hostility in the Milieu

Anger is inevitable in inpatient treatment, and is perhaps more pervasive in treatment settings for children and adolescents than for adults. Cramerus writes that adolescent units usually include a large number of angry rebellious adolescents who treat staff members with hostile devaluation, mockery and negativism. Felicetti distinguishes between noninterpersonal anger and highly interpersonal anger in the treatment milieu, and describes the latter as being more potentially destructive. This anger can be threatening, and can easily target the staff member's own insecurities and uncertainties. It can also be used to manipulate. Felicetti then asks where anger goes. He describes each treatment facility as possessing an atmosphere that, though intangible, can be felt immediately. The anger doesn't happen and then disappear, but it can just sit there, or ripple through the community making staff members feel a little angry, a bit depressed, questioning of their own competence or the competence of others. Anger can be buried or displaced or put on the alert for scapegoats. Felicetti recommends that the staff member back away from anger once it occurs and the problem is resolved, and then try to figure out what issues the patient is raising, what is being said on the surface and what is really being said, and then ask if there is something that can be done better next time [1–2].

UNDERSTANDING HOSTILITY, ANGER AND AGGRESSION

Children and adolescents placed in a treatment center often have rage at being expelled by the family, and rage at the family itself whose neglect allowed this to happen. Anger and aggression also become their normal way to handle a variety of feelings—frustration, inadequacy, depression or hopelessness. Staff members who are the blameless recipients of this anger will feel confused but may also feel angry and punitive themselves. However, they must address it. If the child's anger and the staff members' anger are ignored, they cannot be dealt with effectively. If children are taught not to express their anger, passive-aggressive behavior may replace it, or they may hold this anger until returning to their family where they may express it more violently. This is not to say that anger and aggression must not be controlled in inpatient treatment. Aggressive outbursts can create a chaotic environment and can also lead to premature discharge and no treatment at all. There must be some effective outlet for angry feelings. Children need to be able to deal with anger in the healthiest possible way, and be able to safely process their angry experiences and its effect on others. The treatment program must provide a variety of ways to help children identify, express and finally channel this anger so that it does not stand in the way of the other therapeutic progress that they need to make [3].

Understanding anger and aggression requires work by both staff and patients. Staff members must realize that some of this anger results from the feeling of powerlessness and that ventilating hostility may decrease the person's feelings of vulnerability. Hostility may also take other forms. The person may withdraw, physically or by silence, to protect against rage or destructive behavior. Passive-aggressive behavior is the indirect expression of anger. Noncompliance with treatment may give the patient a feeling of revenge or power. Hostility can also be expressed through somatic illness, or even in exaggerated opposites—being excessively compliant or ingratiatingly polite. Anger is also expressed through displacement or projection, directed to the wrong target or attributed to another person [4].

How should the staff member respond to hostility? Least effective is responding in kind. Keeping in mind that hostility is often a form self-protection may help. When confronted with an angry person, the staff should remove other patients from the area. This can be done by enlisting the help of others through a prearranged code. Staff members should try to learn why the patient is angry, redirecting the focus on the patient's problems rather than on the desire to act out the anger. However, in order to learn this, the staff member should not use questions beginning with the word, "why," since for some reason such questions tend to provoke even more anger. The staff member should give brief and clear instructions to the angry person, but also be willing to discuss options, such as going to another area, making a telephone call, discussing the situation with another person who might help. However, staff members must not make promises they can't keep just to solve a situation; nor should they threaten the patient with further actions or consequences [4–5].

It is best to be personal, stressing acquaintance with the person, using words that anticipate possible cooperation, demonstrating concern and a willingness to listen. Appropriate responses will encourage the person to talk. The patient's problems should not be minimized. The staff member who tries to remain calm must not overreact by being cold and neutral, but should attempt to match the mood, the level of emotional exchange without being angry. Being cold and neutral and not matching the person's mood will serve to merely increase anger because the person may escalate in the absence of an appropriate response. Turnbull and colleagues advise responding to the level of arousal by empathy, but not with anger. The staff member should allow the angry person physical space. Staff members should avoid threatening postures. Hands should be at the side with palms turned outward; they should not be behind the back or in pockets. Avoid folding arms across the chest [5].

Lancee and colleagues demonstrate that it may be possible to prevent some of the patient's anger by improving limit-setting styles. They studied six limit-setting styles using role playing scenarios with 97 patients of varying diagnoses and either high or low impulsivity. The patient's level of anger was measured in response to six styles: 1) belittlement and other responses causing the patient to defend a position; 2) platitudes and generic responses with a lack of attention to the individual's particular circumstances; 3) explaining rules or telling a patient what to do without offering possible courses of action; 4) providing solutions with options; 5) affective involvement without options; 6) affective involvement with options, i.e, expressing care and concern or atttending to subjective experiences with the patient and offering possible courses of action. Belittlement generated the most anger. Affective involvement with options was the most successful limit setting style, generating the least anger. Nonimpulsive patients had a lower level of anger to the last three limit-setting styles, while only one limit-setting style was effective with impulsive patients. Affective involvement with options kept anger at a low level. Empathy alone was never enough to contain anger. It needed to be combined with an offer of options for action. This study is important because most work is focused upon handling anger after it erupts rather than trying to prevent it, while still setting limits [6].

ANGER CONTROL TRAINING

Training the staff member to effectively handle anger is not enough; nor is encouraging the younger patient to talk about anger in individual therapy sufficient to change such firmly established ways of behaving. Some form of anger control training may be an important part of the treatment program for adolescent patients. Aggression in response to annoyance is a learned behavior that psychologists believe to be a function of reinforcement, expected outcomes and modeling influences. Because aggression is learned, it can be modified. However, if patients have learned to fulfill their needs by being aggressive, they will probably feel a decrease in anger and an increase in positive mood after aggression [7].

Ventilating anger may not be as effective as once believed. Suggesting to patients that they scream at those who have caused them difficulty or fight with foam rubber bats to resolve conflict are not necessarily successful. Theories about such activities for venting anger have been criticized by experts in aggression, learning theory and occupational therapy. Patterson has demonstrated that sports do not necessarily decrease hostility but instead may increase hostility and aggression. Baron's review of the literature concludes that the cathartic effect of ventilation is limited. The cathartic approach directly contradicts the use of activities that promote adaptive behavior [7–9].

Barfield and Hutchinson describe anger control training groups designed to help children move from being helpless victims of their emotions to feeling that they could learn to control them. The groups were voluntary and offered to boys who had agreed that anger was a problem that prevented them from reaching their personal goals. Ten boys were selected for a six-week course. They were motivated and willing to work. The first sessions were educational, focusing on discussions of the causes and cycles of aggression. The class explored socially accepted and unacceptable ways of expressing anger [10].

The boys kept weekly anger journals, rating the intensity of their anger, identifying its physical and behavioral signs, and describing situations provoking it. They also recorded how they handled the anger-provoking situation (i.e., by "stuffing," directing it, escalating, or time out). The boys were surprised to learn that their earlier irritations were connected to their later outbursts. Many who completed the course realized that their anger was not fully resolved and requested further training [10].

Dangel and colleagues evaluated six group-training sessions for emotionally disturbed children, ages 10 through 17, 5 girls and 13 boys. The first session was cognitive preparation. The students identified situations and people that had previously made them angry. They learned to make a distinction between anger and aggression. They then examined their own thoughts, self-statements or physical feelings that accompanied the build-up of anger. They learned about the physiology of anger. This was followed by an introduction to anger management, coping strategies, verbal self-instruction on how to break up the pattern of escalating anger. The first session accomplished all of these tasks [11–12].

In the second session the students discussed incidents from the previous week that made them feel angry or be aggressive. They then learned an anger management technique that they could use whenever the physical sensations or thoughts they had previously described built up. They were shown how to covertly order themselves to stop and how to quickly relax upper torso muscles. If this didn't work at first, they tried it again. If it still did not work, they were told to walk away. They practiced relaxation techniques in detail, and then verbal self-instruction techniques were introduced [11–12].

Practice continued in the third to sixth sessions. The boys also continued to review their own anger incidents from the previous week, when they either had begun to control or had continued to lose control of their anger. The sessions were devoted to the practices of thought-stopping and relaxation techniques as well as verbal self-instruction. With this technique, the therapist modeled the performance on the task, talking aloud while the children watched. The children then did it, giving themselves instructions aloud. The therapist then did it again, this time whispering self-instructions. The participants followed. Next the therapist did it again, using covert self-instructions, with pauses and signals to indicate thinking. The participants followed. The verbal self-instructions were a series of questions. What's the problem? What are the alternatives? What will be the consequences of them? The participants learned to reinforce themselves for good decisions, saying, for example: "I did a great job of figuring out everything without losing it." The results of this training were favorable and demonstrated a lasting reduction of the participants' verbal aggression. Just as in the classes Barfield and Hutchinson described, the students wanted to participate in further training [11–14].

Anger in the treatment center will never go away. It seems to be the predominant emotion that all staff will encounter from patients. Because of short-term stays, not all patients can benefit from anger control training. What is striking from most reports, however, is the willingness of so many to recognize that anger is a problem for them and to work toward solutions. Although only two accounts of anger control training are described, many others are available and have proved to be successful.

References

1. Cramerus M. Adolescent anger. Bulletin Menninger Clinic 1990 Fall;54(4):512–23.
2. Felicetti TC. Angry patients in a residential setting: Where does the anger go? How do we cope? Residential Treatment for Children & Youth 1987;4(3):3–8.
3. Barfield C, Hutchinson MA. Observations on adolescent anger and anger control group in residential and day treatment. Residential Treatment for Children & Youth 1989;7(2):45–58.

4. Green CP. How to recognize hostility and what to do about it. American Journal of Nursing 1986 Nov;12:30–4.
5. Turnbull J, Aitken IN, Black L. Turning it around: Short-term management for aggression and anger. Journal of Psychosocial Nursing & Mental Health Services 1990 Jun;28(6):7–10.
6. Lancee WJ, Gallop R, McCay E, Toner B. The relationship between nurses' limit-setting styles and anger in psychiatric inpatients. Psychiatric Services 1995 Jun;46(6):609–13.
7. Taylor E. Anger intervention. American Journal of Occupational Therapy 1988 Mar;42(3):147–55.
8. Patterson A. Hostility catharsis: A naturalistic quasi-experiment. Paper presented at the 82nd Annual Convention of the American Psychological Association. New Orleans, LA, September, 1974.
9. Baron R. Social influence theory and aggression. In: Green R, Donnerstein EL, eds. Aggression: Theoretical and empirical reviews: v. 2. Issues in research. New York: Academic Press, 1983, 173–90.
10. See reference 3.
11. Dangel RF, Deschner JP, Rasp RR. Anger control training for adolescents in residential treatment. Behavior Modification 1989 Oct;13(4):447–58.
12. Novaco R. Anger control. Lexington, MA: D. C. Heath, 1975.
13. McCullough JP, Huntsinger JM, Nay WR. Case Study: Self-control treatment of aggression in a 16-year-old male. Journal of Consulting & Clinical Psychology 1977;45:322–31.
14. Meichenbaum DH, Goodman J. Training impulsive children to talk to themselves: A means of developing self-control. Journal of Abnormal Psychology 1971;77:115–26.

3. Delusions

Delusions are false beliefs that are held even in the face of contradictory evidence or experience. Delusions take many forms and serve many purposes. They may be paranoid, punitive, somatic, or grandiose. They may help the person to cope in the face of anxiety. Grandiose delusions may bolster self esteem. Persons in a manic phase of a bipolar disorder may be driven by delusions of grandeur. Depressed patients may have somatic delusions or delusions of guilt or victimization. These are called mood-congruent delusions and are less puzzling than mood-incongruent delusions. Delusions that arise as part of the schizophrenic process are less easily understood.

More important than considering what staff members should do in response to a patient's delusions, is what not to do. If the staff member treats the delusion as if it is real, it will seriously confuse the patient. Staff members should convey respect and communicate that although they don't share this belief, they know that the person finds it very real. Direct questioning about the reality of the delusion is not recommended. Confrontation, argument, or appeals to logic are never successful and agitate the patient. Staff members should try not to display their frustration or anger with delusions. Even when the delusions are quite bizarre, they should be treated with sensitivity. Any other response will distance the staff member from the patient. Humor will not dislodge the belief and may seem demeaning. However, at times when the delusions cause the patient extreme anxiety, the staff may need to act. If, for example, the person begins to believe that family members are in danger, the staff might provide reassurance by family phone calls or visits. It is not helpful to encourage the patient to go into details about the delusion. It's much more valuable to discuss the person's feelings about it. Opening up to discussing feelings will validate the person's reality and build trust. Instead of encouraging the patient to focus on the content of the beliefs, identifying the feelings and then developing ways to manage them successfully is a long-term goal. Rosenthal and McGuinness report that even persons with persecutory delusions required appreciation of their perspectives and when this was not done, all interventions failed. Validation helps the person develop much more awareness and a better ability to identify what is happening. This awareness decreased anxiety and the need to project internal conflicts outward, making the delusional ideation not as necessary. Although the staff should not go into details of delusional content with the patient, this does not mean that the treatment team should not gather information about the patient to better understand delusions. A final understanding of why the patient distorts reality increases the staff member's success in working with delusional patients and promoting coping strategies [1–3].

Avoiding discussing the patient's delusions does not mean avoiding the patient, since frequent interactions increase safety and trust. Patients should be given positive feedback when they talk about feelings and reality-based experiences. Patients with nonparanoid delusions should be made comfortable in socializing with other persons and staff. Once the delusions have been given respectful attention, it is helpful to divert the patient with other activities and ideas so social interactions can take place [3].

Soon after admission of the delusional patient, the staff should try to learn about the precipitants and the results of the patient's delusional thinking. Justic reports, for example, that if a delusional person refuses medication, it may be because of a fear of being poisoned and the staff member may need to taste the person's food or prepare medication in the patient's presence to provide reassurance. The patient may respond favorably when given a great deal of control over the treatment environment—scheduling personal activities, meals, etc. This will help to develop security and self-esteem. Flexible meal scheduling will allow a frightened patient to eat alone when necessary to avoid anxiety and agitation. Turning over these controls communicates respect and concern that can help avoid the power struggles which diminish trust [3].

Carr speculates that perhaps the timely introduction of a plausible, objective explanation for subjective experiences that aren't easily explained could inhibit the development of delusional beliefs. Other forms of coping may include thought suppression, the deliberate exclusion from awareness of disturbing ideas. Persons subject to delusions may try to cope by not thinking about them, trying to forget them or ignoring them. They may also learn to shift their attention toward neutral, comforting or less disturbing ideas and perceptions [4].

Some research has indicated that group work using cognitive reframing can be effective in dislodging delusions, when done by experienced professionals. Lowe and Chadwick report the collaboration of two patient and clinician teams who examined evidence and lack of evidence for a delusion. Following this work, the patient's preoccupation and delusions were diminished. Milton and colleagues tested the comparative effectiveness of confrontation versus collaborative investigation in two patient groups. Therapists in the confrontational group firmly and politely corrected the patient's delusions, while the group working with belief modification, taught patients to examine other explanations for their delusions. Patients in both groups were able to decrease their social anxiety and the intensity of delusions, but those in the belief modification group experienced a greater decrease in the intensity of their delusions [5–6].

Persons with primary delusional disorders, i.e., not associated with affective disorders or schizophrenia, usually have fragile self-esteem and unusual sensitivity. Staff members should remain empathic and develop a flexible approach that preserves an appropriate physical and emotional distance. These patients are suffering and usually feel isolated and abandoned. Understanding and responding to their suffering is the most helpful approach. Patients with paranoid delusions will feel safer with consistent staff assignments. Staff members working with delusional patients may inevitably grow impatient or angry that they are not getting better or that an appeal to logic won't work. They need to realize that they may be feeling this because of their own struggles with feelings of inadequacy. For some patients delusions are a protective device and more comforting than reality [7–9].

References

1. Rosenthal TT, McGuinness TM. Dealing with delusional patients: discovering the distorted truth. Issues in Mental Health Nursing 1986;8(2):143–54.
2. Manschreck TC. Delusional Disorders: Clinical concepts and diagnostic strategies. Psychiatric Annals 1992 May;22(5):241–51.
3. Justic M. Nursing care for the hospitalized patient with psychotic symptoms. In: Wells LA, ed. A handbook of psychiatric nursing. St. Louis: Warren H. Green, 1989, 245–87.
4. Carr V. Patients' techniques for coping with schizophrenia: An exploratory study. British Journal of Medical Psychology 1986;59:399–52.
5. Lowe CF, Chadwick PDJ. Verbal control of delusions. Behavior Therapy 1990;21:461–80.
6. Milton F, Patwa VK, Hafner RS. Confrontations versus belief modification in persistently deluded patients. British Journal of Medical Psychology 1978 Jun;51(2):127–30.

7. See reference 2.
8. See reference 3.
9. See reference 1.

4. Difficult Patients

Conventional diagnosis does not predict treatment difficulty. In order to learn what patient characteristics make treatment difficult, Colson, Allen and colleagues studied 127 long-term psychiatric hospital patients and produced several analyses of this data. The dimensions of treatment difficulty were derived from the Hospital Treatment Rating Scale, a list of 25 problems or behaviors that patients may display during hospitalization. This problem list was compiled from interviews with senior clinicians in three psychiatric hospitals. These problems were rated for each patient by clinical staff members, who also rated the patient for treatment difficulty, progress, and prognosis. The studies indicate that the staff perceives the following patient behaviors as contributing to treatment difficulty: psychotic withdrawal, severe character pathology, violence and agitation, and suicidal, depressed behavior. These studies of treatment difficulty can prepare the multidisciplinary staff for problems that will arise, both because of staff countertransference and strong differences of opinion. The staff can anticipate difficulties in involving psychotic patients in the social milieu. They can recognize the need for clear planning and communication about violent and agitated patients and prepare to settle the staff conflicts that develop in response to character pathology [1–6].

Colson and colleagues found that treatment difficulty was even more extreme for patients who combined dimensions of severe psychopathology. They describe the most difficult group of patients as "pansymptomatic." Not only did this group have psychotic symptoms, but they were also demanding, manipulative, and hostile. They were potentially violent, suicidal and depressed. Many of this group had organic dysfunctions, but none were schizophrenic. Behavioral dyscontrol associated with organic impairment contributed to treatment difficulty. The pansymptomatic group presented many difficulties. Their progress was slow, they were involved in the greatest number of incidents, and required the greatest number of special controls. Colson and colleagues present a composite picture of such patients, describing them as patients who are in a regressed state at admission, continue to regress, are inaccessible and continue to demand and control staff time and attention, while resisting treatment [1–6].

Colson's 1990 article challenges the conventional wisdom that violent or suicidal patients are always the most difficult. The rankings of difficulty placed the violent group as fourth or fifth after pansymptomatic patients, patients with both psychotic withdrawal and severe character pathology and those with psychotic withdrawal alone. Violent patients are usually difficult because of the risk they pose, but violence may be only episodic. Violent patients may often be described as difficult because the staff tends to avoid them. Reactions to difficult patients include fearfulness, helplessness, and anger. Once such reactions can be expected, staff members can create an environment to contain and process these feelings. Their reactions will help them understand the patient's intrapsychic and interpersonal problems. Such knowledge will brace them throughout the patient's emotional storms, devaluation and inability to find comfort in relationships [6–7].

Staff Members' dissatisfaction and patient characteristics

Staff members accustomed to an interpersonal approach find psychotically withdrawn patients difficult, leaving them frustrated with the effect of their treatment. Staff members can feel helpless, confused and angry that they can't "reach" these patients. This is particularly true in treatment environments where interpersonal involvement is a predominant model for treatment [8].

Patients with character pathology leave the staff feeling frustrated with the inadequacy of the unit's structure and control. Staff members can become polarized about permissiveness or control. These patients inevitably elicit anger, which in turn can influence treatment decisions. The restrictions imposed because of the staff's frustrations and anger may seem punitive to those who feel a need to protect the patient from restrictions that seem too harsh. Violent and agitated patients continually challenge the staff's ability to work as a team. Although suicidal depressed patients are difficult, they apparently do not leave the staff frustrated by any particular aspect of treatment [8].

Colson and colleagues have also devised a scale for assessing treatment difficulty in child and adolescent patients in order to learn whether this difficulty relates to their progress in treatment, how staff/patient and family interactions relate to treatment difficulties, as well as the transference reactions elicited by work with these patients. Staff members will feel alone and helpless if they don't realize that these problems are to be expected, and studies of these difficult young patients provide a shared recognition and anticipation of the problems they present. The staff's belief that a patient is difficult will always affect the patient and the treatment process. The study included 49 boys and 20 girls. Rating scales were completed by the unit director-psychiatrist, a social worker, and child care worker. Higher scores for overall treatment difficulty correlated with higher scores for difficulty in establishing a therapeutic alliance and lower rates of progress in treatment. Higher overall treatment difficulty scores were also associated with lower family progress scores during the patient's hospital treatment [9–10].

Treatment difficulty was related to the following patient behaviors: angry defiance, inaccessibility and self-endangering behavior. Perceived angry defiance was most strongly associated with treatment difficulty. However, it was inaccessibility that produced the weakest therapeutic alliance. While angry defiant and aggressive types of behavior are strongly associated with perception of treatment difficulty, patients who are passive, evasive and isolated tend to make less progress in treatment. Treatment difficulty, the therapeutic alliance and outcome represent a complex set of interacting variables [10].

Neill's 1979 study finds similar categories of difficult patients, but describes other staff reactions. Staff members found it difficult to empathize with these patients and found themselves trying to avoid them. The nonphysician staff found them to be demanding, attention-seeking and manipulative. Physicians were more willing to see these behaviors as part of the patient's illness. Both physicians and nonphysicians conceived of them as angry, needy children who could be dangerous if not satisfied. Neill finds, however, that the treatment program itself may have also contributed to the difficulty. When compared to a control group of patients, those categorized as "difficult" were found to not have documented treatment contracts, a formulated problem description or a treatment plan. They had no clearly designated person responsible for coordinating their treatment programs and had previously been in two or more treatment programs with no coordination. Neill believes that the treatment system had "actively conspired" to enhance their difficult behavior by diffusing responsibility [11].

The type of treatment provided may sometimes be a factor in the patient's lack of improvement. Pardes and colleagues describe a patient group that steadily became worse during their stay in an intensive hospital milieu with a permissive atmosphere. This predominantly female group had several characteristics: uncertainty as to diagnosis, history of acting out which increased in the hospital, and strong reactions to separation. Whereas in 1972, their diagnosis was uncertain, they most likely would have a diagnosis of borderline personality disorder today. This patient group, following transfers to a custodially oriented, authoritarian city hospital, apparently reversed their regression and were soon discharged [12].

Countertransference Reactions to Difficult Patients

Groves indicates that the physician may have the following responses to difficult patients: feelings of helplessness, self-punishment, inappropriate confrontations or unconscious punishment of the patient, or even a desperate attempt to either avoid or discharge the patient from the hospital. Groves, who was writing about both medical and psychiatric patients, described four categories: dependent clingers, entitled demanders, manipulative help-rejecters, and self-destructive deniers [13].

While entitled demanders resemble clingers in their inexhaustible neediness, rather than making staff members feel needed, they may intimidate, devalue, and induce guilt. Their own deep dependency is the motivating factor in this behavior and it may be hard for staff members to realize that their hostility masks a fear of abandonment. Manipulative help-rejecters seem out to prove that no treatment will help. Self-destructive deniers, too, are painfully dependent but seem to glory in their own destruction. Groves believes that the starting point for their care is to honestly recognize that they can provoke in their caregivers a wish that they would "die and get it over with" [13].

Groves finds that what makes these "hateful" patients so difficult is that they evoke such negative feelings in their caregivers. Staff members may want to simply avoid the dependent clinger. Entitled demanders make caregivers fearful but also make them want to counter-attack. Manipulative help-rejecters make the staff feel guilty and inadequate. Self-destructive deniers may initially evoke affection mixed with anxiety, but their repetitive, destructive behaviors may make the staff wish it were all over. Groves advises that over time these behaviors teach the physician that it's how one behaves toward them, not how one feels about them, that is important in their care. This does not necessarily mean swallowing or restraining feelings. The physician, in response to clinging, should set limits on dependency. The staff should resist the urge to counterattack in the face of entitled demand; such entitlement might be redirected, for example, toward becoming an informed consumer. Groves advises that the physician who begins to wish the patient would die should realize that this is a congruent response to the patient's own wish to do so. Groves feels that errors in both diagnosis and treatment can occur when the patient creates feelings that the caregiver must disown or deny [13].

Colson and colleagues studied emotional responses to difficult patients and found five countertransference categories: positive engagement, protective, angry-provoked, helpless-confused, and fearful. They also studied the various professional groups and their most predominant responses. All staff disciplines shared two responses: positive engagement and an angry-provoked response. Psychiatrists and social workers both shared a helpless-confused response, while for nurses and activity therapists helplessness was more often associated with anger [14].

Anger, helplessness and fear were the countertransference feelings associated with treatment difficulty. Patients with character pathology most often made staff members feel angry. Withdrawn psychoticism made the staff feel helpless. The various disciplines differed in their response to violence and agitation. It was associated with helplessness for psychiatrists, fearfulness in social workers and nurses and anger for activity therapists. Suicidal-depressed behavior did not evoke any consistent emotional response from psychiatrists or activity therapists, but evoked a wide range of responses from social workers and nurses [14].

PROFESSIONAL ROLES AND EMOTIONAL REACTIONS TO DIFFICULT PATIENTS

The staff member's primary role with the patient affects the emotional response. The psychiatrists' and social workers' response can be less intense and more distant than those of activity therapists and nurses whose contact with patients is more frequent. The fearfulness experienced by nurses in response to difficult patients is a realistic response to their daily contact and fits with Colson and colleagues' conclusion that nurses are more affected by behavioral dyscontrol than other disciplines [14].

Gallop and Wynn redefine the difficult patient as a sociocultural actor living in a particular environmental context—not simply a victim of intrapsychic conflict. Using semistructured interviews and an adjective checklist with psychiatric residents and nurses, they attempted to learn whether the staff's categorization of difficult patients varied by profession. The nurses described two predominant categories of difficult patients: patients with high affect, intensity, and chronicity who were interpersonally attractive and another group with the same characteristics but who were not interpersonally attractive. Patients with high affect would often scream, hit, moan, or threaten. They demanded attention. They were "draining, demanding, and devouring." They were labeled as chronic because they had made no progress. They seemed to have made a deliberate decision not to improve. There was a subcategory of chronic patients who were called "responsive." This group seemed willing to listen to nurses and to often act on their advice [15].

Psychiatric residents in this study divided difficult patients in two categories: chronic and exploitative. Exploitative patients are difficult because they "disrupt" the treatment system and often place the psychiatric resident in a difficult relationship with the clinical team. These patients are variously described as splitting, manipulative, attention-seeking, histrionic, and noncompliant. Similar to the description of the chronic patient, their behavior is seen as deliberate and somehow within their control [15].

Both staff groups found that these patients left them feeling incompetent and not in control. The nurses' own reactions to such patients were intense and negative. They described themselves as feeling overwhelmed, guilty, helpless, and engulfed. The psychiatrists' reactions were different. They felt frustrated, angry, and irritable. In order to feel competent and in control, nurses needed some response from patients, some signal that their work is making a difference. Psychiatric residents believed that the management of difficult patients generated conflicts with staff psychiatrists. They felt isolated and unsupported and described the staff psychiatrists who attended these patients as not being interested in feelings, avoiding these patients and the unit, and changing their treatment plans without consultation [15].

Gallop, Lancee and Shugar later studied nurses' and resident psychiatrists' reactions to short stay patients, using the Hospital Treatment Rating Scale and a staff rating of management difficulty. Since they were studying a short-stay unit, they placed more emphasis on behaviors rather than personality characteristics. The patients' sabotage of treatment was a contributing factor to the perception of their difficulty. Treatment sabotage usually includes the ability to polarize staff, substance abuse, elopements, and sexual acting out. Nurses found this more difficult than psychiatric residents, not only because it made a treatment alliance difficult but because their constant need to respond to these behaviors made other treatment efforts more difficult. Both psychiatric residents and nurses find that the behaviors that make patients difficult to treat are those that invalidate their special treatment efforts— psychopharmacology and interpersonal relationships. However, in short-term treatment, patients who don't respond to medication have a greater need to establish relationships since such relationships may be the only treatment available to them. In turn, they may not accept medication as treatment until they establish a trusting therapeutic relationship. This study of short-stay patients confirmed that specific professional roles affect the perception of treatment difficulty. Kelly and May also confirm that "problem" patients are those that challenge the nurses' ability to help by rejecting the services they are able to give. The perception of a difficult patient is bound up with the nurse's identity. When nurses judge severity of disturbance they usually do so on the basis of patient behavior that is most disruptive of their task of managing the hospital milieu [16–17].

May and Kelly believe that for psychiatric nurses, difficult or problem patients don't usually constitute an identifiable or homogeneous group. What they hold in common is an unwillingness to acknowledge, either implicitly or explicitly, the legitimacy of the nurses' therapeutic role. They also challenge the nurses' own confidence in their ability to understand, accept, and manage the most irritating and demanding behavior. Nurses must hide real feelings about patients while still trying to interact with them openly and honestly. The nurses' ability to cope with such difficult demanding patients may be central to their concept of themselves as nurses. The ability to cope with a demanding patient may provide the very essence of what psychiatric nursing is all about [18].

May and Kelly feel that nurses might differentiate among problem patients and that the distinction will have to do with whether the behavior is related to the patient's illness. Nurses will usually not reject patients if they understand that their behaviors are a part of their illness. We might, in this connection, regard the diagnosis of borderline personality disorder as a stroke of wisdom to assuage the feelings of helplessness and frustration experienced by psychiatric hospital staff in dealing with extremely difficult patients who frequently looked and acted as if there was nothing wrong with them, other than the severe disturbances they caused on the unit. Once their collection of maddening and destructive behaviors were described as part of their illness, more effective therapeutic work could resume [18–20].

Colson and colleagues found that social workers judged the patients' severity of difficulty by scrutinizing social skills, psychiatrists by judging their peculiarity and alienation, and that nurses judged them by their expressive behaviors. These variations in perceptions explain the difficulties of the multidisciplinary team in reaching consensus, each member using a different language to assess the patient's difficulties. At the same time, Colson and colleagues suggest that these very differences demonstrate the usefulness of the team approach, both for diagnosis and effective treatment [21].

MANAGING COUNTERTRANSFERENCE FEELINGS

Anger, the predominant emotional reaction to character pathology, may be used constructively when channeled into a search for more effective structure, limits, and expectations. The staff members' own experience of anger can help them understand the patient. The staff's helplessness and confusion with psychotically withdrawn patients is a normal reaction. The staff's patience and perseverance are challenged, and they can only look to slow and subtle changes that may inspire them [21].

Since violence and agitation evoked varying responses among disciplines, it may always be difficult for the team to develop a cohesive treatment plan for such patients. Colson and colleagues write that because they have the greatest impact on the nursing staff, the team should concentrate on ways to support the nurses and increase their feelings of safety [21].

Suicidal-depressed behavior elicited a notable lack of dysphoria across disciplines. This behavior seems to elicit positive engagement from others. Patients who score high on this dimension may also be receiving a response that provides a subtle reinforcement for their self-destructive behaviors [21].

Outcome for Difficult Patients

Treatment difficulty does not necessarily point to a poor outcome, but can often signal slow improvement. It is the type rather than the extent of the difficulty which affects prognosis. Those patients with character pathology in Colson's 1990 study, although shown to have difficulties with interpersonal relations, did not have a poorer prognosis than other patients. Those with psychotic withdrawal, however, not only presented great overall difficulty, but also tend to fare poorly. They can make staff members feel confused and helpless and they rarely participate in the treatment milieu [22].

Difficult patients experience treatment impasses more frequently. Staff members should not feel that their countertransference signals poor treatment, for it can be potentially helpful. These emotional reactions do not need to cause interference or destroy alliances with the patient or other team members. Rather than feeling hopeless, staff members must be experienced in handling treatment impasses and know that they can be resolved. Colson recommends that staff education outline how specific patient difficulties affect staff members and make them feel isolated. Since work with difficult patients brings about strong emotions and staff conflicts, the recognition of these potential difficulties can preserve the therapeutic milieu. Team meetings about such patients may not always lead to decisions but can provide staff members with a sounding board for sharing interactions and reactions to difficult patients. This can help them defer decisions about the patient until everyone's experience can provide a synthesis and possible agreement [22].

Treatment difficulty is determined not only by the behaviors of patients but also by the staff members' perception and experience of them. Difficult patients can make the staff feel overwhelmed and helpless and lead to team splitting and disagreements, when staff members have different emotional reactions. An expanding knowledge of staff members' responses to difficult patients will help them use these emotions as a technical instrument helpful in understanding patients and planning an integrated treatment [22].

Colson and colleagues find that it is the difficult patient who calls attention to the absence of a systematic theory of hospital treatment. These patients demonstrate the need for developing concepts of hospital treatment similar to those of psychotherapeutic treatment, such as the therapeutic alliance, transference and countertransference that can outline specific approaches for difficult-to-treat patients [23].

References

1. Colson DB, Allen JG, Coyne L, Deering D, et al. Profiles of difficult psychiatric hospital patients. Hospital & Community Psychiatry 1986 Oct;37(10):720–4.
2. Colson DB, Allen JG, Coyne L, et al. Patterns of staff perception of difficult patients in a long-term psychiatric hospital. Hospital & Community Psychiatry 1985 Feb;36(2):168–72.
3. Allen JG, Colson DG, Coyne L, Dexter IN, et al. Problems to anticipate in treating difficult patients in a long-term psychiatric hospital. Psychiatry 1986;49:350–8.
4. Colson DB, Allen JG. Organic brain dysfunction in difficult-to-treat psychiatric hospital patients. Bulletin Menninger Clinic 1986;50(1):88–98.
5. Colson DB, Allen JG, Coyne L, Dexter IN, et al. An anatomy of countertransference: staff reactions to difficult psychiatric hospital patients. Hospital & Community Psychiatry 1986 Sep;37(9):923–8.
6. Colson DB. Difficult patients in extended psychiatric hospitalization: a research perspective on the patient, staff, and team. Psychiatry 1990;53:369–82.
7. Cornfield RB, Fielding SD. Impact of threatening patients on ward communication. American Journal of Psychiatry 1980 May;137(5):616–9.
8. See reference 6.
9. Colson DB, Murphy T, O'Malley F, Huyland PS, et al. Assessing difficulties in the hospital treatment of children and adolescents. Bulletin Menninger Clinic 1990 Win;54(1):78–89.
10. Colson DB, Cornsweet C, Murphy T, O'Malley F, et al. Perceived treatment difficulty and therapeutic alliance on an adolescent psychiatric hospital unit. American Journal of Orthopsychiatry 1991;61:221–9.
11. Neill JR. The difficult patient: identification and response. Journal of Clinical Psychiatry 1979 May;40:209–12.
12. Pardes H, Van Putten T, Bjork D, Kaufman M. Failures on a therapeutic milieu. Psychiatric Quarterly 1972;46:29–48.

13. Groves JE. Taking care of the hateful patient. New England Journal of Medicine 1978;298(16):883–7.
14. See reference 5.
15. Gallop R, Wynn F. The difficult inpatient: identification and response by staff. Canadian Journal of Psychiatry 1987;32:211–5.
16. Gallop R, Lancee W, Shugar G. Residents' and nurses' perceptions of difficult-to-treat short stay patients. Hospital & Community Psychiatry 1993 Apr;44(4):352–7.
17. Kelly M, May D. Good and bad patients: a review of the literature and theoretical critique. Journal Advanced Nursing 1981;2:147–56.
18. May D, Kelly M. Chancers, pests and poor wee souls: Problems of legitimating in psychiatric nursing. Sociology of Health & Illness 1981;4:279–301.
19. Main TF. The ailment. British Journal of Medical Psychology 1975;30:129–145.
20. Burnham D. The special-problem patient: victim or agent of splitting? Psychiatry 1966;29:105–22.
21. See reference 5.
22. See reference 6.
23. See reference 2.

5. Elopements from the Treatment Center

Greater patient freedom and unlocked hospitals increase the risk of hospital elopements, and runaway patients may be risking accidents or danger. Elopements disrupt the continuity of care and strain hospital-community relations. Frequent runaways may suggest that the hospital staff is irresponsible or that the treatment setting is in a state of instability. Indeed, elopements can occur during periods of staff turnover and deteriorating staff-patient relationships, but they usually have more to do with the person than the treatment milieu. Adolescent elopements receive more attention since they are usually more frequent [1–2].

Reasons for Elopement

Interviews with patients who have eloped may help the treatment staff to anticipate and possibly prevent them. The adolescent's running away may be yet another form of resistance to defeat the treatment staff's efforts or as a way to cope with stressful situations. Many writers note that adolescents will elope when discharge is imminent. Other separations, such as a friend's leaving, a patient transfer or staff disapproval of a relationship will prompt adolescents to leave. Elopements often have something to do with the patient-psychotherapist relationship. McNaught & McKamy find that fear of intimacy and closeness often prompt elopements and that elopement is a means to communicate with staff. They believe that elopement is never an isolated decision and that it may provide information about the treatment program. Benalcazar's study of 15 adolescent runaway patients found that their elopements were not really related to the therapeutic process [2–5].

Adolescent elopements often occur around experiences of separation—therapists' vacations, homesickness and responsibility for family, impending discharge, the end of relationships, discharge of friends. Often elopements represent simple defiance or adolescent bravado. Miller and colleagues describe runaways with varying levels of experience. For the first degree runner, running was a solution to a problem. Second degree runners saw running as a solution, but it also became a problem. For third degree runners, running had become a life choice. While running at first seems like a solution, it becomes a problem in itself. Miller and colleagues reported that the adolescents they studied ran for reactive and impulsive reasons. Runaways were usually in response to house rules. Levy cautions against the therapeutic culture's excessive focus on pathology and feels that running away may be healthy, self-preservative and self-healing. Elopements may be adaptive efforts to increase autonomy, escape from unwanted confinement and search for more stimulating experiences [5–7].

Others may concentrate on the predictors, rather than the explanations for elopement in adolescents. Berman and Goodrich found that previous runaway history, the diagnosis, severity of illness, and adoptive status predicted elopement behavior in adolescents. Prediction can be helpful if those who are at a high risk for elopement could be targeted for interventions designed to prevent their running away but a review for the literature indicates that there are no universal predictors of elopement, other than runaway history [8–9].

Staff Response

When patients run, the staff may feel angry, let down, and defeated, or even feel blamed, incompetent and guilty. Benalcazar reports that psychotherapists may blame the ward staff, particularly if they have no part in administering the unit. Levy notes sometimes the staff does ignore clues, or that there can be splitting on the team, or that staff departures have not been appropriately handled. Falkowski believes that when few if any changes are made in management on the patient's return, further investigation may be necessary. Swindall and Molnar report that when elopements tripled after a hospital changed to an open setting, the solution was to establish an observation sheet to record hourly observations noting the patient's location and activity. This procedure documented the observation process, fixed responsibility throughout the day, and increased staff-patient interactions. Greenberg and colleagues feel that while establishing tighter controls after a return can establish a nurturing and protective environment, it can also lend a prison-like atmosphere to the milieu. Molnar and colleagues report that since elopers usually do not engage in high-risk behaviors during their time away, it might be just as helpful to renegotiate privileges of the elopers who are close to being discharged. If offered a choice patients may prefer to negotiate extensions of privileges rather than elope [10–15].

Levy believes that most staff, at some level, have felt secret delight when thinking about an adolescent runaway as a sign of independence or emancipation. He believes that a psychotherapeutic stance can best be maintained if staff resists the countertransference feelings that the patients are abandoning them, and that responses should be more realistic. Cancro advises the psychotherapist to understand what the elopement communicates and attempt to correct the nature of the therapeutic relationship that may have prompted the escape. He believes that the therapist's extreme involvement with the patient may create a serious countertransference problem, and notes that nurses report that when a doctor can't share a patient with the team, they usually expect the patient to elope. Some patients escape because the therapist's intrusiveness has threatened their autonomy. Professionals and patients do not necessarily agree upon the meaning of hospitalization. McIndoe described patient interviews after elopement that indicated that the patients who eloped placed a low value on their own treatment and made suggestions on how to improve it. They saw their elopements as a positive experience that they wanted to repeat [16–18].

When all efforts at prevention have been made and elopements still occur, the staff must also be open to the possibility of a positive outcome of an elopement. For some patients it seems to interrupt a cycle. From interviews from staff following elopements, Benalcazar reports that they indicate that many patients were able to form a better grasp on relationships and treatment and became more open on return. Benalcazar felt that perhaps some patients had been given an unsupervised status too quickly and were uncomfortable. Elopements sometimes increased the patients' self-esteem because of the staff's attention and this in turn strengthened that relationship. Miller and colleagues feel that effective treatment will turn the problem of elopement into a solution for the adolescent and the larger system at the same time. When they interviewed patients about what were the most helpful things that were done to stop them from running away, five said that nothing would stop them. Four said that talking, increased freedom, and consequences would have helped. However, when asked about the least helpful interventions, they mentioned nagging, and reminders of possible consequences. Molnar and colleagues, once again considering negotiation as an alternative, advise that if the goal is truly the rehabilitation of the patient, negotiating rather than eloping can then give the patient choice and more responsibility [19–21].

References

1. Molnar G, Pinchoff DM. Factors in patient elopements from an urban state hospital and strategies for prevention. Hospital & Community Psychiatry 1993 Aug;44(8):791–2.
2. Kashubeck S, Pottebaum SM, Read NO. Predicting elopement from residential treatment centers. American Journal of Orthopsychiatry 1991 Jan;64(1):126–35.
3. Benalcazar B. Study of fifteen runaway patients. Adolescence 1981;17(67):553–66.

4. McNaught TR, McKamy LR. Elopement of adolescents: Dynamics in the treatment process. Hospital & Community Psychiatry 1978 May;29(5):303–5.
5. Miller AT, Eggertson-Tacon C, Quigg B. Patterns of runaway behavior with a large systems context: The road to empowerment. Adolescence 1990;25(98):271–89.
6. Levy EZ. Some thoughts about patients who run away and the staff they leave behind. Psychiatric Quarterly 1972;46(1):1–21.
7. See reference 1.
8. Berman LB, Goodrich W. Running away from treatment: Observations and admission predictors for hospitalized adolescents. Adolescent Psychiatry 1990;17:29–34.
9. See reference 2.
10. See reference 3.
11. See reference 6.
12. Falkowski IJ. Patients leaving the hospital without the knowledge or permission of the staff—absconders. British Journal of Psychiatry 1990 Apr;156:488–90.
13. Greenberg, H, Blank R, Argett S. The anatomy of elopement from an acute adolescent service: Escape from management. Psychiatric Quarterly 1968;42:28–47.
14. Swindall LE, Molnar G. Open doors and runaway patients: a management dilemma. Perspectives in Psychiatric Care 1985;23(4):146–9.
15. See reference 1.
16. See reference 6.
17. Cancro R. Elopements from the C. F. Menninger Memorial Hospital. Bulletin Menninger Clinic 1968;32:220–38.
18. McIndoe KI. Elopement: Why psychiatric patients go A.W.O.L. Journal of Psychosocial Nursing & Mental Health Services 1986 Jan;24(1):16–20.
19. See reference 3.
20. See reference 5.
21. See reference 1.

6. Firesetting

There are several categories of firesetters that can pose serious threats in the psychiatric treatment center: persons who are fascinated by fire and play with matches or lighters, the "cry-for-help" firesetter, and antisocial children or adolescents who use fire as a weapon against adult authority. The treatment of the firesetter is discussed in Chapter VI.

It is important to clearly outline the staff's role and responsibilities in case of a fire. There should be a continual updating of emergency procedures with full accessibility to fire fighting equipment. It is not possible to predict which patients are likely to set fires while in treatment. It can occur in persons with no past history of the behavior because it provides a dramatic way to get attention. Although firesetting can be associated with a manic disorder or command hallucinations, some patients' desire for a response or for attention may be so compelling as to cause them to light fires. Geller refers to this behavior as communicative arson and finds that persons lacking social and communication skills may resort to this action since it requires absolutely no verbal exchange. Such persons may also have had a history of nonlethal self-injurious behavior. They may even use fire to voice the need for transfer from a less restrictive to more restrictive setting [1–2].

Institutions are vulnerable to firesetting during periods of organizational instability when there are administrative changes, staff conflicts, or blurred lines of authority. There may be early signs of instability, such as poor staff communication or frequent staff absences. It may occur in an adolescent population when patients with histories of poor impulse control, antisocial acting out, and primitively organized personality structure are in crisis situations [3–4].

If a fire occurs, careful management is needed. Those who participated in setting the fire should be separated from each other and from the unit where the fire was set so that an evaluation can begin. Some patients may need to be transferred to another unit or facility. As soon as possible the staff and patients should discuss the event of the fire, what caused it, and together plan all measures to stop it from happening again [4].

The staff should anticipate aftershocks throughout the hospital after a fire. Everything should be done, however, to help the staff to build confidence, regain a positive attitude and return to normal. The staff should remember that any variation from normal routine can cause problems for patients with poor impulse control so that any emergency provisions, such as providing temporary rooms for patients should be evaluated. Firesetting is an extremely dangerous behavior. Although infrequent, it is unpredictable, highly lethal, and not uncommon in the psychiatric population. Firesetting should be handled by rapid, clear, and limit-setting responses [5].

References

1. Geller JL, Bertsh G. Fire-setting behavior in the histories of a state hospital population. American Journal of Psychiatry 1985 Apr;142(1):464–8.
2. Geller JL. Communicative Arson. Hospital & Community Psychiatry 1992 Jan;43(1):76–7.
3. Boling L, Brotman C. A fire-setting epidemic in a state mental health center. American Journal of Psychiatry 1975 Sep;132(9):946–50.
4. Rosenstock HA, Holland A, Jones PH. Fire-setting on an adolescent inpatient unit: An analysis. Journal of Clinical Psychiatry 1980;41(1) :20–2.
5. See reference 1.

7. Hallucinations

Persons with hallucinations may hear, feel, see or taste something that does not exist. The person creates a perception which is purely internal that seems to be coming from the external world and becomes convinced that it is real and not self-created. The most common hallucinations are auditory. Hallucinations may begin when an isolated or anxious person invents an imaginary helper for comfort and begins to interact with helping voices as if they are real. As the person continues to feel bad, the voices may become more threatening than comforting. The person may later come to feel controlled by the voices. Although medication can usually control auditory hallucinations associated with schizophrenic disorders, there will be many instances when persons hallucinate in the treatment setting [1].

Assessment of Hallucinations

The treatment team must identify the sensory modes involved in hallucinations, the length of time they have been experienced, and the person's ability to determine whether or not they are real. It may be helpful to determine the time of day they occur and identify their content and the feelings that are behind them as well as the feelings they produce. The staff should explore strategies that the person has previously used to control them. It is important to learn whether the person experiences command hallucinations and determine how compelling is the need to obey [2].

The Staff Members Response to Hallucinations

If staff members suspect the person is hallucinating, they should not directly ask "Are you hallucinating?" This might suggest that they are mind-reading or can also hear the voices. Rather, a staff member might say something like: "You seem to be paying attention to something other than your own voice or mine. Is something else happening?" Remember, however, that patients may fear punishment from the voices if they tell others about them. If possible, the staff should guide the hallucinating person to a private setting and should remain there. The hallucination should not be ignored; the staff member must realize that the patient's experience is real and frightening. It is not helpful to question the reality of the voices or argue about them. Many patients will feel more secure if the staff member says that although the voices don't exist in reality, they do exist as part of the patient's illness, which can finally be overcome [3].

Approaches to Controlling Hallucinations

The person who hallucinates should be given clear and reassuring explanations that the hallucinations are part of the illness and that the staff understands them. The staff can provide assurance that hallucinations may decrease with treatment, but that there are also other ways to decrease them. Since it is difficult to do two things at once, keeping patients involved will help to control hallucinations. More active mental involvement is more effective than passive mental activity. Competing stimuli reduce the severity and frequency of hallucinations. Reports have indicated that listening to the radio or watching TV can interrupt the presence of hallucinations, and independent recreational activities can take the place of talking to one's self [4–5].

Staff members must be sensitive and aware of the fear and loneliness associated with hallucinations. The development of a therapeutic relationship may help the patient control the hallucinations and eventually replace them with human relationships. In addition to medication, hallucinations may be treated indirectly by therapy that strengthens ego functions so that the person can learn to test the reality of the hallucinatory experience [6].

Self-Regulation

The treatment team may decide that the staff should work toward enabling the patient to increase self-regulation of the hallucinations. This might begin with helping the patient recognize the anxiety that precedes the hallucination and learning other ways to cope with it. There is evidence that many hallucinating persons have developed their own self-regulating devices and with professional support they can learn from each other, develop these capacities, recognize precipitants of their illness and act to prevent relapse. These abilities have been underestimated. Many persons can respond well to therapeutic instruction helping them to understand their illness and monitor and control their symptoms. Patients can explore techniques during inpatient treatment. Humming quietly may diminish hallucinations since it requires some thought, distracts and can also interfere with the cognitive processes that coincide with hallucinations. However, tasks that require other efforts, such as raising the eyebrows or being in groups, do not diminish hallucinations. Field advocates telling the voices to go away. The patient should practice this with staff members to overcome reluctance to do it. A loud and clear voice may be necessary in contrast to the initial mumbling command the patient may first prefer. Field advises that this be done repeatedly in order to make it work [7–10]

Even more innovative solutions have come from those who have suffered from hallucinations. In response to a televised request, 173 persons who heard voices answered with descriptions of their own experiences. Only about 1/3 of the respondents reported complete success. Twenty persons successful at coping were interviewed in depth. They described four main strategies: distraction, ignoring, selective testing and setting limits. Distracting was accomplished by physical means such as meditation or yoga. One woman described how she finally learned to ignore the voices after her husband compared the voice to that of a nagging neighbor and asked her if she would really harm herself if the neighbor had told her to do so. She learned to ignore the voices, gained control, and after that was not readmitted to psychiatric treatment. Another woman described selective listening as an experience of lifting her voices in the air, throwing them as far as possible and telling them that there was no place for them there. This ritual helped her distinguish between good and bad voices and control them. Another woman set limits on the voices by bargaining that they could only be present after 8 p.m. so that she was never bothered during the day. The authors concluded that helping patients to accept the voices and then develop their own coping strategies could become an effective part of psychiatric rehabilitation. Techniques usually involve a form of suppression or distraction. Suppression involves such techniques as "pushing the voice aside," or "avoiding it like static on the radio." The person with hallucinations must not only work toward controlling them but also must find a way to make them less frightening. One person reports using relaxation techniques learned in the hospital, and applying desensitization to hallucinations. This involves sitting down, relaxing completely using relaxation techniques, then considering all the hallucinations that had been frightening, in increasing order of terror. Each time anxiety increased, the person would stop, relax again, and go back to the beginning [11–12].

Arieti suggests the use of preventive expectations. That is, the person develops a state of mind in which the expectation of hallucination arises before it occurs. The awareness of these expectant states of mind gives persons an opportunity to prepare coping techniques which might stop the symptoms from emerging. Brier and Strauss describe the self-control process in three phases: detecting unwanted behavior, evaluating the behavior as a warning, and the use of a control strategy, such as self-instruction or reduced or increased involvement in activity. Falloon and Talbot note that chronic schizophrenic patients can alter their experience of auditory hallucinations by changing their level of activity. It is satisfying to realize, however, that some of the most helpful techniques can come from first-person accounts from those who have suffered from psychotic symptoms [13–15].

References

1. Justic M. Nursing care for the hospitalized patient with psychotic symptoms. In: Wells LA, ed. A handbook of psychiatric nursing. St. Louis: Warren H. Green, 1989, 245–87.
2. Williams CA. Perspectives on the hallucinatory process. Issues in Mental Health Nursing 1989;20:99–119.
3. See reference 1.
4. Margo A, Helmsley DR, Slade PD. The effects of varying auditory input on schizophrenic hallucinations. British Journal of Psychiatry 1982 Apr;140(4):515–6.
5. Wong SE, Wolsey JE, Gallegos F. Behavioral treatment of chronic psychiatric patients. Journal of Social Service Research 1986–7 Win-Sum;10(2–4):7–33.
6. See reference 1.
7. See reference 2.
8. Green MF, Kinsbourne M. Subvocal activity and auditory hallucinations: Clues for behavioral treatments. Schizophrenia Bulletin 1990;16(4):617–25.

9. See reference 5.
10. Field WE. Hearing voices. Journal of Psychosocial Nursing & Mental Health Services 1985 Jan;23(1):8–14.
11. Romme MAJ, Honig A, Escher AD Coping with hearing voices: An emancipatory approach. British Journal of Psychiatry 1992 Jul;161:99–103.
12. Carr V. Patients' techniques for coping with schizophrenia: an exploratory study. British Journal of Medical Psychology 1986;59:339–62.
12. Rollin HR, ed. Coping with schizophrenia. London: Burnett, 1980.
13. Arieti S. Interpretation of schizophrenia. New York: Basic Books, 1974, 573–80.
14. Brier A, Strauss JS. Self-control in psychotic disorders. Archives of General Psychiatry 1983;40:1141–5.
15. Falloon IRH, Talbot RE. Persistent auditory hallucinations: Coping mechanisms and implications for management. Psychological Medicine 1981;11:329–39.

8. Manipulation

Manipulation is essentially a purposeful behavior. The person placed in treatment has diminished power and must look to others to fulfill many needs. If they can't be expressed directly or effectively, the patient may resort to manipulation. A patient who has been able to succeed in meeting certain needs despite initial staff resistance is often called manipulative. While the psychiatric hospital often strives to train patients to be assertive, their own success and ingenuity in achieving their goals at the expense of staff is usually not met with admiration. Hoffman and Singer believe that such pejorative labeling allows the system to maintain itself when the community fails to achieve conformity in one of its members. Staff members must be extremely careful when labeling the patient's behaviors as manipulation since the accusation that a patient is manipulative can signal a breakdown of the helping process [1–3].

It is helpful for all staff members to pull back and consider what behaviors and what persons they are calling manipulative. Although manipulation is an interpersonal strategy intended to get a given response, it is rarely met with objectivity or sympathy. The anger it arouses in staff members often marks a shift from helping to adversary behaviors. The adaptive uses of manipulation are rarely recognized. But when manipulation becomes the primary method to get needs met, when the rights and feelings of others are so disregarded that they are treated as objects whose only purpose is to fulfill needs, then manipulation is maladaptive. The strategy becomes so habitual that it may eliminate other forms of interpersonal influence, and the person becomes known as manipulative. These persons manipulate the self-esteem of others, both negatively and positively. They are not sincerely close to others although they may develop pseudo-intimate relationships with them. Because they have no relationships or because relationships make them feel too vulnerable, they must use manipulation. They may flatter and compliment staff members, tell them what they know they want to hear, even to the point of sharing personal or private thoughts. After laying the groundwork for such relationships, they then begin to ask for exemption from rules or special privileges. They seem to be able to perceive and take full advantage of the weaknesses of others. Other manipulative maneuvers include refusing to talk, acting helpless, suicidal gestures for attention, temper tantrums or anger when denied [3–5].

RESPONDING TO THE MANIPULATIVE PATIENT

Making decisions with these patients is always difficult. To simply deny all requests because of the fear of manipulation will produce constant power struggles. If the staff member fears angry responses when limits are set, the temptation is to allow manipulative actions to succeed. If manipulative patients seem to have inexhaustible needs, the staff will put up barriers for protection. They may find themselves completely avoiding the patient, thereby reinforcing the pattern and decreasing their own self-esteem. Ignoring manipulative behaviors may only increase them. Diamond and Factor write that patients who are called manipulative are really unskilled at dealing with people and therefore cause others to feel angry and resentful. If the staff can understand that their demands arise from deficits in interpersonal skills, then helping patients to develop better skills may allow them to get their needs met without producing so much anger [4–5].

Chitty and Maynard recommend that when the staff member is confronted with the manipulative patient, interventions should center on increasing the patient's trust, security and control. Anticipating the patient's needs before manipulative behaviors occur can increase trust. This can best be achieved by examining previous patterns of manipulation. In building trust, it is helpful to assist the patient in discovering what needs manipulation is expressing and find other ways to meet them. It becomes important for the staff member to confront the patient every time manipulation occurs and describe what it feels like to be the recipient of it [5].

These patients may be manipulating others in order to make their own surroundings secure and predictable, and they may be crying out for more security. Therapeutic limit setting will provide temporary boundaries and set limits. The patient will always test limits, since when they are lacking, the manipulative patient's anxiety will rise and manipulative behavior will increase. Setting limits will involve establishing consequences and enforcing them without denying all of the patient's requests. Control is also vital to the patient who manipulates. The patient should participate in the treatment plan, in goal setting and evaluation. Some of these abilities to influence might eventually develop into leadership skills. Hospitalization increases the feelings of powerlessness, and the patient may begin to manipulate as a natural response to the loss of power [5].

Manipulation and Antisocial Personalities

Manipulation is a technique used not only by helpless patients but also by persons with antisocial personalities. Their manipulation uses aggressiveness, cleverness and deceit to influence others. Even when the motivation to manipulate is unconscious, manipulation itself can be conscious and planned. For some their behavior is so entrenched that they can be described as manipulative personalities. They exert influence by employing a deception of some sort and take pride in putting something over on another person [6].

What can be done in response to manipulation? Peer supervision can be helpful in trying out staff responses. Helping staff members reframe manipulation as a means to influence people, and following this by helping the patient develop more appropriate ways to influence others can be very helpful. Reframing manipulative behavior so that one conceives of the manipulator as a masterful artist may provide an opportunity to rid oneself of negative feelings and assume a wider perspective and an objective stance. An analysis of manipulation as an interactional sequence can provide insight to the treatment team. Initially the patient and the staff member agree to certain defining conditions of a relationship. The staff member imposes certain restrictions on the manner that treatment will be administered. Rather than respecting the limits the manipulative patient tries to exceed them. Manipulation may illustrate the poverty of the patient's strategy rather than deceit. When the term manipulation is used, it is time to scrutinize the treatment relationship, since this is an indication that it has shifted from therapeutic to adversarial grounds [7–8].

References

1. McMorrow ME. The manipulative patient. American Journal of Nursing 1981;82:1188–90.
2. Hoffman J, Singer PR. The incompatibility of the medical model and the therapeutic community. Social Science & Medicine 1977;11:425–31.
3. Mackenzie TB, Rosenberg SD, Bergen BJ, Tucker GJ. The manipulative patient: An interactional approach. Psychiatry 1978 Nov;41:264–71.
4. Diamond RJ, Factor RM. Taking issue: Treatment-resistant patients or a treatment-resistant system? Hospital & Community Psychiatry 1994 Mar;45(3):197.
5. Chitty KK, Maynard CK. Managing manipulation. Journal of Psychosocial Nursing 1986 Jun;24(6):9–13.
6. St. Clair H. Manipulation. Comprehensive Psychiatry 1966;4(4):248–58.
7. Johnson GB, Werstlein PO. Reframing: A strategy to improve care of manipulative patients. Issues in Mental Health Nursing 1990;11:237–41.
8. See reference 3.

9. Peer Contagion and Negative Influence

When the adolescent retreats from the family, the peer group makes up for the loss. Unless there is a stronger influence from nonparental adults, the peer group's influence grows in strength. When adolescents in treatment come together, they find much in common, including a general distrust of adults. The reactions of adults toward them may merely confirm their perception of a society that is hostile to them. Female patients are vulnerable to peer influence in other ways, particularly by imitative acts. This becomes evident in epidemics of wrist-cutting in hospitals. It is difficult to know whether such acts stem from a pathological identification with others or from the need to be one of a group [1].

Although there may be groups of patients who are strong enough to become leaders in supporting treatment, it is more common for adolescents to form groups that resist treatment and support one another's negative self-defeating attitudes. These groups may eventually dominate all other patients who, even if they support treatment, cannot risk the group's disapproval nor prevent its destruction. Redl breathlessly describes peer group phenomena in such colorful terms as "group psychological intoxication," "group psychological role suction," "contagion clusters," "subclique formation," and "mascot cultivation." He describes these processes as forces that every resident will experience. Peer groupings then remove the benefits of individual staff relationships with patients, since the staff begins to see the patients as a group or a gang and loses touch with them as persons that they know and like [2–3].

An appreciation of the importance of groups rather than trying to destroy them is usually called for, respecting the influence of groups and enhancing their sense of responsibility rather than ignoring it. The most successful way to turn this peer influence into beneficial treatment is illustrated by the positive peer culture model, a form of treatment used in many residential treatment centers. Lewis and colleagues discuss a early form of this technique, a protreatment group process for adolescents that relies on making the group accountable for the behavior of each member and each member responsible to the group. The group participates in destructive behavior by passively allowing it to happen. If some members of the group seem near to destructive acting out, the staff members encourage members of the group to give support and offer the opportunity to talk rather than act out these feelings. At first, many of these patients will simply "play the game" and pretend to be honest and concerned. Many, after acting in new ways, find themselves incorporating these behaviors into their lives [4].

The protreatment group can lose its power and influence when several adolescents are discharged at the same time or when well functioning patients are replaced by resistant adolescents. If the protreatment process becomes part of the ongoing culture and each new patient who enters it is "outflanked" by committed peers regression may be prevented. A well-formulated unit culture and structure will also help to modify peer contagion and negative influence. This early article provides only one, not the ultimate answer, to peer contagion and negative influence. The protreatment process had definite power because group privileges could be withdrawn because of the action of one peer. Subjecting an entire unit to restrictions because of one person's actions often stimulates anger and violence, and is no longer recommended [4].

Formation of Adolescent Gangs

Even more serious than peer contagion is the development of antitreatment groups or even "gangs" in residential treatment or in the psychiatric hospital. These groups can destroy treatment for themselves and others, threaten the safety of other patients and staff, and often leave the hospital after little progress. Gangs exclude others, making patients and staff members into nonpersons. They will usually be extremely provocative toward staff members, cause many splits between patients and staff, and their behaviors are primarily negative [5].

Interventions for Gangs

Obviously, the best intervention is to learn how to prevent gang formation. The selection of patients and the ability to distribute them in separate units can be helpful, avoiding a critical mass of antisocial patients in a single unit. Yet errors in diagnosis, administrative directives, and optimistic beliefs in the hospital's effectiveness with such patients may bring more than the desired number of antisocial patients together. The most common response to gang formation may be paralysis of the treatment team [5].

If possible, preventive interventions should not include threats to discharge the gang members. Berland and colleagues suggest several ways to intervene. The first involves a kind of joining with the gang on the part of the staff. They write about a unit director who spent evenings interacting with two or three gang members, talking about their problems and later about their difficulties with each other. The director and other staff members were able to help develop more positive interactions among the boys, decrease the gang activity, and increase requests for group help with drug problems. The staff member finally became a facilitator working within the group to resolve conflicts [5].

The second intervention suggested by Glenn is a protreatment process, similar to that described by Lewis and colleagues. Glenn looked to the literature on street gangs for knowledge on how to work with delinquent subgroups in hospitals. The literature suggests that the staff member be casual in initial contact since members will need time to size up an adult. The adult staff member should be honest about motives in approaching the group and should also respect the group's leadership. Early in the group's development the staff should remain neutral toward the antiestablishment attitudes expressed. The gang will undoubtedly test how judgmental, critical or punitive the staff member will be [6].

These approaches view the hospital and the gang as two cultures and try to "infuse" the culture of the gang with the culture of the institution. In *Cottage Six*, Polsky describes the way in which adolescents formed a group subculture with specific values and attitudes toward the institution and staff. Polsky finds that a central task in treatment is the insertion of staff values into the resident's daily lives. The person is treatable to the extent that there is an identification and emotional commitment to staff values. Glenn worked with a group of late adolescents and began her influence by telling a gang that had formed that she had something she wanted to talk to them about. When they became curious and asked to meet with her, they asked her to help them make the unit more fun. This led to further meetings, where she was able to let the members know that she knew that they were important to each other and expressed her surprise that they got along so well. This helped them to begin to share their insecurities with each other and to step back to examine their need to cling to each other for support. Glenn believes that direct work with adolescents in their natural groupings can prevent them from displacing their fear and hostility to staff members. If adolescents can risk expressing their feelings directly in the group and feel a good sense of belonging they may be less defensive with staff and more active in seeking new alliances, both with other peers and staff [7–8].

If staff members continue to simply see gang formation as sociopathic, they will probably respond in a tough rather than empathic manner and unintentionally contribute to an unruly climate on the unit. If, instead, they recognize the defensive nature of gang formation, they may respond with an understanding that will allow approaching gangs from another perspective [9].

References

1. Caplan LM. Identification, a complicating factor in the inpatient treatment of adolescent girls. American Journal of Orthopsychiatry 1966 Jul;36[(4);720–40.
2. Hartocollis P. Aggressive behavior and the fear of violence. Adolescence 1972;7:79–80.
3. Redl F. The concept of a "therapeutic milieu." American Journal of Orthopsychiatry 1959;29:721–36.
4. Lewis JM, Gossett JT, King JW, Carson DI. Development of a protreatment group process among hospitalized adolescents. Adolescent Psychiatry 1973 Nov;2:351–62.
5. Berland DI, Homlisch JS, Blotcky MJ. Adolescent gangs in the hospital. Bulletin Menninger Clinic 1989;53:41–3.
6. Glenn KL. Gang work in a psychiatric hospital. Bulletin Menninger Clinic 1969;33:122–43.

7. Polsky HW. Cottage Six: The social system of delinquent boys in residential treatment. New York: Russell Sage, 1962.
8. See reference 6.
9. See reference 5.

10. Physical and Sexual Abuse in the Treatment Setting

There is now no question that sexual or physical abuse of patients can occur within psychiatric facilities. The treatment center staff should develop preventive measures and establish set procedures in the event of such occurrences. The communication network of the treatment center is one safeguard that does not exist in other institutions. Since behavior is always being observed, recorded and evaluated for its meaning, it would seem that few behaviors will escape scrutiny [1].

When staff members are trained to deal with anger and with physical aggression and have crisis management training, they are usually prepared to abstain from any behaviors that could be interpreted as physical abuse. They should also be trained to refrain from questionable sexual behaviors with patients. It happens too often that the need for training becomes important only when a charge of inappropriate behavior has been made. Male staff members who work with female adolescents may not know how to set limits. Others may so fear accusations of sexual abuse that they cannot act naturally. They need to be able to develop helping relationships without being misinterpreted or falsely accused of sexual harassment or abuse, as well as how not to succumb to their own feelings of sexual attraction [2].

The male worker should attend to the message he conveys and the way his relationship with the patient is defined. He must not only be aware of his own messages but also anticipate how they can possibly be interpreted. If the staff member begins to look at all communications as an attempt to define relationships, he will be more aware of their meaning. Patients who have previously been sexually abused present a special problem. Although one may question whether male staff workers can work with them, they would benefit from experiencing a helpful nonexploitative relationship with a male and learn new ways of relating [2].

Staff members must develop sufficient self-awareness to set appropriate personal and professional boundaries. Even an understanding of the concept of boundaries should be helpful. They must first recognize that patients often have poorly marked boundaries and attempt to mark their own. A clear setting of limits will reduce personal vulnerability. Even something as innocent as keeping secrets can point toward a boundary violation or nontherapeutic relationship. Boundary discrimination must be spelled out clearly. While physical contact is not appropriate in many situations, touch may be therapeutic. Averill and colleagues write that there is a long tradition of the laying on of hands in the medical profession, but staff members should understand what limits should be placed on physical touching. Prohibiting physical touch is usually not warranted [3].

COUNTERTRANSFERENCE

In an article disturbing in its frankness, Ponce describes both conscious and unconscious erotic countertransference in psychiatric settings. Staff-induced erotic countertransference is the most problematic. This erotic countertransference can result in both benign and projective exploitation. Benign exploitation becomes obvious in a staff member's compelling need to help, be needed or to be indispensable. Projective exploitation is the projection of the staff member's unconscious erotic needs. This exploitation has the most tragic outcome since it eventually can lead a staff member to somehow justify overt sexual behavior, in the guise of being therapeutic. Patient-induced erotic countertransference is the sexual stimulus that comes from the adult, child, or adolescent's ways of relating. As an example of patient-induced countertransference, Averill and colleagues describe the sexual exploitation of male adult patients whom female staff wish to rescue from despair. They also discuss the staff's tendency to exploit children's sexual behavior, by sometimes condoning sexual behavior that provides a vicarious gratification of their needs. Ponce believes that erotic countertransferences are understandable responses to children's developmental and psychopathological issues [3–4].

There must be clinical and administrative procedures available that will help staff identify and deal therapeutically with these reactions. It is much easier for staff members to discuss their anger at patients than their sexual countertransference. Fear of open discussion can eliminate staff education and prevention [3–4].

STAFF EDUCATION AND SUPERVISION

All staff members will eventually encounter patients who stir up troublesome feelings and they will need the help of trusted colleagues. Staff education should address the question of inappropriate relationships and interactions; profiles and discussions about vulnerable patients and staff members will be helpful. An atmosphere of open discussion in staff meetings and supervision about difficult feelings that arise in treatment are effective preventive measures. Supervisors should be able to comfortably raise issues about sexual feelings and dangers of exploitation [3–4].

If Abuse Occurs

All accusations of abuse must be investigated. Physical examinations are necessary. All persons who participated in the incident or were witnesses must be interviewed. If there are witnessed accounts, the staff should conduct individual and separate interviews. When there are no witnesses and an immediate physical examination shows no confirmation, interviews may still provide useful clues. The personal consequences for staff members are extremely serious [5].

The staff must quickly respond to the feelings of patients, parents, and other staff. Meetings with patients, both individually and in groups will help the staff understand what has happened. Even before this, the staff should meet to process its own feelings and investigate the best ways to transmit this information to patients and their parents. A guiding philosophy is to be as honest as possible and encourage the patients and parents to express all of their feelings, no matter how upset they may be [6].

Bloom believes that an institution's first response to accusations may be similar to reactions to abuse within a family: denial, attempts to "cover-up," and defensive behaviors. The institution must overcome denial and take allegations seriously, with full acknowledgment that abuse can happen. When an accusation is made, the institution has three responsibilities. The first is to protect the child victim and the other children. The second is to provide support for the alleged perpetrator and all other staff members. Last, but critical, is to protect the institution itself [7].

Supporting the child

The child must be listened to, carefully and nondefensively, and the incident explored with empathy and openness. Supporting information should be gathered, such as where the event occurred, what else was happening at the time, and who else might have been nearby. Everything should be done to help the child from feeling guilty or responsible for what occurred. Bloom advises that the child be "flooded with support" during the investigation process and after. The child should be helped to tell the story to parents, to child protection workers, and legal authorities. Increased therapy time and interaction with the child's significant adults will be helpful. The staff should also reach out to the child's parents, inform them immediately of the allegations and tell them what steps are being taken to help the child through the crisis [7].

Supporting the Staff

The institution must protect the rights and dignity of the alleged abuser. Bloom recommends that accused staff members be allowed to tell their story in the same manner and with the same interviewing techniques that were used with the child. The accused staff member is initially suspended, and the suspension explained as necessary because it is the institution's primary responsibility to protect the child. The staff member should be informed of rights to due process as well as help to use them. The entire staff should then be told what has been done. There should be time devoted to allowing the staff to challenge what has been done, ask questions and ventilate feelings. These feelings of anger, frustration and vulnerability must be validated. Administrators should maintain an open door policy. After the staff discovers ways to take care of itself, it should prepare to deal with the expected feelings and behaviors of the children. Inservice training should be available to handle the children's anger toward the staff and toward the victim as well as respond to the reawakening of some of the children's previous abuse experiences. The staff should continue to be informed as events happen [7].

SUPPORTING THE OTHER CHILDREN

The alleged victim's treatment team should meet with unit peers so that they can ask questions and express their feelings. The team asks for support for the child and assures the other children of their own safety. There should be similar meetings in all other units in order to make the children feel safe and to gain empathy and support for the victim. A child who makes such allegations is often scapegoated by peers, and sometimes by staff members. The alleged abuser is often popular with children, and they will be angry. They may isolate the child, and some may blame the child for being seductive. There must be a consistent focus on supporting the children and continuing treatment [7].

SUPPORTING THE INSTITUTION

The administration should avoid efforts to deny, cover up, or defend. One person should be in charge of managing the information process. The media should be provided with information about steps being taken. All revelations should be completely honest and cooperative. Bloom writes that it is not a breach of confidentiality to discuss matters that have already been made public. The next step is to analyze the factors that may have made the abuse possible. This would include a review of hiring policies, orientation, training, and supervision. Since the communication network is often a safeguard, the staff should evaluate its openness and the whether it still works [7].

Krantz writes that child abuse typically has been studied in isolation, as an aberration unrelated to the operating structures of the institution. He recommends looking not only at the person who abuses but also at the work organization where the abuse occurs. The features of organizational life have a powerful effect on the workers' ability to manage themselves effectively. What aspect of the staff's behavior achieves expression depends on the conditions that inhibit or reinforce certain attitudes or potential. Krantz gives examples of how organizational factors influence the emergence or suppression of abusive relationships. If the organization has no clear channels for communication, the stress of work can lead to splitting and projection, polarization, and mutual blaming. Organizational problems, such as lack of structure, unclear goals and inconsistent procedures are exposed in those positions that are subject to the most stress and anxiety. There must be structures and support that will help the staff to contain and manage its anxieties. Those persons lower in the hierarchy are the most vulnerable to the frustration and alienation that comes with powerlessness. Averill and colleagues write that passivity and lack of agreement among administration and staff about sexual boundary crossing may bring about abuse [8–9].

Powers and colleagues also believe that institutional abuse of patients can originate in the system, and compare it to familial abuse. Some causes of institutional maltreatment include stressful working conditions, unclear behavioral expectations, minimal training of front-line staff, conflicting demands on child care workers and lack of response to their concerns. Blatt also looks at the institution and believes that management must continuously assure that both the children and the staff are valued and treated with dignity. Staff members not consulted about decisions or given appropriate responsibility will feel forgotten and unappreciated. The administration must provide experienced, approachable supervisors who can monitor the actions, stresses, and concerns of the staff [10–11].

Thoms argues against the use of the word "abuse" to describe peer-to-peer victimization. He calls for a more precise definition of institutional abuse and argues against an interpretation that the abuse is in the system. He writes that if two or more staff members have behaved in a similarly unacceptable manner with children, the system is described as abusive. Thoms feels that doing this makes it difficult to hold anyone responsible and does not change the reality that real people did real harm [12].

False Allegations

Sederer and Libby discuss how the treatment center should respond to allegations of sexual abuse that may be false. They recommend the formation of a clinical investigative team and a physical examination. Since a claim may be a symptom of the patient's pathology, every claim must be confidential and approached promptly, seriously, and with total respect. There should be standard procedures for a response, which should include an established person to be contacted to report abuse and a team to investigate the charges. A clinical inquiry should follow the allegation. Sederer and Libby write that false claims may be detected when the story or evidence seems implausible, where there is no evidence, or when the patient has a history of false allegations. The investigative process must be well documented. If the charge is not supportable, protecting the investigation from public information is advisable because of the destructive results of a false charge. If the charge is supportable after peer review inquiry, reports should be made to appropriate regulatory and licensing boards. Staff members should be advised to seek legal counsel if external investigations proceed. Patients who make false allegations deserve thoughtful attention and support. The staff member who has been falsely accused will also require extreme clinical support and the opportunity for an open discussion of the incident with the staff in order to recover [13].

The effects of abuse allegations on any treatment center will always be severe and the center itself is seen as guilty for having housed the perpetrator. Vigilance is necessary so that the staff's own fear, guilt, and sense of helplessness will not affect the residents.

References

1. Matshushima J. Interviewing for alleged abuse in the residential treatment center. Child Welfare 1990 Jul/Aug; 49(4):21–31.
2. St. Germaine EA, Kessell MJ. Professional boundary setting for male youth workers with female adolescent clients. Child & Youth Care Quarterly 1989;18(4):259–71.
3. Averill SC, Beale D, Benfer B, Collins DT, et al. Preventing staff-patient sexual relationships. Bulletin Menninger Clinic 1989 Sep;13 (5):384–93.
4. Ponce DE. Erotic countertransference issues in a residential treatment center. Residential Treatment for Children & Youth 1993;11(2):107–23.
5. See reference 1.
6. Rosenbaum J, Rosenberg KF, McDonnell C. Treatment staff as perpetrator: Sexual abuse within an agency. Residential Treatment for Children & Youth 1990;7(3):87–94.
7. Bloom RB. When staff members sexually abuse children in residential care. Child Welfare 1992 Mar-Apr;71(2):131–45.
8. Krantz FC. Institutional approaches to child abuse. Journal of Child & Youth Care 1990;4(6):35–44.
9. See reference 3.
10. Powers JL, Mooney A, Nunno M. Institutional abuse: A review of the literature. Journal of Child & Youth Care 1990; 4(6):81–95.
11. Blatt E. Staff supervision and the prevention of institutional child abuse and neglect. Journal of Child & Youth Care 1990;4(6):73–80.
12. Thoms G. Institutional child abuse: the making and prevention of an un-problem. Journal of Child & Youth Care 1990;4(7):1–22.
13. Sederer LI, Libby M. False allegations of sexual misconduct: Clinical and institutional considerations. Psychiatric Services 1995 Feb;46(2):160–3.

11. Privacy: Confidentiality and Privacy in the Treatment Milieu

Privacy should be supported in the psychiatric milieu with every means available. Patients need an appropriate private living space from which to construct their own boundaries. The milieu's architecture can carefully mark those spaces that are private and those which are public and those which lead from privacy to relating with others [1].

Confidentiality and Privacy for Patients

The hospital setting creates unusual problems about patients' rights and privacy. It should be established from the very beginning who will have access to information about the patient since some sharing of information among staff members is necessary for a coordinated treatment effort. While in outpatient therapy, a transaction between therapist and patient is completely confidential. In the hospital, what happens between a patient in one part of the milieu cannot justifiably be kept from another part. In residential settings, the team is the treatment [2].

The primary therapist should tell the patient exactly how therapy sessions will be recorded and whether or not they will be shared with other members of the staff. In order to prevent a split between psychotherapy and the milieu, most hospitals have redefined confidentiality to mean that information from the patient is not shared with the family and other patients but is shared with staff members. The staff is considered to be essentially one person with the right to know anything of significance involving the patient [3].

One form of privacy that is not always considered is the privacy that is violated when staff members talk about children or adolescents in front of them. This reduces the value of confidences but it also objectifies the children, reducing them to a set of problems to be solved [4].

Privacy among Staff Members

Therapeutic relationships are often built by private one-to-one relationships between the staff member and the patient. It is important not to intrude into the private space of a therapeutic relationship. Such encounters happen frequently in the therapeutic milieu and to not be aware that they are happening may be to accidentally disrupt them. One suggested rule to follow is to not interfere with another staff member working with a patient unless the situation presents danger or requires assistance. If a staff member disagrees with what is being done, such disagreements are better saved for staff meetings [4].

Confidentiality with Family Members

The staff's interaction with the patient's friends or family members requires respect for confidentiality. The staff should regard the details of the patient's problems and treatment as confidential and patients should decide for themselves what information to share with friends or family. In order to preserve the therapeutic alliance with the patient as well as obey the ethics of confidentiality, the staff must not discuss the patient's care without getting permission and giving advance knowledge. Inviting the patient to be present during conferences with family or others will help to prevent misunderstandings [5].

Patients must feel absolutely secure that their privacy and confidentiality are protected. In addition to conferences or social meetings, there are also phone calls from the family. There should never be a reason for the patient to believe that the staff is communicating with friends or family in secret. In the event of a phone call giving or requesting information about a patient, the staff member should let the caller know that the patient will be informed of the conversation in its entirety. The staff should fully inform patients of any conversations, discussions, or chance meetings which happen in their absence. Respecting these policies will build a trusting therapeutic alliance. These guidelines may not apply to young children but should be considered for adolescent psychiatric patients as well [5].

SECRETS IN THE THERAPEUTIC MILIEU

Privacy and confidentiality must be distinguished from secrecy. Secrecy in the milieu can result in disruption and distress. The inappropriate keeping of secrets can stem from the person's all-too-human need to know something that no one else does and an unconscious identification with the patient. Having a secret may help an insecure person feel valuable in the milieu. Secrets among staff about patients can recreate a family psychopathology. Szajnberg believes that by its very nature, a secret in the milieu is not valuable to its functioning as a caretaking environment. Keeping a patient's secrets within the milieu is destructive and anti-therapeutic [6].

What should happen when the staff member becomes the chosen recipient of the patient's secret? If the patient is discussing difficulties concerning psychotherapy, emotional support and encouragement to work it out with the therapist is important. If treatment is to be effective for the patient, only one person can be the primary therapist [7].

There are other situations where the patient's secret causes isolation from the community and has made meaningful involvement with peers impossible. Because of the secret, peers have a generally distorted impression of the patient. The staff member who knows this secret also becomes isolated from the patient community and may feel a strong need to reveal the secret to end this isolation. The secret might be the patient's homosexuality or an illness, or a previously publicized tragic event [8].

PRIVACY AND SAFETY

There are times when confidentiality will threaten the safety of other patients. For example, what can be done if a patient has previously committed a sexual offense? Staff interventions that provide safety while still maintaining confidentiality are preferred, if they can assure protection. However, patients with a past history of offenses should not be admitted to a program unless they understand that an open discussion of problems with the milieu is a necessary part of treatment [8].

BODY SEARCHES

Body searches create a different kind of problem about privacy. Body searches involve the visual inspection of the patient's body, including orifices, clothing, and personal belongings. The search is to find substances deemed harmful to the patient and to the treatment center. Many treatment centers have policies that permit body searches at admission, on return from leaves of absence, and at other times when deemed necessary. Others now confine body searches to times when they are absolutely necessary. *The Patient's Bill of Rights* indicates that body searches require informal consent, congruent with hospital policy, and should be well-documented. The issue of body searches will continue to be controversial. The treatment staff should continue to review pending legislation and be aware of psychiatric trends specific to patients' rights. Patients should learn about all of their rights when admitted. They should be given the chance to express their opinions about body searches by being provided with constructive information. Staff members should try to ensure that such searches are carried out only when necessary [9–10].

References

1. Szajnberg N. The developmental continuum from secrecy to privacy in a psychodynamic milieu. Residential Treatment Center for Children & Youth 1989;6(2):9–28.
2. McGlashan TH. Residential Treatment. In: American Psychiatric Association Task Force on Treatments of Psychiatric Disorders. Treatments of mental disorders. v. 2. Washington, DC: American Psychiatric Press, 1989, 2689–2706.
3. Berman E, Segel R. The captive client: Dilemmas of psychotherapy in the psychiatric hospital. Psychotherapy 1982 Spr;19:31–42.
4. Felicetti TC. Privacy, infant lessons and therapy. Residential Treatment for Children & Youth 1989;6(3):3–10.
5. Milliner EK. An introduction to psychoanalytic theory. In: Wells, LA, ed. A handbook of psychiatric nursing. St. Louis: Warren H. Green, 1989, 34–67.
6. See reference 1.
7. See reference 5.
8. Schwartz RS. Confidentiality and secret-keeping on an inpatient unit. Psychiatry 1984;47:279–84.
9. American Hospital Association. The Patient's Bill of Rights. Chicago: American Hospital Association, 1972.
10. Alexis A. Body searches and the right to privacy. Journal of Psychosocial Nursing & Mental Health Services 1986 Nov;24(11):21–5.

12. Scapegoating

Scapegoating can be a difficult problem in psychiatric settings. It may be a way to displace conscious or unconscious bad feelings onto another person in order to feel better. It also becomes a way to build group unity, producing a "us and them" kind of security. In order for a scapegoating cycle to be complete, the victims must accept the feelings directed toward them and accept expulsion from the group. Staff members, too, may find themselves using a patient for a scapegoat. If not aware, they may displace negative feelings toward a fellow staff member onto the patient [1–2].

It is not easy to intervene in the scapegoating process, but it is important to do so since many patients do not have the ability to cope with it. Brodie discusses the therapist's stance as trying to "increase the thickness of the patient's skin" while poised between overprotection or standing by while the patient is verbally destroyed. The overprotective therapist can irritate other staff members and any obvious infantilization risks more negative stereotyping and scapegoating of the patient. Yet a staff that remains aloof leaves the patient without any protection. The predominant and long-term task is to explore the reasons why the patient provokes scapegoating and work toward helping the person fit into the group [3].

References

1. Steel E. Scapegoating: Manifestation and intervention. Journal of Psychosocial Nursing & Mental Health Services 1981 Apr; 19(4):11–5.
2. Felthous AR. Preventing assaults on a psychiatric inpatient ward. Hospital & Community Psychiatry 1984 Dec;35(12):1223–6.
3. Brodie RD. Some aspects of psychotherapy in a residential treatment center. American Journal of Orthopsychiatry 1966 Jul;36(3):712–9.

13. Self-Wounding

This section will concentrate on self-wounding, particularly wrist-cutting or burning. Although the terms are often interchanged, self-wounding differs from self-mutilation, which is usually more extensive and on other parts of the body. While self-mutilation as an inclusive term includes all forms of self-wounding and wrist-cutting, it can also refer to even more serious forms of mutilation. That type of self-mutilation is a psychotic symptom and an isolated incident. Self-wounding is often repetitive. This section concentrates on wrist-cutting, the most prevalent type of mutilation in inpatient treatment [1].

REASONS FOR SELF-WOUNDING

Self-wounding is a primitive communication, expressing self-hate, frustration, anger, and anguish as well as a hunger for contact. Patients who cut their wrists often describe a feeling of unreality, with self-wounding making them feel real again. Favazza describes self-wounding as an irresistible urge, a way to influence others and establish control. Walsh and Rosen believe that these patients do not have the verbal ability to deal with emotions and that expressing emotions verbally does not give them relief. Self-wounding, however, is a concrete, dramatic, highly visible expression with a powerful message [2–5].

Sequence of Events

Self-wounding often occurs in response to loss or abandonment. Tension becomes a primary affect. Patients need to express feelings but can't seem to do it in words. They seek solitude. Tension becomes unbearable and they begin to feel numb or unreal, absorbed, withdrawn, isolated. And suddenly they cut. Those who cut often seem unaware that they have cut themselves, and yet the depth of the wound and the site chosen would indicate that they had made some decisions about it. The act of cutting provides a release. It is experienced as a way to recover from a feeling of deadness and unreality. The act is also used to change the behavior of others and it usually has a dramatic impact. Persons may also threaten wrist-cutting if their demands are not met [6].

Staff Countertransference to Self-Wounding

Control of countertransference is central to effective milieu management of these patients. Countertransference takes many forms: labeling the patient as a "cutter," as manipulative, or seeking attention, avoiding the patient, expressing extreme nurturance, or wanting to punish. After wrist-cutting occurs, the staff feelings will vary from sympathy and solicitude to guilt, rage, and an urge to retaliate [7–8].

If the patient continues this behavior, extreme staff conflict often results. Conflict may center on the amount of supervision needed. Staff members may feel that the therapist is too permissive and that they know how to handle the patient. The therapist will feel guilty and may retaliate by blaming the patient for lack of progress and want to transfer the case. The staff may also begin to distance itself and describe the patient as manipulative or attention seeking. The self-wounding patient has the power to polarize the community. The patient may seek out a few specific staff members to confide in or will form a dyad with another patient. Self-cutting provokes a profound emotion from staff members. They may see the patient as bad and may devalue the patient's real distress and even justify indifferent treatment. They may transfer their frustration to anyone with whom the patient has formed a relationship. In order to minimize conflicts, staff members must try hard not to accept the good or the bad projections of the patients and discuss their own differences about them in private [8–9].

Staff members will need to stay attached to these patients without feeling exhausted by their needs. No staff member should be deemed responsible for the patient's self-cutting, but this does not imply that such incidents should go unexamined. A review of each incident should develop an understanding of the patient's dynamics [10].

Staff Communication

Communication about ways to manage these patients is very important. Night staff must know the patient and the policy of the treatment team. The team must accept phone consultation for these patients in order to help avoid mistakes. Although detailed summaries and agreements appear in the notes, personal contact with night staff is often necessary.

EPIDEMICS OF WRIST-CUTTING IN TREATMENT CENTERS

A patient who self-wounds often confides secretly in another patient, forming a covert patient dyad, which may represent a rescuer-victim pattern. Secrets need to be directly confronted. Pawlicki and Gaumer advise that frequent reports by one patient that another is going to self-wound should be confronted as dysfunctional for the "rescuer." Other patients need to learn what constitutes positive and what constitutes negative support for the self-cutter. An outpouring of attention and nurturance following cutting will only reinforce it [11–12].

Although many persons self-wound without any knowledge of others doing it, many patients begin to self-cut in inpatient treatment without ever having done it before. It occurs frequently for the first time in corrective institutions, adolescent treatment centers, and psychiatric hospitals. Wrist-cutting can be very contagious in a psychiatric setting. One person will begin, and others will take it up. It can even happen that two or more patients will get together and cut simultaneously. The staff's efforts to stop it are usually not effective, whether they try to analyze it, give medication, sympathy, or even punishment. Patients can learn this way to relieve tension from others in the hospital. Staff reaction to it helps it continue. Simpson describes an epidemic on a general hospital unit that finally involved 12 patients and two nurses. These cutting behaviors disturbed the nurses so much that they then began to cut themselves. Simpson believes that the conflict and guilt that wrist-cutting arouse in the staff can serve to sustain it. Self-wounding can increase as patients perceive staff resources decreasing [12–15].

When patients begin to self-wound, the normal prohibitions against such behavior are substantially reduced. Patients who self-wound receive a great deal of attention, and the behavior can seem to be attractive. There may even be hierarchies of status for patients who mutilate themselves, with higher status afforded by the severity of the self-mutilation [15].

Periods of contagious wrist-cutting heighten the intensity of the milieu for these patients to the point that real life begins to appear dull or unreal. Walsh and Rosen describe the bonds between wrist-cutting patients as similar to that found in soldiers during wartime. Some writers have found that patients who learned wrist-cutting in the hospital stopped their wrist-cutting behaviors after transfer to more custodial institutions. They analyzed this change as due to frustrating transference relationships with staff in treatment-oriented institutions. There are no definitive solutions to this contagion, although separating patients in different units will help. Walsh and Rosen found that labeling self-mutilation as an imitative behavior reduced its prevalence. Adolescents wanted to defy this prediction and did not want to be seen as followers [15].

Treatment

An Addiction Model

Favazza uses an addiction model to conceptualize treatment. Repetitive wrist-cutters cannot resist the impulse to disfigure themselves. Although these acts are usually not lethal, they are a repeated response to internal or external stimuli. When this mutilation is out of control, they are often hospitalized. For these patients, coercive self-wounding brings the response they want from others and removes their dysphoria. Using the addiction model, Favazza reports that the treatment goal is to eliminate this behavior for about 30 days. Favazza finds that many patients will have withdrawal similar to that from substance abuse. The model uses behavioral techniques such as taping gloves on patient's hands when the impulse increases and 24-hour nursing observation. The treatment is a kind of detoxification and will include observation, encouraging the patient to ventilate feelings, and consistent and predictable experiences from the staff. Medication to suppress feelings is contraindicated. Favazza cautions that only highly motivated persons succeed with this treatment [16].

Excessive controls upon the patient are not recommended. When the staff lifts controls, the patient usually begins to cut again. These controls take away the person's own controls and put them in the hands of the staff. Moreover, there is no evidence that punishment is of help. Punishment seriously affects the relationship between staff and patient. For some patients it may even be rewarding, and at least more desirable than indifference. It is hard to decide whether self-cutting should be "rewarded" by special attention or concern. Some writers advise staff members to make clear to these patients that their expression of feelings will bring appropriate concern and that their self-wounding will be taken care of with medical treatment but no other response. Although it would be helpful for the staff to express their own criticism about self-cutting to the patient, this is ill-advised. Self-mutilation can be a form of emotional blackmail, but patients rarely self-mutilate for the dramatic effect it has on others [16–17].

Cognitive Therapy

Cognitive therapy techniques can be used to change the pathological thinking that precedes self-wounding. When self-wounding becomes a way of communicating feelings, it becomes the currency of the person's relationships. The person needs to begin to change communication and relationships with others. Reinforcing social skills is the first step toward building relationships. Cognitive therapy explores the connection between thoughts and self-wounding. The therapist helps the person to examine the thoughts that precede cutting and monitor thought patterns that lead to this behavior. Labeling and describing the feelings brings more control over them. Cognitive therapy can demonstrate that self-wounding is incompatible with self-respect. Since self-wounding often represents a splitting of mind and body, this must also be restored through therapy so that the person comes to see mind and body as one, with mind controlling the body [18].

A Nursing Model for Self-wounding

Pawlicki and Gaumer outline a model of nursing for the self-wounding patient, which focuses upon helping patients become aware of their feelings and acquire cognitive and emotional skills for affect regulation. Patients are also taught self-soothing techniques such as taking warm baths, listening to relaxation tapes, holding a teddy bear, and discovering a safe and secure place. The safe place might simply be a comforting image rather than a physical space. The patient should not continually turn to staff members for soothing, since the ability to soothe the self is necessary for a successful transition from the hospital [19].

The patient must learn to interrupt the state of arousal that culminates in cutting. Awareness of these stages will be new to some patients who often describe the urge to cut as coming "from nowhere." They can be helped to recognize times of high risk as well as what triggers such incidents. They can begin to notice early warning signs and times when they feel especially vulnerable. The next step is to devise a plan of action to develop control and safety. This plan might involve increasing interaction with others, turning to physical activity, processing feelings by talking or writing in a journal or using self-soothing techniques [19].

This plan of action should not only be placed in the patient's room, but should be carried at all times. Staff members, too, should become familiar with it. The plan should be tried out, reviewed and periodically revised. It should help the patient to control impulses and build coping skills to replace self-wounding. Pawlicki and Gaumer believe that short-term contracts, giving such promises as "I will not cut myself while in the shower" can help the staff and give the patient a feeling of success at controlling impulses for an agreed-upon time. They don't find long-term contracts to be realistic. Not only can such contracts cut off communication, but patients may also be tempted to test them [19].

Attention to the wound

A behavioral therapy technique is recommended when the self-cutter's wound is sutured. It has been suggested that it be done with minimal verbal concern and that the person be asked to apply the gauze and tape. Pawlicki and Gaumer recommend a consistent approach to caring for the wound, with the hope of replacing self-wounding with self-healing behavior. One week after admission, patients with a history of self-cutting are taught how to care for the wound. They learn how to cleanse the wound, how to look for infection, and nutrition for wound healing. Pawlicki and Gaumer recommend that after a wound is inflicted, the nursing staff's attention should be minimal and the patient should be expected to care for the wound. The reality of HIV-infection now calls for safety precautions and protective gloves for those who attend the self-mutilating patients [19].

Responding to the Person's Threats

When staff members respond to threats of self-mutilation with insecurity, it strengthens the patient's attempt to control others. The therapist's attempts to protect the patient depends on the patient's diagnosis, impulse control, and history of self-destruction. If staff and therapist take too much responsibility for the patient, regression is predictable. Patients will threaten self-wounding when discharge is imminent so that they can stay in the hospital. The therapist must give the patient confidence that discharge will not lead to abandonment, but also continue to shift responsibility to the patient [20].

Treatment Goals

Milieu treatment should help the patient make and keep relationships. The patient should be able to learn to stay calm and develop more understanding. The staff may choose to reframe self-wounding as an expression of feeling that the patient must learn to express in words. In addition, the patient must develop self-responsibility and must finally learn not to use threats. The patient must learn to stick to the limits and the staff must be able to stick with the patient through the fluctuations and frustrations of treatment. The addiction model would indicate that the patient must be helped with withdrawal symptoms and increase determination to change. Changes must be recognized by rewards for the new behaviors. The patient must be guided in the attempt to learn how to resolve conflicts and develop intimacy with others [21].

There is a general belief that self-wounding should not be treated in the same way as suicidal behavior. Pawlicki and Gauman describe the goal of self-mutilation as actually feeling alive, concretizing emotional pain into physical pain, in contrast to the goal of suicide, which is to end all pain. But one must be cautious about firmly believing that such patients are not suicidal. Wrist-cutters are not exempt from other types of self-harm. Favazza has challenged the conventional wisdom that self-mutilators do not make serious suicide attempts. In his sample of several hundred patients, 57% had taken a drug overdose, and a third expected to be dead within five years [22–23].

The goal of treatment for self-wounding patients is to help them develop responsibility for the self. This will require the patient's full awareness of what leads to self-wounding and what comes after. The patient finally must develop alternative ways for releasing tension, expressing anger, self-soothing, and gaining nurturance and support.

References

1. Lion JR, Conn LM. Self-mutilation: Pathology and treatment. Psychiatric Annals 1982;12(8):782–7.
2. Pawlicki CM, Gaumer C. Nursing care of the self-mutilating patient. Bulletin Menninger Clinic 1993 Sum;57(3):380–9.
3. Close HT. Wrist-cutting. Psychotherapy 1974;22(3):254–5.
4. Favazza AR. Repetitive self-mutilation. Psychiatric Annals 1992;22(2):60–3.
5. Walsh BW, Rosen PM. Self-mutilation: Theory, research and treatment. New York: Guilford, 1989.
6. Simpson CA, Porter GL. Self-mutilation in children and adolescents. Bulletin Menninger Clinic 1981 May;45(5):428–38.
7. See reference 2.
8. Feldman MD. The challenge of self-mutilation: A review. Comprehensive Psychiatry 1988;29(3):252–69.
9. Tantam D, Whittaker J. Personality disorder and self-wounding. British Journal of Psychiatry 1992;161:451–64.
10. See reference 2.
11. See reference 5.
12. See reference 2.
13. Winchel RM, Stanley M. Self-injurious behavior: A review of the behavior and biology of self-mutilation. American Journal of Psychiatry 1991 Mar;148(3):306–17.
14. See reference 6.
15. See reference 5.
16. See reference 4.
17. Figueroa MD. A dynamic taxonomy of self-destructive behavior. Psychotherapy 1988 Sum;25(2):280–5.
18. See reference 5.
19. See reference 2.
20. See reference 7.
21. See reference 8.
22. See reference 2.
23. Favazza AR. Suicide gestures and self-mutilation (Letter). American Journal of Psychiatry 1989 Mar;146(3):408–9

14. Separations in the Treatment Milieu

Hospitalization detaches the person from a known space into an unknown one. The first emotional experience in hospitalization is one of separation—the separation from earlier relationships, behaviors and from the self. Because of the change in social setting and relationships, the person experiences a change in self-perception and perception of others—a break in the continuity of self that was once very familiar. Albert and Gallagher believe that if the patient can develop sufficient ego strength, mastering the repeated separations that occur in treatment can be a valuable therapeutic task. The realization that there is a self that survives the separations allows the patient to prepare for changes in the self and those relationships that once supported the illness. The staff, however, must distinguish between the patient's original illness and the emotional reactions that accompany separation [1].

Homesickness

The younger patient usually always experiences a deep longing to go home during inpatient treatment. These feelings can create a serious crisis if not handled properly. The child may deny all problems in an attempt to leave the hospital or begin to act out dramatically with the hope of being discharged, bringing the parents' own guilt into play. They then wonder whether the child couldn't be treated at home or they become angry at the treatment center. The child, in this painful stage of separation, will need active staff intervention. Meeks advises imposing firm limits with a careful explanation of their therapeutic purposes. The child or adolescent will require honest support and confirming praise during this difficult time. The therapist should give complete support to the limits and inform the parents that staff and administration are in agreement that the child should remain in the hospital. Parents must be informed of the measures that are planned for such situations and be told that with parental cooperation, they can be effective. Both parents and staff must come to see that resolving such crises can provide therapeutic opportunities and that in no sense do they indicate that treatment is not progressing [2].

Staff Separations

The separation produced by the rotation of psychiatric residents occurs so often and with such predictable results that the lack of proper planning cannot readily be excused. Ravenscroft describes the phases of resident turnover. In the anticipatory phase, patients begin to sense that they are being "pushed" to make progress or that they are being left more on their own. Rather than relating, both psychiatric residents and nurses begin to turn inward. Despite behaviors so mystifying that they should be explained, there is often no honest discussion of the staff's new behaviors during this time [3].

After the residents leave and during the turnover, it is as if the patients are without doctors. They begin to act out to handle their tension and anxiety. The instability becomes contagious, resulting in angry outbursts, elopements, and a danger of suicide attempts. Sometimes these feelings of abandonment are not addressed until patients verbalize them at unit meetings. It may take a major confrontation or dangerous acting out to refocus staff on the patients. Ravenscroft makes several recommendations, among them the staggering of resident entry and departures. He recommends that permanent and experienced staff should not take vacations during transitional times. The new residents should gradually, not immediately, assume responsibility. Staff meetings and staff therapy groups can process the emotional issues of the transitions and the staff should develop the self-awareness to analyze its own reactions and possible dysfunctions during these difficult periods [3].

O'Reilly describes the hostility that the patient often directs toward the new resident, including verbal abuse and unfavorable comparisons with the departing resident. These behaviors, if not skillfully managed, can threaten the therapeutic alliance. The patients' earlier symptoms will reappear or they may go through a depressive stage. The new residents will need strong direction to handle these intense and potentially dangerous feelings of abandonment in the patients [4].

There may be a limit on the number of staff changes that the unit can successfully manage at one time. The results of staff's separation are often profound for both patients and other staff. Patients can seriously regress in response to a staff member's leaving. The predominance of treatment team functioning becomes even more important at such times [5].

PATIENT TRANSFERS

Transferring patients brings about another kind of separation. Eisen and Grob studied the results of transferring patients to another unit within a psychiatric hospital. Results suggested that such transfers are not necessarily negative experiences. Satisfaction was positively correlated with being informed ahead of time about the new unit. Patients reported that more information about the new unit, advance notice, and better communication all helped [6].

Shugar and colleagues developed a model for patient transfers based on interviews with transferred patients and their families. They outline four stages to an effective transfer process: planning, preparation, transfer, and adjustment [7].

The planning phase. If patients have early and active involvement in planning a move, it will reduce the negative effects of a sudden change and give them a greater sense of control. The staff should carefully consult the family and involve them in the transfer process. Early involvement with full explanations will bring about acceptance and compliance with recommendations [7].

The preparation phase. This phase should begin from two to five days before transfer. Treatment issues should be resolved so that the patient can attain a sense of closure with patients, staff, and therapists. The patient will have many questions. The staff should carefully review the reasons for transfer, give the patient and family complete information about the new setting as well as assurances about its quality. A pretransfer interview with a nurse and psychiatrist from the new unit will provide assurance about the continuation of treatment and will help the patient feel more secure. Staff members can give support by helping the patient pack. They should give the patient and family full details about the transfer, including the time, the location of the new unit, and the staff members in charge. The staff can fully assist with all practical arrangements [7].

Transfer phase. The transfer phase, although brief, produces the greatest anxiety with its need to disconnect and reconnect. Patients can feel reassured and supported if a "home" staff member accompanies them to the new unit, providing a link between settings. If the patient can tour the unit and meet key staff members and patients, an easier adjustment may follow [7].

Adjustment phase. The last phase, the adjustment phase, will be complete when the patient becomes comfortable in the new unit. The new staff should be sensitive to the patient's fears and loss of previous relationships [7].

The Patient's Discharge

The patient's separation from the treatment center must be carefully handled, not avoided nor denied. There should be formal good-byes between the patient and staff members, preferably in individual meetings that will enable both to discuss their relationship and provide closure. Staff members must be equipped to handle their own sadness over the patient's separation and not yield to the temptation to withdraw when separation is imminent. They must be willing to express to the patient their own sad and happy feelings about the discharge. Unit and community meetings should also address separations and patients should be encouraged to share day-to-day feelings about upcoming departures [8–9].

References

1. Albert RS, Gallagher EB. Separation phenomena as a basis for resistance to hospitalization. International Journal of Social Psychiatry 1966–67;12–13(1):59–66.
2. Meeks JE. Homesickness and the homesickness crisis in residential therapy. Journal American Academy of Child Psychiatry 1968;7:360–3.
3. Ravenscroft K. Milieu process during the residency turnover: the human cost of psychiatric education. American Journal of Psychiatry 1975 May;132(5):506–12.
4. O'Reilly R. The transfer syndrome. Canadian Journal of Psychiatry 1987;32:674–8.
5. Bouras N, Trauer T, Watson JP. Effects of staff changes on psychiatric patients. Journal of Nervous and Mental Disease 1982;170(2):107–10.
6. Eisen SV, Grob MC. Patient outcome after transfer within a psychiatric hospital. Hospital & Community Psychiatry 1992 Aug;43(8):803–6.
7. Shugar G, Smith IJ, Katz G, Zilbert DE. Moving experiences: A model for inpatient transfer based on interviews with patients and their families. Hospital & Community Psychiatry 1986 Nov;37(11):1035–40.
8. Shields JD, Choras PT. Treatment of the hospitalized adolescent: Management of regression during discharge. Adolescent Psychiatry 1982;10:407–24.
9. Zaozirney J. Separation in the adolescent therapeutic community. Journal of Psychosocial Nursing & Mental Health Services 1988 Jan;26(1):20–7.

15. Sexual Behavior in the Treatment Milieu

The small body of periodical articles addressing sexuality in inpatient settings is evidence that there are simply no clear answers to the management of sexual relationships between psychiatric patients. Patients deserve a normal life, privacy, and should be treated as mature and responsible; yet patient sexual liaisons are not usually therapeutic and can seriously distract from the psychotherapeutic relationship. Patients may engage in sexual relationships for many reasons other than love: to prove masculinity or femininity, to act out transference, to meet dependency needs, and to offset feelings of loneliness and emptiness. Sexual feelings may be distorted and used to express aggression, anger toward staff, or even to act out staff expectations. Patients may act out sexually during a manic episode, in response to delusions or hallucinations, or form rapid, intense sexual involvements with disastrous results. Sexual relationships can create an emotional symbiosis that inhibits independence and recovery. Acute decompensation or even suicide can follow the end of a relationship. Sexual relationships should be discouraged if the patient is nonconsenting, is psychotic, is a minor or mentally retarded. The hospital has a serious obligation to protect minors and the elderly from sexual and emotional exploitation by others. The function of the hospital is treatment and protection, and families may press legal charges for sexual exploitation, pregnancy, or disease. The patient's marital status is also a factor in the assessment of hospital responsibility for adults [1–3].

ADOLESCENT SEXUALITY

The problem of adolescent sexuality in the hospital demands special attention. Easson believes that adolescent patients lack sufficient ego strength to deal with sexual impulses. Their emotional dependence easily becomes symbiotic, and threats to separate them can bring emotional decompensation. He states that the adolescent capable of real love probably does not belong in treatment. Adolescents may use sex to play at growing up, to receive nurturance, or to feel cared for. Unless their emotional disturbance is treated, their sexual acting out will remain dysfunctional. The treatment setting has many characteristics that stimulate sexual acting out. Issues get acted out in the intensity of these environments that are not acted out in the outside world. Feelings are experienced with even greater intensity because there are fewer distractions posed by real life. Adolescents in the treatment setting experience a family environment but are really living with strangers. This living situation builds tension and desires and patients need protection. All other patients must be considered when adolescent psychiatric patients are sexual, since such sexuality is rarely private and can create discomfort and anxiety in other patients. If the sexually involved patients are breaking the rules, it will make others wonder if the staff can truly care for them and keep them safe from their own destructive tendencies [4–6].

Levy's humane discussion of adolescent sexuality may be too soothing, but it provides a humane perspective for those who work with adolescent patients. He advises that the adolescent patients' sexual behavior be responded to as part of their total being, and that the response should help them to grow to develop a way of life that includes their sexuality within a good human relationship [7].

Sexual Language and Sexuality in Children's Treatment

McNeil and Morse present an intelligent discussion of the management of sexuality in a treatment setting for emotionally disturbed children, where sexual references were contagious and frequently used as an expression of regression, resistance, and rebellion toward adults. They recommend that staff not act shocked by sexual language, but instead help the child understand the motivation behind it and suggest replacing it with more acceptable expression. Powers writes that children use profane sexual talk for many purposes: to attract attention, cover up fears, to test what the staff can tolerate. Children on home leaves may use it to get back at the staff. The staff can't completely stamp out sexual language, but can help the children to recognize the feelings it expresses and help them find more socially acceptable ways to express them. Most children will learn what is appropriate and will need this language less as they improve. McNeil and Morse report that sexuality was classified as a private activity in the treatment center and sexual information was given to the children whenever it was requested. The staff helped reduce the children's exposure to sexual temptations by being ever present during their waking hours. McNeil and Morse regard complete suppression as self-defeating since it covers up symptoms rather than dealing with causes. At the same time, the treatment center must provide protection, since the unsophisticated child introduced to sexuality without a way to understand it cannot put it in a normal perspective. They believe that there is no "neutral zone" for adults who must deal with children's sexuality. If the staff ignores sexual expression, it will escalate. They view adult neutrality as most often a defensive avoidance of sex [8–9].

The age and developmental stage of the child will help to determine whether the incident is normative. Issues of power, role confusion and the confusion of nurturance with sexuality, are all factors to consider when examining the child's sexual behavior. An assessment of the child's social skills is necessary since the child may be turning to sexual interactions to make up for an inability to normally engage others [10].

Staff members often make inappropriate responses to children's expressions of sexuality, such as withdrawal, avoidance, disgust, punishment or over-protection. Child care workers should also be alert to their own innocent but sexually provocative behaviors. St. Germaine and Kessell address the difficult question of how male child care workers can set appropriate professional boundaries with female patients. They caution the male worker to develop awareness to the message he conveys, the definition of his relationship with the patient (as helper, as father, as brother, therapist, or rescuer) and his possible sexual expressions toward the patient. The male must recognize his own needs for intimacy and realize that they should not be satisfied by patients, even when the relationship is innocent. Professional boundaries can be set verbally by commenting on what is appropriate, clarifying what the patient means by words or behavior, and nonverbally by standing at an appropriate distance with appropriate eye contact [11–12].

MASTURBATION

Most writers agree that the patient's solitary autoerotic activities should be handled discreetly and with "benign neglect" if they are private and appropriate. Continual or public masturbation can be a problem if the child simply disregards social conventions or is unaware of them.

STAFF RESPONSES TO SEXUALITY

The treatment team's response to patient sexuality is often one of silent approval, since there is a high level of staff anxiety, denial of the situation, or even a vicarious overinterest. However, there are many responses available once the staff recognizes its evasion: confrontation, moving patients into separate units, meetings for staff members to explore their own feelings and plan responses, group discussions and community meetings. If a sexual relationship does develop between patients, some writers recommend conjoint therapy with the patients and their therapists as a way of managing the difficulties that such relationships may bring. They suggest that these sessions can be as potentially informative and valuable to patients as individual or family therapy (13–15).

In an honest and disturbing article, Weisbrot points out that the same institution that has rules prohibiting sexual behavior also dispenses birth control to patients. She reports that those who make rules assume that some patients will ignore them and that they can't be enforced. Many clinicians are apparently able to make peace with these contradictions by making analogies with family rules. A good parent will tell a child not to have sex but will provide counsel about birth control in case it should happen. Weisbrot believes that the staff must ask if the sexual relationship is harmful to the patient and to treatment within the institution. If a patient's sexual behaviors are forbidden without full understanding of how they disrupt basic ego functioning and cause symptoms, then Weisbrot feels that such restrictions are not ethical. Gochros argues that by trying to eliminate sexual behavior, the institution may be depriving the adolescent of the right to an important behavioral expression and exploration and also is failing in its duty to teach and promote development. Weisbrot writes that if a careful psychodynamic evaluation indicates that a sexual relationship would be injurious, the staff must help prevent it. She finds this quite different from creating a rule that everyone knows will be broken. This does not mean that staff should abdicate responsibility simply because youthful sexual behavior is normal. It can still be injurious to growth and development. Adult neglect can lead to exploitation and trauma [16–18].

Staff Training

Realmuto and Erickson recommend a training program for staff to develop knowledge about the interaction between normal sexual development and psychopathology and to promote staff members' awareness of their own feelings and how these influence their observations and interactions. Commons and colleagues found that staff decisions about patients' sexual activity were more influenced by its nature, location, sex of the initiating patient and the partner, than by professional norms or an assessment of the patient's competence. They recommend that staff members reexamine their attitudes, particularly those that are homophobic. Training should also help develop the staff's mutual support in their stance toward patient sexuality [19–20].

Staff Guidelines

Institutional policies can be realistic, unrealistic, rational or irrational, or out of touch with what actually happens. A survey of 130 psychiatric units in Ontario by Keitner and Grof found no written guidelines for handling patient sexuality in any hospital, and that most psychiatrists reported that the hospital prefers to deal with patient relationships on a case-by-case basis. Keitner and Grof describe varied staff reactions to sexuality: anger, disbelief, denial, embarrassment. They report that these attitudes may have a critical influence on the emergence and development of these relationships. They believe that these patient relationships often highlight current conflicts on the unit. If patients feel that the staff is ignoring ongoing problems they will create incidents based on emerging relationships to draw the staff into setting clear limits. If the psychiatrist takes a passive and laissez-faire attitude toward relationships, each team member will then take an individual stance which may contradict all others. Keitner and Grof make a strong case for written guidelines, for making patients and staff aware of them, and recommend that they be discussed and applied. Guidelines do not prevent cases from being treated individually. The hospital guidelines described by Keitner and Grof were completed with patients' assistance. The guidelines recognized that patients were likely to develop emotional and sexual attachments. Patients were asked to respect the feelings and moral standards of other patients by not engaging in sexual activity. They were then advised that if they did develop a relationship, they could meet with the staff to discuss the advisability of continuing it. With these guidelines, the hospital recognized that such attachments were normal, but made it explicit that it was the staff's role to consider the therapeutic or nontherapeutic aspects of the relationship [21].

PATIENT EDUCATION

Education can also address patient sexuality. Steiner and colleagues describe an adult program initially involving both male and female therapy groups, that progressed to a mixed group with a structured format that helped to provide essential information. There was a cycle of four topics discussed in a weekly rotation. A 1/2-hour didactic presentation was followed by 15 minutes of discussion. The four topics presented were sexually transmitted diseases, birth control, intimacy and relationships and sexual myths [22].

The values and expectations of the treatment community regarding sexual behavior should be clearly expressed. There should be a set of shared assumptions about how to understand sexual behaviors and the needs they are expressing. The staff should be equipped to discriminate between sexual behavior that is benign and developmentally appropriate and that which is pathological. Children and adolescents will need adults to define the limits for physical touch. The treatment community must protect the patients while still respecting normative development [23].

References

1. Binder RL. Sex between psychiatric inpatients. Psychiatric Quarterly 1985;7:121–6.
2. Akhtar S, Crocker E, Dickey N, Helfrich J, et al. Overt sexual behavior among psychiatric inpatients. Diseases of the Nervous System 1977;38:359–61.
3. Keitner G, Grof P. Sexual and emotional intimacy between psychiatric inpatients: Formulating a policy. Hospital & Community Psychiatry 1981 Feb; 32(2):188–93.
4. Easson WM. Adolescent inpatients in love: A therapeutic contradiction. Archives of General Psychiatry 1967;16:758–63.
5. Striar SJ, Ensor PG. Therapeutic responses to adolescent psychiatric patients' sexual expression: Beyond a restriction/permission stance. Journal of Social Work & Human Sexuality 1986 Fall/Win;5(1):51–69.
6. Stevenson JE, personal communication. 1985. In: Striar SJ, Ensor PG. Therapeutic responses to adolescent psychiatric patients' sexual expression: Beyond a restriction/permission stance. Journal of Social Work & Human Sexuality 1986 Fall/Win;5(1):51–69.
7. Levy EZ. Understanding sexual behavior in a therapeutic setting. Menninger Perspective 1974;5(3):20–6.
8. McNeil EB, Morse WC. The institutional management of sex in emotionally disturbed childen. American Journal of Orthopsychiatry 1964;34:706–11.
9. Powers D. Some medical implications of sexuality in residential treatment center. Residential Treatment for Children & Youth 1993;11(2):23–36.
10. Hargrave MC. Sexual incidents in residential treatment. Child & Youth Care Forum 1991 Oct;20(5):413–20.
11. Carrey NJ, Adams L. How to deal with sexual acting-out on the child psychiatric inpatient ward. Journal of Psychosocial Nursing & Mental Health Services 1992 May;30(5):19–23.

12. St. Germaine EA, Kessell MJ. Professional boundary setting for male youth workers with female adolescent clients. Journal of Child & Youth Care 1989;18(5):259–71.
13. See reference 4.
14. Collins, R. An effective therapeutic intervention with adolescent patients in love. Canadian Journal of Psychiatry 1984; 29:428–30.
15. Levy J, Trossman B, Kravitz H, Robertson B, et al. Inpatients in love: Conjoint therapy of two adolescents. Canadian Psychiatric Association Journal 1973;18:35–38.
16. Weisbrot DM. The politics of sexuality in adolescent psychiatry. International Journal of Adolescent Medicine and Health 1986; 2(1): 27–35.
17. Gochros H. Social work and the sexual oppression of youth. Journal of Social Work & Human Sexuality 1982;1:37–49.
18. Schimmer R. Dangerous development: Considerations concerning the governance of sexual behaviors in residential treatment center. Residential Treatment for Children & Youth 1993;11(1);23–35.
19. Realmuto GM, Erickson WD. The management of sexual issues in adolescent treatment programs. Adolescence 1986; 21(82):347–56.
20. Commons ML, Bohn JT, Godon LT, Hauser MG, et al. Professionals' attitudes towards sex between institutionalized patients. American Journal of Psychotherapy 1992 Oct;66(5):571–80.
21. See reference 3.
22. Steiner H, Lussier RG, Maust GC, DiPalma LM, et al. Psychoeducation about sexual issues in an acute treatment setting. Hospital & Community Psychiatry 1994 Apr;45(5):380–1.
23. Johnson TC, Aoki WT. Sexual behaviors of latency age children in residential treatment. Residential Treatment for Children & Youth 1993;11(2):1–22.

16. Smoking

Psychiatric facilities have not immediately joined other hospitals in instituting no-smoking policies. Cigarette smoking among psychiatric patients has always been higher than in the general population. It has been estimated that from 52 to 88% of patients smoke. Patients may smoke because they believe that smoking self-medicates disturbing symptoms, counteracts the sedative effects of medication, or because they find that cigarettes help them to relax or concentrate. The belief that psychiatric patients were less able to cope without cigarettes caused many to believe that the treatment problems of nicotine withdrawal and the resulting behaviors far outweighed the health benefits. Many fear that psychiatric patients will become increasingly irritable, anxious, confused and unable to concentrate when trying to withdraw from nicotine. Still, the information on the effects of passive smoking provides a stronger need to change the smoking policy in any facility that works toward improving health [1–3].

Smoking can be very dangerous behavior for many psychiatric patients, with serious risks of fire and self-inflicted injuries, as well as high costs of hospital maintenance. It also causes many patient-staff disagreements, such as aggressive incidents when some initial limits are put on smoking behavior or disruption of milieu and therapy meetings. Others feel, that with the establishment of a smoking ban, the issue of smoking would tend to displace more central conflicts, such as those which had brought the patient to the hospital [4–5].

It is even more crucial to establish smoking bans in psychiatric units for children or adolescents. It is possible to establish a nonsmoking policy for this population, despite initial patient and staff opposition. In addition, reports from many institutions that ban smoking indicate that it did not produce an increase in aggressive incidents or an increased need for seclusion or restraints. Eliminating cigarettes as a source of conflict can eventually free the staff to deal with more significant treatment issues [6].

While many staff members initially will be against a smoking ban, Dingman and colleagues report that they are usually in favor once it is in operation. Parks and Devine report that a survey at 11 state hospitals indicates that staff had greater difficulty with smoking bans than patients, primarily because of the stress of having to enforce the rules. Staff response ranged from predictions of doom to overt resistance or sabotage. When smoking bans are discussed, it must be remembered that many hospitals allow smoking away from the unit or outside the hospital, and that the smoking ban is applied to smoking in hospital areas, not banning the actual smoking of patients or staff. Thorward and colleagues report, for example, that patients could take cigarettes with them if they went outside on their own. Patients with off-unit privileges could smoke. This motivated patients to work very hard to get such privileges. Although many attempts were made to not allow off-unit privileges to be labeled as smoking privileges, this was difficult to do [6–8].

PREPARATION FOR A NONSMOKING POLICY

Erwin and Biorid suggest that the following preparations should be made before establishing a smoking ban:

1. Insure the entire staff's support and cooperation.
2. Elicit staff's concerns, expectations, and ideas on how to successfully carry out the ban.
3. Familiarize the staff with symptoms that result from smoking cessation and withdrawal.
4. Insure medical support, the help of a physician when needed, and decide whether to use medical aids such as nicotine gum.
5. Organize a professionally led smoke cessation group for both staff and patients.
6. Review all fire safety procedures with both staff and patients since patients will find hidden areas for smoking.

The policy will also require specific procedures with patients. Admission procedures should be rewritten to include the need to remove all tobacco, store it on admission, and return it after discharge. Patients going on activities or on a pass should not be given tobacco or have it returned to them, since this weakens the no-smoking message. Positively worded no smoking signs, with messages such as "Thank you for not smoking" have been found to be slightly more effective than negatively worded ones. Verbal prompts, gently telling patients that smoking was not allowed, were also helpful [9].

Gralnick stresses strong educational efforts and a gradual process to prepare for a no-smoking policy. He began by sending out educational information, research and newspaper clippings, to staff members and patients as well as posting them on bulletin boards. A value system against smoking increased in influence. Nonsmokers were encouraged to know that they were entitled to a smoke-free workplace. Patients who smoked had to weigh their own desires against providing a healthy environment for others. Signs prohibiting smoking were placed in the dining rooms. The process was gradual. Cigarette machines were removed. Staff were instructed to no longer order cigarettes for patients. Both groups were encouraged to attend a smoking cessation program, and many completed it successfully. Later, patients who were admitted were told that they would be taken off smoking, and they did not refuse to come. It was finally decided that the hospital had really been allowing patients to use and administer a dangerous drug to themselves. With this framing of the issue, it was then decided that patients should not own cigarettes, but the hospital would stock them as they did other drugs. During the withdrawal period they would be dispensed as other drugs [10].

Although much of the literature describes a surprising success in changing smoking policies, it is probable that the problems associated with trying to do this have been underreported. Freeman and McClellan report that when a smoking ban was established in a VA hospital, up to 25% of the patients who smoked had difficulty adjusting and some patients experienced major disruptions in treatment. Some were too impaired to understand the reasons for a ban, to respond to counseling or to use nicotine gum. A great deal of staff time had to be spent assessing the patient's ability to safely leave the unit to smoke, and there were many fears that clinical misjudgments would occur and that an impaired patient would be in danger. Freeman and McClellan recommend that patients be aware of smoking restrictions early in admission so that alternative arrangements can be made if necessary. Within a hospital system, such as the VA, administrators might consider developing a unit at one facility where smoking is permitted so that patients who have proven unable to abstain can be accommodated. This would be needed for patients who are held involuntarily for extended period of time. Freeman and McClellan also found that off-unit smoking breaks were practical for even seriously disturbed patients if accompanied by another patient who served as escort. They also believe that patients who cannot leave the unit should still be able to smoke, with a well-ventilated area on a psychiatric unit. This would be only a temporary measure, however. Lavin believes that an institution cannot defend imposing smoking bans on unwilling psychiatric patients. The argument that smoke can harm nonsmoking patients can be solved, according to Lavin, by providing smoking rooms or letting patients with privileges smoke on hospital grounds [11–12].

There should be no illusions about long-term individual benefits from a smoking ban in the hospital. Jonas and Eagle found that the involuntary ban on smoking had no effect on the long-term abstinence from smoking in psychiatric patients following discharge. Despite patient education and the help of nicotine gum, there was a high relapse rate and patients were really not motivated to stop smoking. Smoking was taken up almost immediately after discharge. If the final goal is to completely stop persons from smoking, more structured programs will be required. Future rehabilitation programs may need to use other techniques to reduce addiction, such as relaxation training and support groups as well as the standard smoking cessation training. Smith and Grant found that controlling the urge to smoke was converted into a therapeutic opportunity to learn and practice impulse control skills, such as self-directed talk, relaxation, stimulus substitution, and distraction [13–14].

Glassman examines the possible effects of smoking and nicotine withdrawal on psychiatric illness. Anxious patients usually report that smoking decreases anxiety, although experimental evidence has not supported this impression. Glassman writes that the great number of patients with schizophrenia who smoke suggests the possibility that this heavy use of nicotine may serve some therapeutic purpose. Smoking cessation can bring on depression. Glassman reports that 75% of smokers with a history of depression described a depressed mood after the first week, as compared to 30% of smokers without such a history. Glassman concludes by asking whether pressure to stop smoking may produce some risks for psychiatric patients. Smoking cessation is not only more difficult for these patients, but for some, it risks exacerbating their pathology. Breslau and colleagues, studying the association between nicotine dependence and major depressive disorder, find that either depression influences or causes nicotine dependence or that nicotine dependence brings on depression, or that there is a common factor in both disorders. Effects of withdrawal are more severe in smokers with depression. They may require specific attention. Hall and colleagues report that smokers with depressive histories did better after cognitive interventions designed to enhance affective regulation than smokers provided with health education classes and nicotine gum. The long-term effects of being without nicotine are not known [15–17].

The solution might be redefined in adult facilities by providing a smoke-free environment, but continuing to provide secure outside areas for smoking. However, providing staff escorts for patients to smoking areas is not recommended since it takes staff away from more urgent tasks. Parks and Devine believe that the effectiveness of smoking bans will depend on administrative commitment, staff support and patient access to outdoor areas for smoking [18–19].

References

1. Hughes JR, Hatsukami DK, Mitchell JE, Dahlgren LA, et al. Prevalence of smoking among psychiatric outpatients. American Journal of Psychiatry 1986 Aug; 143(8):993–7.
2. Erwin S, Biorid D. A smoke-free environment: Psychiatric nurses respond. Journal of Psychosocial Nursing & Mental Health Services 1991 May;29(5):12–8.
3. Kaplan SI, Busner J, Rogers E, Wassermann E. Patient, parent and staff attitudes toward allowing adolescent psychiatric inpatients to smoke. Journal American Academy of Child & Adolescent Psychiatry 1990;29(6):925–8.
4. Geller JL, Kaye N. Smoking in psychiatric hospitals: A historical view of a hot topic. Hospital & Community Psychiatry 1990 Dec;41(12):1349–52.
5. Thorward SR, Birnbaum S. Effects of a smoking ban on a general hospital psychiatric unit. General Hospital Psychiatry 1989;11:63–67.
6. Dingman P, Resnick M, Bosworth E, Kamada E. A nonsmoking policy on an acute psychiatric unit. Journal of Psychosocial Nursing & Mental Health Services 1988 Jan; 26(1):11–14.
7. Parks JJ, Devine DD. The effects of smoking bans on extended care units at state psychiatric hospitals. Hospital & Community Psychiatry 1993 Sep;44(9):885–6.
8. See reference 5.
9. Dawley HH, Williams JL, Guidry LS, Dawley LT. Smoking control in a psychiatric setting. Hospital & Community Psychiatry 1989 Dec;40(12):1299–1301.
10. Gralnick A. Nicotine Addiction: Coping in the psychiatric hospital. Carrier Foundation Letter 1988 May;134:1–4.
11. Freeman M, McClellan TA. Negative effects of a smoking ban on an inpatient psychiatry service. Hospital & Community Psychiatry 1991 Apr:42(4):408–12.
12. Lavin M. Let the patient smoke. (Letter). Hospital & Community Psychiatry 1989 Dec;40(12):13–102.
13. Jonas JM, Eagle J. Smoking patterns among patients discharged from a smoke-free inpatient unit. Hospital & Community Psychiatry 1991 Jun;42(6):636–7.
14. Smith WR, Grant BI. Effects of a smoking ban on a general hospital psychiatric service. Hospital & Community Psychiatry 1989 May;48(5):497–502.
15. Glassman AH. Cigarette smoking: Implications for psychiatric illness. American Journal of Psychiatry 1993 Apr;150(4):546–53.
16. Breslau N, Kilbey M, Andreski P. Nicotine dependency and major depression. Archives of General Psychiatry 1993;50:31–35.
17. Hall SM, Munoz R, Reus V. Depression and smoking treatment: a clinical trial of an affective regulation treatment. NIDA Research Monograph 1982;119:326.
18. Richardson M. Nursing implementation of smoking bans on psychiatric wards. Journal of Psychosocial Nursing & Mental Health Services 1994 Jun;32(6):17–9.
19. See reference 7.

17. Splitting

Splitting is a defense that causes the patient to see the self and others as either all good or all bad. The patient presents varying self-representations to the staff. After receiving both good and bad part-object representations the staff becomes a collective representation of the patient and responds in kind. When team members begin to describe their experience with a patient and everyone begins to wonder if they are all describing the same person, splitting is alive and well. One staff member may seem to be the only one who understands the patient. Another may feel that the patient needs a great deal of love and indulgence for the first month, while another feels that the patient should be immediately placed on room restrictions. Another staff member defends the patient against staff criticism [1].

Splitting becomes more serious when staff members are not aware of what is happening to them and begin to act on their kind or punitive impulses without thinking. It can result in explosive staff disagreements and can sabotage consistent treatment for the patient. Even when all staff members are aware of the dangers of splitting, it can still occur with great immediacy because it is an unconscious process. Splitting occurs through projective identification. The patient projects either the good or bad parts of the self and the person receiving these projections identifies with that particular aspect of the patient [1].

Staff members then find it difficult to believe that their judgment about a patient can be so misguided. They find it hard to believe that they are not right or that everyone else is not wrong. It may be hard to predict which staff members will receive the good projections and which the bad. Early in the patient's treatment the psychotherapist is often idealized and the unit staff devalued. Splitting can also result in secrecy in hospital treatment, since the patient who splits may confide everything to a specially chosen staff member and hold all others in contempt. Rosnick describes patients who are completely silent with their therapists but share their private emotions with the psychiatric technician on the night shift. The concept of splitting has become so commonplace that it may be simply labeled but not explored or understood. Splitting must be monitored so that it does not threaten the patient's treatment, lower morale, or permanently destroy staff relationships. The team can provide many safeguards against its effects. A team norm that encourages the discussion of countertransference feelings can build a milieu that will detect splitting. If during the team process, staff members provide information about their experiences with the patient, including their own feelings, and if the therapist shares information about what has been learned in individual therapy, good work can begin. All decisions about privileges should be made by the team, not the therapist. Patients should know that their therapists are members of the treatment team, but that the team makes all decisions. The therapist should also be responsible for compiling the staff's observations about the patient and later sharing them with the patient with the hope of finally integrating these varying representations [1–3].

Staff members should empathize with the patient's use of splitting; it is a defense mechanism developed for emotional survival. Not all staff splitting can be blamed on the patient. Silver and colleagues point out that previous staff conflicts always play a role in intense disagreements, which are not really related to the patient in question. Nor can staff be expected to always agree on questions of treatment. Staff splitting frequently centers on decisions about setting limits. One group may see the patient as hostile, demanding, or manipulative, while another group recommends negotiating privileges to shore up the patient's predominantly competent ego functioning. The staff may split on how much gratification a dependent patient should receive. Dependent and disorganized patients can cause staff members to argue whether they can control their maladaptive behaviors or whether they are simply manipulating. Green and colleagues advise that solutions to staff splitting can be sought in examination of the patient's pathology, the family's dynamics, and the intrastaff processes that cause the conflicts. Both the patient's and the staff's contribution must be examined. This would include a review of the administrative structure and the unit's clinical and administrative leadership. Leadership should be directed toward forming a cohesive group representing an integrated authority figure that the patient who uses splitting may have never had in the past [4–6].

Although the results of staff splitting can finally be corrected, Freeman believes that the patient's splitting cannot be eliminated in short-term treatment but requires long-term intensive psychotherapy. Gabbard recommends that the patient be asked to meet with the therapist, the staff member who has received the good projections and the staff who have received the bad projections so that they can frankly discuss what has been going on. The patient can then reexperience these polarized views and come to recognize the staff is acting reasonably. Gabbard believes that the patient's own internal splitting can begin to mend when the staff comes together as one. The split-off parts of the patient can be modified and reintrojected with further integration [7–8].

Splitting is particularly characteristic of borderline patients, but strong contradictory feelings toward people are sufficiently prevalent to be called normal. Patients should be helped to recognize their own opposite emotions, and be led to realize that many persons are a balance of good and bad qualities. They must be able to finally recognize that conflicting emotions do not destroy the relationships or the image of self. Milliner believes that it may be a helpful experience to guide the patient toward empathy for the persons they hate. For example, they may finally be able to see their parents as victims of their own early upbringing. It is not a question of searching for repressed, unconscious material but the integration of two or more alternatively active ego states that will ameliorate splitting.

Silver and colleagues believe that splitting can sometimes be a positive indication for successful treatment. If a few staff members disagree with a general staff assessment of the patient's extreme difficulty, then the patient's ability to gain an advocate is an early favorable prognostic sign [9–11].

References

1. Gabbard GO. Splitting in hospital treatment. American Journal of Psychiatry 1989 Apr;146(4):444–61.
2. Gallop R. The patient is splitting: Everyone knows and nothing changes. Journal of Psychosocial Nursing & Mental Health Services 1985 Apr;23(4):6–10.
3. Rosnick L. Use of a long-term inpatient unit as a site for learning psychotherapy. Psychiatric Clinics of North America 1987;10(2):309–23.
4. Silver D, Cardish RJ, Glassman EJ. Intensive treatment of characterologically difficult patients: a general hospital perspective. Psychiatric Clinics of North America 1987;10(2):219–45.
5. Green SA, Goldberg RL, Goldstein DM, Leibenluft E. Limit setting in clinical practice. Washington, DC: American Psychiatric Press, 1988.
6. Carser D. The defense mechanism of splitting: Recommendations for nursing care. Journal of Psychiatric Nursing & Mental Health Services 1979 Mar;17(3):21–8.
7. Freeman SK. Inpatient management of a patient with borderline personalty disorder: A case study. Archives of Psychiatric Nursing 1988;2(7):360–5.
8. See reference 1.
9. Milliner EK. A introduction to psychoanalytic theory. In: Wells, LA, ed. A handbook of psychiatric nursing. St. Louis: Warren Green, 1989, 34–67.
10. Schulz CG. The struggle toward ambivalence. Psychiatry 1984 Feb;47(1):28–36.
11. See reference 4.

18. Suicide

Hospitalization of suicidal patients will not guarantee the preservation of life. Of the approximately 30,000 suicides that occur in the United States., 5 to 6% take place in the hospital. A similar figure was found in the United Kingdom, with inpatient suicides accounting for 5% of all known suicides. There are many ways available to prevent hospital suicides, but the first step is making the physical environment safe [1].

Suicide Prevention

SUICIDE-PROOFING THE PHYSICAL SPACE.

The first step in making the physical space suicide-proof is to remember and anticipate the various ways that patients can use to commit suicide. Hanging can occur with the use of many materials: wire hangers, ties, clothes, belts, yarn, electric cords, bed linens, guitar wires, clothing and string. These can be attached to shower rods, grates, bedposts, door handles, clothing hooks, or other fixtures. Cutting can be done with scissors, knives from the kitchen, light bulbs, and mirrors. Benensohn and Resnick advise that knives and silverware should be counted. All windows should be shatterproof. Poisoning can be accomplished by ingesting medicines, perfumes, cleaning compounds, and lighter fluid. Patients can also drown in the bathtubs, use plastic bags to smother themselves, bang against walls, and even set themselves on fire. Many reports list jumping as the most prevalent method, so that the quality of windows and impenetrability of screens are important. New psychiatric units should be designed on the lower floors [2].

The bathroom has been a common site for suicide attempts. Curtain and shower rods should be of the "breakaway" type, breaking at under 50 pounds. Shower nozzles should be set into wall or ceiling and never protrude. There should be no exposed pipes, and ventilating ducts should be at floor levels. Bedrooms are also a common site. Benensohn and Resnick recommend that suicidal patients should not have private rooms and should be allowed minimal time in bedrooms [2].

Other parts of the physical environment should not be forgotten. All windows should have screens that are impenetrable and cannot be removed except by special keys. Utility and storage rooms should not have windows and should remain locked. All electrical appliances and lamps should be near an outlet with minimum-length cords. Visitors may unknowingly bring items that could be dangerous for the suicidal patients, and they should report all gifts to the nursing station. Patients should be searched on admission or on return for such objects and suicidal patients should be searched on return from passes. The importance of locking doors and windows should be stressed to all who have access to the unit. The staff should also be aware, however, that suicides can happen somewhere near the unit, not necessarily on it [2].

Both patients and staff know that a unit cannot be made completely invulnerable but all attempts to suicide-proof the unit will decrease the possibilities open to the patient who contemplates suicide. Suicidal patients will inevitably test the physical limits of their ward. Suicide prevention does not necessarily require a locked unit. When the open unit manages suicidal patients, the 1:1 staff arrangement will become primary and the suicide-proofing of areas beyond the unit should also be considered. Benensohn and Resnick believe that suicidal patients are reassured by external controls and all of these precautions will provide a message of care [2].

Suicide Risks

Suicidal risks are highest in males, in depressed patients, and in the first week of hospital admission. Patients are at the highest risk of suicide during the time when the hospital staff members are trying to get to know them. Suicidal patients do not always express their thoughts. A Menninger study revealed that only 1/4 of the patients who made serious attempts were not even known to be actively suicidal at the time [3–4].

SUICIDE ASSESSMENT

When a patient discloses suicidal thoughts, an assessment of risk must be done. The degree of suicidal risk takes precedence over all other treatment problems and therapeutic issues. It is important to know whether the patient has a suicide plan beyond suicidal ideation. The more lethal the means the patient plans, the greater the risk. When assessing adolescents for possible suicide risk, denial should have no place in the evaluation. The staff member needs a high degree of suspicion and skills at interviewing to discover the nature and severity of suicidal intent. The existence of a specific plan and the availability of any means to execute it presents a dangerous combination. From the beginning patients should be helped to understand that the staff will sincerely invite and accept their talking about disturbing feelings. If the patient can share suicidal ideation with the staff, express it, and be willing to talk about it, the treatment in a locked unit can continue. A distinction must always be made between idea and threat. If the patient doesn't believe that suicidal impulses can be controlled, the staff will experience the patient as a suicidal threat. As long as the staff is faced with the suicidal threat it will be vulnerable to the patient's manipulation. The security measures staff members must provide will make them much less able to help the patient tolerate grief and pain. If idea can be distinguished from action and threat, the patient can remain in an open unit. The staff must be able to examine the environmental reinforcers for the patient's suicidality. A suicide threat can empower a patient, turning the once helpless victim into a person who completely controls the staff [5–6].

SUICIDE PRECAUTIONS AND PREVENTION

When a patient is at risk for suicide, precautions to prevent self-destructive behavior are put into place. This can include restriction to the unit, assignment to a nonprivate bedroom near to the nursing station, removal of all potentially dangerous objects, and close surveillance. Suicide precautions should be interpersonal, with the focus being a one-to-one relationship between staff member and patient. The staff member encourages communication and helps the patient work through conflicts and problems. Since the suicidal person is often alienated from the support of significant others, the staff member must enter the social world of the suicidal patient to learn the meaning and consequences of the person's action. The suicidal person is fearful and hopeless with an extremely narrowed perspective to the point that suicide seems to be the only reasonable solution to end the pain. The primary staff can help the patient expand the narrow definitions of self and the world. If the staff member begins to learn about and share the patient's suffering, the patient has the opportunity to expand and try out new ways of interacting with others [7–9].

Wolk-Wasserman describes deficits in social interaction in the treatment of suicidal patients on a nonpsychiatric intensive care unit. Insecurity and anxiety allowed the staff to be "nice" but reserved in conversation with suicidal patients. Staff members were really afraid to listen to the patients or to talk about suicide. Unfortunately, the patients interpreted this failure to discuss the suicidal acts as punishment. Their feelings of being left out increased, and this certainly did not help to reduce their guilt and shame. The fearful staff did not know how to draw closer to the patient in order to motivate the patient for future care. Their own powerlessness and helplessness made the staff members seem as if they were rejecting the suicidal patient. Stotland and Kobler write that a fearful and helpless response to the patient may indicate that suicide is likely to occur while a hopeful active response indicating the possibility of change can avert it [10–11].

Without meaningful confirmation, important information for further treatment will be seriously lacking. Patients need as much interaction as possible. A Menninger study that examines the suicide rates and the frequency of patient attendance at the first morning activity reveals that hospitals with the highest suicide and suicide attempt rates had the lowest average patient attendance. They also report that patients who made serious attempts showed a gradual withdrawal from activities over a period of several weeks, probably reflecting a depressive withdrawal from the external world [12].

Staff interactions and mutual support can also play an important part. An investigation of suicide attempts in a teaching hospital revealed that high rates of suicide often followed a decrease in interactions between resident physicians and their supervisors, turnover among top-ranking psychiatrists or when there was a low ratio of older to new resident physicians. These were times when the psychiatric residents lacked the support they needed to feel competent in dealing with patients. Those who treat suicidal patients need support from each other to sustain them in feeling competent and suicide risk is higher under conditions of weakened staff relations [13].

The Suicide Observation or Suicide Watch

Patients who are in danger of suicide are placed on maximum observation. Suicide observation provides an unfortunate message that the staff and hospital take responsibility for the patient's life that could lead some to believe that the patient can abdicate all responsibility. Blythe and Pearlmutter write that staff should conscientiously try to prevent a patient's suicide by its presence and actions, but must also realize that despite its best efforts there is no way that one person can prevent another from killing himself, at least not indefinitely. The patient should not become a passive recipient of control and management. The most effective suicidal precautions are interpersonal. Maximum observation should be considered as an opportunity to build an alliance with the patient the goal of being able to finally return control. Since suicidal patients vacillate between the wish to die and the wish to live the staff member must come down on the side of living. As soon as possible, the staff member should shift emphasis from saving the patient to supporting the patient in the desire to live [14–15].

Every effort should be made to engage the patient in conversation. The staff member must listen carefully if the patient is willing to talk, since listening will begin the process of reestablishing human ties, the breaking of which had caused the patient to be suicidal. Listening helps to decrease the patient's feelings of alienation. The staff member's concern should be apparent. All attention should be focused with the patient, and any indication of "guarding" the patient or inattention (such as reading a magazine) and not being emotionally present are contraindicated. The interactions may not be harmonious, and the staff member may become the target of abuse and hostility. This should not be taken personally. Blythe and Pearlmutter suggest that to simply inform the patient that such behavior should stop immediately often produces a rapid result. Setting limits is helpful. Patients are often relieved when told when told firmly what is expected of them. In a suicidal crisis, rules seem to evaporate and firm consistency and external limits will communicate safety to the patient [14–15].

There are some patients whom staff members find it difficult to work with. Many may find such great difficulties with the suicidal patient that they should be offered other assignments. rather than face the task with dread or condemn themselves for negative feelings. Taking care of the patient who has already attempted suicide may be even more difficult. The patient who has attempted suicide threatens the staff member's professional identity and reactions may include a lack of empathy, fear of involvement, and even anger. These feelings result in an avoidance that maintains the patient's isolation and feelings of worthlessness. The staff's response may reinforce the patient's own negative views and increase the risk of another attempt. Staff members may be afraid of talking to the suicidal patient, feeling that if one talks too much about it, the patient may be tempted to do it again. Most patients are willing to talk about their experience. This means, however, that the staff member must deal with the patient's most difficult emotions: depression, ambivalence, loneliness, hostility, hopelessness and helplessness. The staff should become familiar with the unit's philosophy and guidelines about suicide precautions. Staff members should be encouraged to discuss their fears and concerns about being with suicidal patients [14–16].

CONTRACTS WITH THE SUICIDAL PATIENT

Contracts with the suicidal patient can ensure that communication will continue to be open and they encourage the nurse or therapist to form mutual relationships with the patient. The collaboration involved in contracting can provide the patient with feelings of competence and mastery. The most important statement in a suicide prevention contract is that the patient will tell the staff member immediately about suicidal thoughts. The language of the contract should be clear and specific. The exact nature of what is to be done and not done should be spelled out in simple language. "I will not kill myself. I will not kill myself without talking to you first." The ideal contract is the client's agreeing to the statement: "I will not kill myself accidentally or on purpose, no matter what happens." The suicide prevention contract is a bilateral commitment. The contract provides a balance for the staff member between expressing care while at the same time expressing concern for patients and protecting them against themselves. Professionals must strike a balance between overestimating the risk and becoming alarmed and unnecessarily restrictive and underestimating it so the patient has an opportunity for self-harm [17].

The second component of the suicide prevention contract is the open expression of caring. The feeling that someone cares is fundamental to the patient's belief that life is of value. The patient is vulnerable to suicide when isolated or when there is no help or response from others. A crucial element in preventing suicide is the alleviation of the person's pain of aloneness [17].

The final component is reinforcing the suicide prevention contract. The professional witnesses the contract as the patient states its terms out loud. This process seems to increase its chance for success. Assey believes that when a patient verbally repeats or acknowledges the terms of the contract, what will be done and not be done, it is rare that the contract is breached [17].

Crisis-Intervention Techniques for Suicidal Patients

Crisis-intervention techniques can provide longer protection for the suicidal patient than suicidal precautions. Crisis intervention provides problem-solving techniques which helps the patient move through the suicidal crisis. There are six steps which the staff member can use with the patient.

1. Help the patient identify the describe the problem. The patient should be helped to focus solely on the immediate problem. Writing it down will also clarify it. The staff member should express conviction that resolving the problem is possible.
2. The patient is then helped to consider possible solutions and list these in writing. The staff member should try to learn what the patient has done about problems before.
3. The next step is to evaluate the possible consequences of each solution, listing every alternative with pros and cons.
4. Then the patient chooses which solution to use. The patient must be the one to make the decision.
5. The plan should be put into action.
6. The staff member will help the patient evaluate the results [18].

Intervention by this method is very active but remains focused on the crisis.

Client safety must be assessed, and this assessment should include a determination of depression and/or alcoholism, history of previous attempts, and feelings of hopelessness. In addition, the client's coping mechanisms and strengths as well as the nature of the support system should be determined [18].

SUICIDE CONTAGION

If a suicide occurs, special precautions should be taken with those who were continuously associated with the victim. Sacks and Eth warn the staff not to forget other patients who may have made pathological identifications with the victim because of their similarities in past experiences, especially if both had had a suicidal or abandoning parent. The staff should be aware of the strong but undetected intimacies that take place between patients, even in a brief hospitalization. Depressed patients become more vulnerable to suicide after they learn that this has happened on the unit, and their own reality testing may be so impaired that they may not realize that suicide means the end of life [19–20].

Ponce and Smith describe the management of adolescent patients following a suicide. The adolescents were brought together in small unit groups, rather than in the large milieu. The unit supervisors described as factually as possible what had happened. They had decided not to go into discussion of the motivation or analyze the suicide attempt since speculations would merely perpetuate uncertainty and anxiety [21].

SUICIDAL CHILDREN AND ADOLESCENTS

Although suicide is rare before puberty, many disturbed children have suicidal ideations and may make threats and attempts, with the full range of suicidal behaviors more evident in institutional settings. A chart review of 200 patients on an adolescent psychiatric unit revealed that 34% had made a suicide attempt. A significant number of this group had displayed major depression, aggressive behavior, or alcohol abuse. Borst and Noam examined the evidence of suicidality in 110 hospitalized 6- to 16-year olds. Seventy per cent showed evidence of suicidal ideation, threats or attempts. One-third had made at least one attempt. These patients did not differ on demographic or family psychopathology variables and no diagnostic differences were indicated [22–23].

All psychiatric patients should be repeatedly assessed for suicide risk, and suicidal preoccupations should be taken seriously. The child should be asked compassionately and directly about suicidal thoughts. Even very young children can talk about them, although some may find it easier to express in play. The primary goal is to keep the child safe with all objects which could hurt the child removed. One staff member should be assigned to continuous supervision of the patient as well as an around-the-clock therapist, even though the child may have another therapist as well. This staff member should encourage the child to express feelings and assure safety. The child's therapist will be immediately informed about any increase in the child's suicidal behavior. A treatment plan will be put in place once the acute danger of suicide has passed. Some children may need exploratory work to help them understand their thoughts and feelings about suicide while others may benefit most from a behavioral management plan which rewards self-protective behaviors [23–25].

RESPONDING TO A SUICIDAL ACT IN RESIDENTIAL TREATMENT

The suicidal act in residential treatment is traumatic for the child, the family, the staff on duty and other patients in the unit. Maas and Ney advise that after attending to the victim's medical needs, the staff must immediately support other residents. Structure must be restored to contain the emotions and anxiety of residents and staff. One person should be placed in charge to coordinate all activities related to the victim, family, staff and community, and to shield the unit from extraneous concerns. Another person should be in charge of answering phone calls to reassure those concerned that everyone is safe and that the situation is under control. A support group of staff can be called in for assistance, but each member should be given a role, since too many staff can be as destructive as too few [25].

Maas and Ney warn that the suicidal act will create a feeling of loss of control, so supportive activities should help everyone regain control through organizing, planning ahead, and resuming meaningful work and activities. The treatment team should meet as soon as possible, from 24 to 48 hours after, to work through the crisis and to understand the event from a clinical perspective. A psychiatrist or psychologist may be called upon to help clarify the meaning of the act from a psychodynamic perspective. All members should be encouraged to share their feelings and reactions in a nonjudgmental manner. The team must identify staff members and residents who need special attention. They should be prepared for many reactions, including minimization or denial of the event, physiological reactions, and expressions of long-term unresolved anger. Some will experience reactions similar to post-traumatic stress disorder [25].

The meetings should help the staff prevent a reoccurrence of the act and prepare to help residents work through their own feelings until life can return to normal. The staff must gather strength to support the victim, family, and residents in the process of healing. There will be a critical period of 90 days after any suicidal act [25].

"SUICIDAL" CONTAGION AMONG CHILDREN

Sokol and Pfeffer describe instances of suicide contagion when children feel needy for attention or when suicide precautions somehow grant status to patients. The staff managed this by keeping these children apart and restricted to their rooms with staff supervision. The nonsuicidal children were allowed to have special activities. The suicidal children earned their way back to normal status by following restrictions and demonstrating self-protective behaviors. Within a week only one child remained on precautions [26].

THE STAFF

Working with suicidal children and adolescents is difficult, and staff members can feel overwhelmed and pulled into depression by such close contact and extreme responsibility. These feelings should be discussed in staff meetings. Rotation of staff is also recommended. There should also be an open dialogue in team meetings about the transference and countertransference feelings toward these children since this will enable the staff to work well together. Some staff will feel overly protective and cautious. Others will feel angry at dealing with attention-seeking or manipulative behaviors. Sokol and Pfeffer warn that there is really no guarantee that staff has previously been trained in the treatment of suicidal patients [26].

DISCHARGE PLANNING FOR CHILD AND ADOLESCENT PATIENTS

Children who are about to be discharged may very well react with anger and depression at abandonment, and suicidal behavior may occur again because of this stress. Specific criteria for discharge and long-term care must be planned. Once a child has made an attempt there is an increased chance that another will be made [26].

STAFF BEHAVIORS THAT MAY CONTRIBUTE TO SUICIDE

Staff conflicts and morale can create an environment for suicidal behavior. There are times when staff members become preoccupied with personal matters or with staff disagreements. They communicate poorly with each other and make poor judgments. There may be times when morale is so low or staff conflict so intense that patients and staff may temporarily reverse roles. The staff's own pathology does not create these situations. They are often brought on by external circumstances, during times of major change in the hospital. When changes threaten the primary values of the institution, a coherent and positive view of meaningful treatment may not be possible, and both staff and patients lose hope [27].

Response and Rehabilitation following Patient Suicide

Despite all careful precautions and interventions, suicides may occur completely without warning on inpatient units. The staff must prepare for the possibility of suicide so that everyone will not be plunged into unmanageable despair. A patient's suicide brings catastrophe to the hospital unit and to the several groups of survivors: family, other patients, the therapist, and staff. Bartels finds that suicide survivors pass through four predictable stages: shock, recoil, post-trauma and recovery, and each stage requires specific management [28].

The first few hours after a suicide are critical. The staff must be prepared to meet the serious needs of the other patients on the unit, contain destructive behavior, and address the possibility of suicide contagion. When containment is assured, the staff and patients can begin the process of mourning and recovery. The family is informed and the psychiatrist meets with them as soon as possible. If at all possible, the news of the death should be given in person. An administrator is also made available to work through all other arrangements following a suicide [28].

The Stage of Shock

The first step following a suicide is to call a staff meeting to inform the staff, make an appropriate strategy and assign tasks. The staff should be reminded of the patient's right to confidentiality. All staff will take special measures to prevent destructive behavior, and special precautions and staff assignments will be given to any patients who may be at risk. All passes off the unit should be suspended and there should be no new admissions [28].

A patient-staff meeting, scheduled as soon as possible following the suicide, can introduce the shock of the event in a controlled fashion and assess the patients' response. It serves as a crisis-oriented group therapy. The leader and the staff must convey effective command of the situation and competence to respond to any future dangerous situations. This meeting will bring about many emotions—disbelief, numbness, fear, blame, anger, guilt. Each patient may experience the suicide as a personal crisis. Bartels reports that some patients may feel responsible for the suicide or guilty because they may have had some knowledge of the patient's thoughts about it. Validating the emotions of the community will help deal with the shock of the event, particularly if the staff can describe the varieties of emotions and fears that suicide evokes and convey confidence that it can absorb them. This meeting should create an atmosphere that opens up further discussion. The staff needs to reassure patients that it will act to contain any further destructive behavior and that the unit will be safe. The staff must carefully observe any patient who leaves the meeting or who is currently suicidal or depressed and review treatment plans in order to work individually on the suicide's effect on each patient [28–29].

The Phase of Recoil

This stage is devoted to processing the feelings brought about by the suicide. The team that treated the patient will need the most support when the initial shock is transformed into intense feelings. The unit leadership should review details of the treatment and suicide with the team and the team should describe their work with the patient. The unit leaders should also listen to the team's concerns, fears and feelings, and share their own personal experiences with suicide. The staff will have feelings of guilt or blame which can lead to serious self-doubt and depression. Even simple decisions may be hard to make because of the loss of confidence in clinical judgment. Team meetings must be designed to collectively work through these feelings. Scapegoating, blaming accusations and self-blame should be addressed and prevented. Informal peer contacts will provide valuable support. Cotton and colleagues note that the strength of an inpatient unit is in the combined emotional capacity of its members, so that is not surprising that staff have found that simple, informal relationships provide the most valuable support for coping [28–29].

When suicide occurs in an adolescent unit, there must be ways to help patients who have suffered many losses. Ponce and Smith outline the three E's of dealing with loss. For these patients, the loss must be experienced, expressed, and finally endured. The experience of loss means to allow the adolescents to feel the impact in their own special way, in a manner that is clinically appropriate for them [30].

Staff and patients should both be involved in the formalized rituals of mourning and memorial services. Staff members will find that sharing grief with the family will help them to express feelings that remained closed off in their hospital work. There can still be dangerous periods for the staff following the funeral and later. As days pass the outpouring of support and the feeling of being together will decrease, and staff feelings can affect patients in serious ways. Suicidal patients may come to be treated with close restrictions because of the staff's intense fears, and decisions about treatment may still be very difficult for the staff to make [31].

SUICIDE REVIEW CONFERENCE

Bartels recommends a suicide review conference to clarify the events of the suicide and provide a retrospective analysis. It should not be called immediately after the suicide because of the immediate vulnerability associated with the loss. An external consultant should chair the review, but it must be clear that it is not done to assign blame. At the same time, if errors in judgment occurred they should be addressed. Bartels indicates that it should be clarified that a clinician's mistakes in the management of a case did not cause a suicide, but may have increased the probability of its happening [31].

THE POST-TRAUMATIC PHASE.

Cotton and colleagues call this phase one of new growth around emotional scars. After an easing of depression and demoralization, there should be a review of the unit's policies, structure, and dynamics, particularly if there has been a history of suicide epidemics. The unit staff should also maintain continual outreach to the family survivors, giving comfort and support. Bartels describes the last stage of the aftermath as a return to the daily routine of caring for patients and facing future clinical challenges. This will include the anticipation of possible suicide, and may include special patients-at-risk meetings. Cotton and colleagues belief that the staff can renew their commitment to work and develop mature coping strategies [31–32].

All attempts to help patients and staff through this process must correspond to the sequence of staff reactions. For example, to confront staff members' denial of feelings would be destructive when they are shocked or numb and need protection. Interaction on the unit can provide support and healing. Cotton and colleagues report that the staff members who attended meetings and shared their feelings were greatly helped by peer support and recovered more quickly [31–32].

Times of Vigilance

When the patient is informed of a recent loss, there is an extreme danger of suicide. The Menninger Suicide Research Project found that losses were associated with 94.3% of the suicides they studied, and in 42% of the cases death occurred within three days of the communication. Apparent improvement in the patient should not bring about decreased vigilance, since it may mean that the patient has resolved the conflict with the decision to die. Despite an assortment of studies and facts, there is no special theory which will help deal specifically with suicide in mental hospitals [33–34].

References

1. Busch KA, Clark DC, Fawcett J, Kravitz HIM. Clinical features of inpatient suicide. Psychiatric Annals 1993 May;23(5):256–62.
2. Benensohn HS, Resnick H. Guidelines for "suicide-proofing" a psychiatric unit. American Journal of Psychotherapy 1973 Apr;27(2):204–12.
3. Copas JR, Robin A. Suicide in psychiatric inpatients. British Journal of Psychiatry 1982;141:503–11.
4. Smith K. Research-informed comments on the treatment of suicidal inpatients. Psychiatric Hospital 1986;17(1):21–25.
5. Slaby AE, McGuire PL. Adolescent suicide: Recognition, treatment and prevention. Residential Treatment for Children & Youth 1989;7(1):23–43.
6. Sederer LI, Thorbeck J. Borderline character disorder. In: Sederer LI, ed. Inpatient psychiatry. Baltimore: Williams and Wilkins, 3rd Ed.,1991, 108–40.
7. Hradek EA. Crisis intervention and suicide. Journal of Psychosocial Nursing & Mental Health Services 1988 May;26(5):24–27.
8. Busteed EL, Johnstone C. The development of suicide precautions on an inpatient psychiatric unit. Journal of Psychiatric Nursing & Mental Health Services 1983 May;21(5):15–19.
9. Fiske M, Snyder MD. Symbolic interactionism: A framework for interventions with the hospitalized suicidal patient. In: Rogers CA, Ulsafer-Van Lanen J, eds. Nursing interventions in depression. New York: Grune and Stratton, 1985, 111–23.

10. Wolk-Wasserman D. The intensive care unit and suicide. Acta Psychiatrica Scandinavica 1985;7(6):581–95.
11. Stotland E, Kobler AL. Life and death of a mental hospital. Seattle: University of Washington Press, 1965.
12. See reference 4.
13. Coser RI. Suicide and the relational system: A case study in a mental hospital. Journal of Health & Social Behavior 1975;17:318–27.
14. Blythe MM, Pearlmutter DR. The suicide watch: A re-examination of maximum observation. Perspectives in Psychiatric Care 1983;21(3):90–93.
15. Gibbs A. Aspects of communication with people who have attempted suicide. Journal of Advanced Nursing 1990 Nov;15(11):1245–9.
16. See reference 8.
17. Assey JL. The suicide prevention contract. Perspectives in Psychiatric Care 1985;23(3):99–103.
18. See reference 7.
19. Sacks M, Eth S. Pathological identfication as a cause of suicide on an inpatient unit. Hospital & Community Psychiatry 1981 Jan;32(2):36–40.
20. Olin HS. Management precautions for surviving patients after a ward suicide. Hospital & Community Psychiatry 1990 Jan;34(1):348–349.
21. Ponce DE, Smith JP. Adolescent suicide in a residential treatment center: A clinical and administrative post-mortem. Residential Treatment for Children & Youth 1989;79(1):45–59.
22. Pfeffer CR, Newcorn J, Kaplan B, Misruchi MS, et al. Suicidal behavior in adolescent psychiatric inpatients. Journal of the American Academy of Child & Adolescent Psychiatry 1988;27(3):357–61.
23. Borst Sr, Noam GG. Suicidality and psychopathology in hospitalized children and adults. Acta Paedopsychiatrica 1989;52(3):165–75.
24. Sokol M, Pfeffer C. The suicidal child and adolescent. In: Lyman RD. Prentice-Dunn S, Gabel S, eds. Residential and inpatient treatment of children and adolescents. New York: Plenum, 1989, 325–339.
25. Maas K, Ney D. Suicide in residential care: implications for child care staff. Journal of Child & Youth Care 1992;7(3):45–57.
26. See reference 24.
27. Kroll JL. Self-destructive behavior on an inpatient ward. Journal of Nervous and Mental Disease 1978;166:429–34.
28. Bartels SJ. The aftermath of suicide on the psychiatric inpatient unit. General Hospital Psychiatry 1987 May;9(3):189–97.
29. Cotton PG, Drake RE, Whitaker A, Potter J. Dealing with suicide on an psychiatric inpatient unit. Hospital & Community Psychiatry 1983 Jan;34(1):55–9.
30. See reference 21.
31. See reference 28.
32. See reference 29.
33. Goh SE, Slamons PH, Whittington RM. Hospital suicides: Are there preventable factors? British Journal of Psychiatry 1983;154:247–49.
34. Kahne MJ. Suicide research: A critical review of strategies and potentialities in mental hospital. International Journal of Social Psychiatry 1966;12(3):177–86.

19. Violence

Violent acts against patients or staff lower morale, threaten the social order, and transform nurturance into vigilance. Assaultiveness breaks down trust in the community. Therapeutic relationships cannot develop if staff and patients do not feel comfortable and safe in the hospital. All milieu staff should have some knowledge of the literature about aggressive patients and the countertransference feelings they can trigger. They should also learn techniques to manage violent patients in emergency situations [1–2].

Prediction of Violent Actions

Patient characteristics, staff and patient relationships, and the unit's physical, temporal, and social structure all influence the frequency of physical assault. Investigations of assaults in psychiatric hospitals reveal that a small percentage of inpatients are responsible for a large percentage of the violence that occurs [3].

Patient Characteristics

The best single predictor of aggressive behavior is past aggressive behavior. Blomhoff and colleagues, in attempting to distinguish between patients who were violent and those who were not, found that the best single predictor of violence was a history of previous violence, which classified 80% of the patients. The only demographic variable that discriminated between the two groups was violence in the family of origin. Men and women with less than seven years of education commit assaults more frequently. Young persons commit the majority of assaults, particularly young men between 15 and 20, who commit five times more assaults than the general patient population. Convit and colleagues write that since a small percentage of patients are responsible for about half the violence in psychiatric hospitals, further research should concentrate on this group [3–5].

Diagnosis and Violence

Violent patients are likely to be young and schizophrenic with a history of preadmission violence. Binder and McNiel reviewed the records of 253 patients hospitalized in a locked university-based psychiatric unit and found that patients with schizophrenic and manic disorders were more likely than patients with other diagnoses to be assaultive before admission. Manic patients are also likely to be assaultive during hospitalization. At one moment they may seem in control of behavior and at another moment they can be explosive and out of control, especially if they feel that their needs are not met. Data show that during the first 24 hours of hospitalization the staff needs to pay particular attention to the violent potential of manic patients. The frequency of violence of schizophrenic patients decreases after admission, demonstrating that treatment can modify it. Violent behaviors are characteristic of persons with personality disorders such as explosive, passive-aggressive or antisocial disorders [6–7].

GENDER AND VIOLENCE

Binder and McNiel's examination also revealed that a significant number of women engaged in physical attacks in the hospital. There may be less adherence to gender role expectations in the hospital environment. Staff members may be less likely to expect violence from females and therefore give them more opportunity to be violent. Staff should be aware of this finding so that they can take preventive measures at the earliest stage of agitation and escalation by female patients [7–8].

PERSONALITY CHARACTERISTICS OF VIOLENT HOSPITALIZED PERSONS

Those who commit violence have lower empathy and insight and concern for others. They can be highly defensive, guarded, vigilant, and distrustful. Personality characteristics of violent males include hostile ideation, a compulsive sense of masculinity and feelings of powerlessness. Physical violence can also be predicted by verbal hostility. Patients who are verbally assaultive also tend to be physically assaultive. Assaults rarely occur in the absence of verbal threats or abuse. Morrison suggests that violent behaviors be seen on a continuum, with verbal aggression at one end and physical violence at the other. Verbal threats should be taken seriously since they often occur before physical violence [9–11].

THE TIMING AND LOCATION OF VIOLENT INCIDENTS

Garrison and colleagues completed a one-year study of 887 aggressive incidents and counteraggressive stategies in a child psychiatric unit. Incidents were more likely to happen during the first five days of a patient's stay than during any other 5-day period. A beginning honeymoon period was often followed by a sharp increase in aggression and counteraggression on the unit. Aggressive incidents were significantly more likely to occur during evening hours, after 4 p.m., with incidents very infrequent during the night shift, 11 to 7. Incidents were more likely to occur during unstructured activity periods, such as sleep hours, room confinement and evening study time as opposed to school, occupational therapy and unit meetings. Transitional times during the hospital day appear to be characterized by elevated levels of aggressive behavioral interactions. Edwards and colleagues found that assaults occurred at most times of day although most took place during the mornings, that is, when activities are less structured than usual. However, lack of structure is only one of many variables. Those assaulted were predominantly staff members rather than other patients [12–13].

PHYSICAL SITES FOR ASSAULTS

More incidents of all types occurred in sites for which behavioral expectations were less clear, such as hallways and patient rooms, than sites for which behavioral expectations were more specific, such as in school and in occupational therapy rooms. Once again, structure is a key. Violent incidents occurred during activities and locations and activities which were relatively less structured [12–13].

Environmental Conditions

The ward's social environment, the staff's behavior and the organization of activities affect the presence or absence of violence. Violent incidents are more common in overcrowded wards. Palmstierna and colleagues found that an increased number of patients on the ward significantly increased the likelihood of aggressive behavior, especially by patients with schizophrenia or schizophreniform disorder. Stronger patients will assault those who are weaker. There are often "chronic victims" as well as chronic assaulters. Chronic assaulters are usually younger, stronger, and more mentally ill than their victims. Durivage believes that not only overcrowding, but a lack of privacy is threatening for many patients. Administrative changes were associated with dramatic rises and falls in violent behaviors. Violence is also likely to occur when the facility is understaffed. The interaction of overcrowding, understaffing, poor staff-patient relationships and an inadequate therapeutic atmosphere increases aggression and violence. Periods of time when many patients are together with little therapeutic activity can also lead to frustration and violence [14–18].

Staff Factors and Provocation

Interactions between patients and staff are major determinants of assaultive behavior. Quinsey notes that staff members and patients often give different reasons for an assault. While the staff member can find no reason for the assault, other witnesses may confirm the importance of frustrating stimuli such as teasing or staff sanctions. Unconscious staff attitudes can trigger aggressive behavior in certain patients. The principal countertransferential emotions when facing aggressive behavior are fear, anger, a sense of frustration and impotence. Staff members who do not feel secure may reflect their own helplessness and fear in hostile countertransference. An authoritarian inflexible attitude is known to provoke an aggressive response. The same can be said for an unnecessarily confrontational approach. Some persons find touch upsetting and require a greater area of personal space. The denial of privileges often triggers a violent retaliation. However, Conn and Lion note that 28% of assaults seemed unprovoked with no warning even when viewed retrospectively. In other cases a provocation was identified: 32% occurred during a seclusion procedure; 20% followed a verbal arguments between patients; 26% followed the denial of a privilege. Armond describes 40 violent episodes and writes that in 32 of the 40 incidents the aggressor was not noted to be greatly altered in mental state or behavior prior to an episode, although violence was typical of the patient's previous record. However in many incidents there were warning signs of impending violence such as irritability or shouting at auditory hallucinations [18–21].

Preventing and Managing Violence

PATIENT ASSESSMENT

Since evidence suggests that assaults are most likely to occur within the first few weeks of hospitalization, early assessment is essential for preventive treatment. The patient should not be asked too many questions that arouse anxiety if there has been no suggestion of previous violence. But when aggressive acts have occurred in the past, interviewers should have pertinent information before admission. Such information should include the kind and frequency of assaults, the type of people the patient behaved aggressively toward, the nature of any provocations, prior diagnoses, effective medications and interventions that were helpful in quelling mounting agitation [22].

PREDICTORS OF IMMEDIATE VIOLENCE

The cornerstone of managing violent patients is the recognition of the clinical indicators of impending violence, i.e., violence that is likely to occur in 30 to 60 minutes. An awareness of these predictors allows the clinician to defuse escalating behavior before it culminates in a violent episode. While diagnosis and a past history of violence have been cited as having predictive value, the patients' behavior as reflected by posture, speech and motor activity may be the most valuable in predicting immediate violence. Postural indications include an increased tension state. Patients literally have their backs up in the air, clenching fists or jaws and have visibly pulsating temporal arteries. Speech may be verbally abusive and profane. Motor behavior is the most important predictor. The majority of assaults begin with a period of mounting tension and agitation and increased hyperactivity [23].

Werner and colleagues studied the relationship between verbal hostility and assaultive behavior. One-third of the patients who were verbally hostile also committed assaults. Verbal hostility thus clearly outlines risk. This study also showed that 80% of patients who committed assaults expressed hostility verbally before it. Staff members must act quickly when patients become verbally hostile as this is often a way patients ask for control [24].

THE QUESTION OF ALLOWING VIOLENT OR FOUL LANGUAGE

Should the treatment center prohibit foul language or verbal threats of violence? Federn believes that it may sometimes be better to let adolescents express all their anger in words because words are replacing fists. They have learned not to act but to talk. If the staff interferes with their talk for moral reasons alone, it may be a therapeutic error. But the talk may be a starting point for violence. The question is knowing the child or adolescent. The question of words is really a question of what the words mean to the person and what they mean to the staff member [25].

PATIENT-RELATED CAUSES OF VIOLENT ACTION

The first and probably most frequent cause of patient violence is frustration. The second most frequent cause is a deficiency in the ability to express ideas in words. Adults with this deficiency more often resort to body language. Other patients start to be disturbed because they have difficulties in relating. A third reason for violence is inability to empathize with the victim. Another reason for violence is fear or anxiety. Individuals, whose earlier life experience have made them afraid of being hit, are violent because the one who hits first is safer [25].

Boettcher presents a theoretical model. Assuming that all humans have an innate potential for violence, Boettcher describes the sequence of events leading to it. There is a threat to the self-system. This is followed by a state of arousal. Severe anxiety emerges with feelings of helplessness and entrapment. The person is then compelled to reduce anxiety and overcome these feelings of helplessness and resorts to behaviors which have successfully given mastery and control in the past over intense feelings of anxiety, helplessness, or estrangement. However, several behavior outcomes may occur: constructive aggression, constructive disengagement, destructive disengagement to destructive aggression. The dominant learned response in the patient's repertoire will be utilized. Boettcher advises that interventions be made before severe anxiety erupts. The patient should be taught and encouraged to recognize and report mounting tensions and these needs can be therapeutically addressed by the staff [26].

First level interventions are important. Prevention can still be possible by attending to subsequent steps of the model—namely by strengthening the self-esteem of the person, actively reducing severe anxiety and engaging the patient in a strategy of unlearning destructive dynamics through carefully structured role playing and role modeling over an extended period of time [26].

If the staff member can come to see violence as a communication that can be responded to and related to personally, fear and anxiety may be prevented. Karin Bar-Zeev speaks of violence as a communication of pain that she can relate to, a communication that indicates that the patients' needs have not been met and a view of the world that dictates that they must protect themselves. Bar-Zeev believes that the way to work with violent persons is to create a nonthreatening situation that alleviates the need for violence, to accept them and not be afraid of them. When staff members begin to see the person not as predominantly violent but as frightened and threatened, then they can deal with understanding. The patient's behavior may serve as a defensive stance against overwhelming feelings of fragility or helplessness. The staff can intervene to help patients control the violent behavior which they, too, find frightening [27–28].

Carney finds that aggressive patients have the following four inabilities:

1. Inability to trust. Violent persons have no lasting sense of self but change from one situation to another.

2. Inability to feel. Violent persons are often free of remorse. They defend against pain through action to decrease tension.
3. Inability to fantasize. A normal person can use fantasy instead of acting out angry thoughts. Abnormally aggressive persons cannot empathize. Aggressive adults have less ability to use fantasy and imagination. Persons with an active imagination can produce a variety of responses to situations, most of which are nonviolent.
4. Inability to learn or profit from past mistakes [29].

Brunstetter and colleagues write of the vigilance necessary for dealing with violence in adolescent patients. Retrospective examination of physical assaults by adolescents usually point to a series of escalating behaviors, beginning with either verbal assault or damages to property, unnoticed or unheeded by staff. The physical damage might be small, such as writing on a desk, but it may be the adolescent's way of communicating that destructive impulses are getting out of control. According to Marohn there is a close correlation between the verbal violence, damage to property and physical assault. The unit staff must develop skill in recognizing impending loss of control before the patient begins to strike out. In addition, adolescents can be swept up in a contagion of violence because of the blurring of their boundaries and the fact that they readily merge psychologically with others. Another person's emotions become their own [30–31].

The purpose of any intervention is not simply external control but to help the patient regain self-control. There are may different interventions: talking with the patient, staying neutral and trying to resolve the problem, accompanying the patient back to the room, helping the patient to sit in the room and calm down. If these are not successful, the final intervention is seclusion or restraint. In working with adults, there may be a greater opportunity to appeal more to cognition. The person should be given help in developing alternative perceptions of situations. The emotion of anger must be discriminated from the behavioral response of violence. Skills for coping with anger can be taught [30–32].

SOCIAL LEARNING THEORY AND VIOLENT BEHAVIOR

The violent person is violent because aggression often pays. When it accomplishes desired goals, there is little need to learn other strategies such as interpersonal skills, negotiation, conflict resolution, compromise or delay of gratification. Davis and Boster turn to social learning theory to explain violent persons. Violent persons find that aggression pays. Social learning theory suggests that aggression is learned primarily through social experience, dependent upon specific instigating factors and made more probable when certain environmental circumstances support continued aggression [32].

Morrison finds Patterson's use of social learning theory and writings on coercive interaction to be the most helpful in explaining aggression. Patterson believes that children develop antisocial behaviors through the reinforcement that comes with disturbed parenting, and that children then know how to train those in the environment to continue to reinforce them for antisocial acts. Two additional reinforcers also maintain aggression: positive reinforcement provided by both positive and negative attention and negative consequences. Morrison has applied Patterson's coercive interaction theory to aggressive patients, and uses it to reexamine five myths about violent behavior: 1) the violent person is out of control; 2) aggressive actions such as hitting a punching bag can release aggression; 3) the staff that can control patients is doing a good job; 4) unconscious staff attitudes result in patient aggression and 5) fearful staff members are most often assaulted [33–34].

THE BELIEF THAT THE VIOLENT PERSON IS OUT OF CONTROL

Rather than subscribing to the biological approach that emphasizes the patient's lack of control, coercive interactional theory proposes that violence is a functional behavior used to control others. When Morrison interviewed patients to explore reasons why they had been violent, they most often responded that they simply wanted to "get the staff off their backs." She concluded that their violence was a conscious attempt to get what they wanted. Morrison finds that a coercive interactional style is the strongest predictor of violence, stronger even that a history of violence which is usually cited as the strongest predictor in the literature [34].

THE BELIEF THAT VIOLENCE-RELEASING ACTIVITIES WILL DECREASE VIOLENCE

This myth is based on the belief that violence is a catharsis for anger. A social learning perspective suggests that using a punching bag would merely reinforce the likelihood that violence would be repeated. Punching a bag maintains aggression, which can be generalized to other situations. Morrison writes that even when patients are encouraged to talk about their anger with a variety of staff members, continuing to talk about anger reinforces it. She suggests that learning techniques of conflict resolution would be more effective. Rather than aggressive catharsis, there should be clear expectations that violence is unacceptable and that patients should be held responsible for their actions [34].

Morrison suggests two interventions based on social learning theory, contracts, and brief time-outs. She believes that a contract changes the reward system and gives some control to the patient. Patients should help write the contract and add their own versions of rewards into it. For example, if the patient likes an afternoon nap, this can be put into the contract as a reward. Time-outs can actually reinforce violence, through the attention given and the chance to avoid ongoing activities the person may not like. Morrison finds that patients often use seclusion and time-outs for unscheduled naptimes. She recommends brief time-outs, for less than five minutes, with no staff attention provided before or after [34].

KEEPING PATIENTS UNDER CONTROL MEANS DOING A GOOD JOB

Morrison finds that a philosophy that emphasizes control can result in rigid staff behaviors that provoke patients into behaving aggressively. A patient with a coercive interaction style will find a controlling environment fertile ground for using violence to control others [34].

PATIENT VIOLENCE RESULTS FROM STAFF CONFLICTS

Morrison believes that a small proportion of violent behavior does result from staff conflicts, but believes that other sources of instability make stronger contributions [34].

THE FEARFUL STAFF MEMBER IS ASSAULTED MOST FREQUENTLY

Morrison believes that this myth developed from the psychoanalytic concept of countertransference, which assumed that the staff's unconscious fears are projected upon the patient who then becomes assaultive. Morrison finds that both tough and vulnerable staff members are assaulted, but that the staff members without peer support are the most vulnerable [34].

Morrison presents a new direction for understanding violence as a social problem, not primarily medical or psychological. The coercive interactional style that these patients have found rewarding is more significant than their mental illness in producing violence. Patients derive many rewards for being violent: staff attention, status and prestige from other patients, being left alone. Once these rewards are understood, effective ways to decrease violence can be planned. The final goal will be to encourage patients to assume more control over their lives so that the use of violence is no longer needed [34].

Other writers have also argued that behavioral contracts with patients can decrease violence. Rumpler and Siegerman describe five essential elements in a good behavioral contract used in a token economy.

1. The contract must be explicit about benefits or privileges each person will receive as a result of fulfilling responsibilities.
2. It must be possible to monitor whether activities required are actually completed.
3. There must be a system of sanctions for failure to meet terms of the contract.
4. There must be reinforcement for compliance with the terms of the contract.
5. There should be a record-keeping system so that it will be clear exactly when a benefit is earned.

Both parties should agree on all terms [35].

Contingency management techniques can also be applied to various settings where aggressive behavior may occur and where staff must frequently employ methods to keep residents from injuring themselves or others. This brings up the ethical issue of control. But it must be remembered that no one is coerced or forced to behave in a particular way. Control is used by behaviorists to mean predictability, not coercion [35].

VIOLENCE AS DEFENSIVE BEHAVIOR

Dubin believes that aggressive behavior represents a defensive stance against overwhelming feelings of helplessness and fragility. These feelings are often exacerbated prior to a violent episode when the staff reacts to a patient in an authoritarian rather than an authoritative manner. Dubin describes an hierarchical approach to treating violent patients, beginning with verbal interventions. Patients are terrified of losing control and welcome therapeutic efforts to restore it and prevent their acting out. Approaching patients in a human and respectful manner conveys the attitude that the clinician intends to help reduces the anxiety and fear that the patient feels. Talking allows patients an outlet for the tension that is being generated. Rapport can be further facilitated by offering the patient food and drink. An offer of food, symbolic of love and concern, frequently weakens the most hostile and angry affect. Verbal interventions also include the use of a form of active listening in which staff may make brief summarizing or directive comments designed to help the patient break a crisis down into a series of small problems and to recognize nonviolent problem-solving alternatives. Staff members learning these techniques are encouraged to give patients appropriate explanations but not to make promises they can't keep. They are reminded that setting a physically safe distance between themselves and an agitated patient can decrease both staff and patients' anxieties and they are encouraged to call for assistance without hesitation. They must also be warned to avoid inappropriate forms of intervention such as reacting inconsistently or with hostility. Staff members should not attempt to calm an angry patient by using reason or logic since this approach will only intensify a patient's anger. The key to verbal intervention is to help patients recognize their intense affect and enable them to verbalize these feelings. By recognizing these feelings the staff member not only conveys an understanding of how the patient feels but also helps to guide the patient to an alternative way to vent emotions [36–37].

Staff members must also know when to call a therapist or psychiatrist for help. One reason for not calling the psychiatrist in is the fear that a manipulative or demanding patient, having once received this attention, will continue to make threats. The staff may fear that the psychiatrist's attention will positively reinforce aggressive acts. Felthous believes, however, that a psychiatrist's quick response to threatening or destructive behavior dampens escalating agitation and may prevent future aggression. The psychiatrist can observe the patient's psychopathology at a time when defense mechanisms are not operating as they do in admission interviews. The psychiatrist can refine the admitting diagnosis by observing whether the agitation is a result of psychotic disorganization, catatonic excitement, or manic behavior. When a patient acts violently out of fear, the responding psychiatrist can assure the patient of safety and teach more adaptive ways for gaining security. For those patients who act out aggressively, the psychiatrist can clearly set limits and strengthen the community norm against violence, understanding the patient's rage and emotions but firmly disapproving of the way they are expressed [38].

PREVENTIVE ATTITUDES

Staff members must acknowledge their reactions to aggressive patients and understand how their own feelings will affect treatment. Their communications can often reinforce violence. When staff members are fearful, this fear can be communicated by hostility, and the patients then respond back to the unconscious violence in the staff member. Staff members need to learn how to communicate a nonviolent message to the potentially violent person, role modeling trust and acceptance rather than fear and anxiety. Morrison, using learning theory, examines the staff's usual response to categories of violent persons and finds that many responses may actually increase rather that decrease violent behavior [39].

Adler and colleagues write that a strong belief that physical aggression has no place in the hospital social system can be of crucial importance. A belief in individual autonomy does not require a permissive attitude toward violence. The patients and staff on a given unit make up a community of persons who are brought and held together by a common purpose. Prevailing social norms within this small but dense community can have either promote or inhibit a patient's potential for assault. Certain assumptions can foster an increased level of physical aggression. An inexperienced staff and staff who have trouble dealing with their own aggressive feelings may unwittingly give patients cues that they expect them to behave violently. Patients may exercise less control over their impulses if they assume that hospitalization protects them from the consequences. Patients who fear attacks from others may strike preemptively [40–41].

A clearly articulated, universally supported hospital norm against violence is required to combat it. The norm against violence can be instilled in a variety of ways: a patient orientation manual, treatment meetings, or staff contacts with individual patients. The norm should not be announced and forgotten. It will need repeating. However, depending on how it is developed and enunciated, there is a risk that it will create rather than prevent aggression. If patients view it as a heavy-handed approach by staff to maintain absolute control, they may regard it as a challenge and will act to test its strength. If a pronounced split exists between patients and staff the norm can become a target for contention. To avoid splitting, hospital staff should involve patients as much as possible in establishing and maintaining the norm against violence. For example, patients can be directly involved in writing the patient orientation manual. Discussion of the norm can take place in patient government meetings and in treatment meetings [41].

Patient-staff meetings should not focus narrowly on the issue of control. Discussions should stress the reasons for establishing and observing the norm: creation of a living and working environment that is sufficiently safe and trustworthy to allow patients and staff to work effectively on treatment issues. It is not possible for patients to deal with inner conflicts while they are frightened of being assaulted. Any dangerous act must be regarded as calling for community attention. Even though only one or two persons have acted violently, a violent incident rushes swiftly and powerfully through the community. If staff try to handle violence alone and not as it affects the community, patients will always leave prevention of violence to the staff and disclaim all community responsibility [41].

The violent act must become a group issue and community meetings should address all serious acts. The meetings should not be held to condemn, punish, or shame the perpetrators but to use the community to understand what happened and why. The staff can energize the community to find more successful ways to deal with tension. Discussion of violent incidents in the community helps the staff to teach the value of nonviolence in preserving an environment where patients can feel safe. If the group instills these beliefs in a sensitive and caring way, both patients and staff will welcome the norm against violence. There is a risk, however, that staff will unknowingly carry this belief too far. Verbal expressions of anger should not always be repressed. Staff must attend to patients who have committed violent acts and cannot simply choose to treat only the less troublesome [41].

Consistent staff management and good team communication support the norm against violence. Medical supervision and support is also necessary. Underinvolvement on the part of the medical staff creates insecurity within the nursing staff which may lead to overstructuring, authoritarian and inflexible attitudes. Team cohesion is necessary to prevent splitting by patients. When patients succeed in creating splitting this causes instability that facilitates aggressive behavior [42].

One of the fears of aggressive patients is that of not knowing if someone can provide protection in times of crisis. It is important for the patient to know that control will be available and that the staff will not let allow the person to be either self-destructive or hurt others. Often aggression arises out of psychotic terror, anxiety and rage and the patient is relieved to experience adequate control. It is also important to actively inquire about the contents of delusions that could lead the patient to act out. Command hallucinations and delusions and their association with suicidal and homicidal behavior must be assessed [42].

Organizational Factors that Prevent Violence: the Sociocultural Environment

Katz spent 38 months in participant-observation in three state mental hospitals in order to compare the interpersonal processes and organizational structure in violent and peaceful wards, which had a similar diagnostic mix. Violent and peaceful wards differed in five organizational characteristics: staff organization, management of staff-patient relations, use of therapeutic procedures, psychiatric leadership and use of schedules and routines. Violent wards had unclear staff expectations, irregular and unpredictable events and schedules, and unpredictable staff-patient encounters. Violence was less frequent and severe on wards with strong psychiatric leaders, well-defined staff roles, and scheduled, predictable activities. This study demonstrates than an ordered social climate supported by strong leadership and predictable events can provide security against violence for staff and patients [43].

Katz and Kirkland provide detailed information about the sociocultural climate of peaceful wards. Meals and activities followed a regular schedule. Team meetings were regularly scheduled, goal-oriented, and encouraged active participation. Staff members made constructive use of their own countertransference. When tensions increased, the staff was able to remain calm and coordinated, turning to established procedures. These included making it clear to the patient that violent behavior was not allowed, and helping to mobilize the patient's own resources to gain control. Staff members were able to communicate that although violence was the patient's problem they could help the patient manage it and could protect the other patients as well [43].

Staffings, which followed every violent incident, reviewed the events which led to escalation and devised further procedures for prevention and management. Psychiatrists who trained, respected and supported the staff helped to create a sociocultural climate which provided a therapeutic environment for the patient [43].

Handling Violent Behavior

The work of Katz and Kirkland demonstrates that interventions with aggressive patients can be planned before violence happens. Roles and assignments for handling future violent incidents should be so well planned that staff can be in control to minimize the risk of injury. A well-managed violent incident is distinguished from a poorly managed one by the presence or absence of teamwork. The staff's trust and confidence in each other also plays a part. The most important person is the team leader, but this will vary with the patient. The team leader should be the person who best knows the person or situation most thoroughly. The team leader makes all necessary decisions and directs the other members. It is no time for democracy. The person who is the logical team leader communicates to others who will serve as leader and determines whether there is sufficient staff to manage the incident. If not, others get additional help. Each treatment center should have a mechanism for summoning extra help [43].

The leader must be able to gauge the intensity of emotions of both patients and staff, and use verbal or nonverbal techniques to reduce this intensity. These will include moving calmly and deliberately, speaking clearly, demonstrating self-assurance, maintaining eye contact with the patient, and presenting a calm expression and posture. The leader should be identified to the patient and the patient should be informed that the leader is there to help. The leader should then become the one person who communicates with the patient. If the incident has not become physical, the leader will try to talk the patient down and help the patient to focus on ways other than physical violence to deal with the distress [44].

Allowing the patient to ventilate can sometimes prevent physical violence. The more the patient is able to talk out the distress, the less likely is the patient to act out. If a period of talking occurs, it allows the staff members to position themselves in case physical intervention is needed. It will be the leader who determines if talking has failed to deescalate the situation and when physical intervention may be needed. When possible, the leader should not be directly involved in the physical control of the patients [44].

The physical environment must also support the management of violent behavior. An adequate, well-padded seclusion room to allow patients to let out physical tension safely should be available. An alarm system should be present in offices unless other members of the staff are very close [45].

Weapons

If a person has a weapon or an object that can serve as one, staff should use a lightweight mattress as a shield. If a more serious threat is perceived such as a gun or knife it is best to try to isolate the patient and send for skilled security personnel [46].

Handling the violent incident after it occurs

Soon after a violent outburst, clinical staff should make a thoughtful attempt to understand its significance. The staff should interview the patient and anyone else involved in the aggressive act. Any major changes in the patient's treatment should be based on two overriding considerations, what would be best for the patient and how others on the inpatient service can be protected. Staff countertransference feelings must be shared and dealt with. Any major changes in the patient's treatment should be shared with the entire patient community in a timely fashion [47].

Violence can often result in a predictable cycle: physical aggression, seclusion, staff's response and then social distancing. The institution must have ways in place for the staff to deal with their feelings after aggression has taken place.

Countertransference issues should be addressed so that the staff can freely discuss feelings of anger and fear that they have toward the violent patient. Awareness of the physical aggression cycle and a procedure for dealing with staff feelings will make it easier later for the staff to approach a previously aggressive patient and refocus on the patient's humanity. This will help decrease social distance to and prevent the cycle from beginning again [48].

HELPING EMPLOYEE VICTIMS OF VIOLENCE

Hospitals have developed a wide variety of techniques to manage patients who assault staff but have often ignored the plight of the victimized employee. Although professional staff who have been assaulted resist seeing themselves as victims, Engel and Marsh believe they experience the feelings and reactions typical of other victims and therefore may need help in dealing with emotional trauma. Verbal abuse and menacing behaviors, although not categorized as violence, are hard on the staff. Some of the literature seems to even blame the victim, particularly literature with a psychoanalytic tinge, suggesting that staff members unconsciously provoke violence through personality traits that irritate the patients or through lack of training and experience. Victims of violence need medical attention, trauma-crisis counseling, legal advice and information regarding insurance, workmen's compensation benefits and rights pertaining to health and safety in the workplace. They should receive medical and psychological care like any other victim—confidential, objective, and impartial care given away from the workplace [49].

Lanza observes that some staff felt they would be overwhelmed if they allowed themselves to admit their feelings. For this reason employees deny the very feelings that are so normal to victims and then become more isolated. It goes against the cultural norms for staff to admit to feelings of vulnerability about their work and their patients. They have difficulty accepting that they too have rights at the workplace. Staff has a self-image of being strong and in control, not showing weakness [49–50].

A permanent committee of persons involved in the care of patients and employees is needed to guarantee patient's and employees' rights. The committee must monitor the effectiveness of an on-call team and ensure its ongoing education. It must guarantee that protocols for treating both violent patients and employee victims are carried out, maintain incident reports, and keep accurate statistics. The committee investigates the causes of each violent episode, make recommendations and monitors outcome [49–50].

Storch reports on a hospital support group for staff victims of violence. Assault victims in the group often felt let down by other staff on duty and needed to reestablish trust in their co-workers and the institution, as well as trust in themselves. Those who came to the group tended to blame themselves for the assault. Lanza writes that the institution that assumes that the assault is the staff member's fault, can deny the problem of patient violence and will take no restorative action. Blaming apparently helps everyone to feel safe and more in control of the environment [50–51].

Supportive counseling can also be made available by forming a victim assault support team, to aid victims upon their request. Staff victims will require more than one meeting. During the first interview they will need to be able to talk about the emotions and symptoms they are experiencing, ventilate, and understand that what they are experiencing is part of what most victims experience following an assault. Lanza advises that there be counselor-led meetings between the victim and staff and victim and assailant, to review the incident and explore how they felt at the time of the assault and afterward. Issues of support are discussed, and it should be realized that the victim often experiences underlying anger toward co-workers and feels unsupported by them. These meetings between the victim and the assailant are important because both will probably continue to be on the same unit [50–51].

The Physical and Emotional Effects on Staff

Fottrell writes that chances of sustaining physical injury as a result of violent behavior by psychiatric patients are usually remote. Edwards and colleagues examined physical assaults and rated them on an 8-point scale ranging from no physical injury through various degrees of injury through death. Most incidents involved only slight contact between assaultive patient and victim and led to no injury in 22 of 37 incidents studied. Although injuries were slight, the assaults frightened patients and younger staff members. They felt they had little support from others in recovering from their upset and welcomed the opportunity to ventilate their feelings. Some of the older and more experienced staff thought minor assaults were just part of the job [52–53].

One of the stumbling blocks that staff members have all had with the violent patient is the paralyzing sense of anger they feel but can't express. It can lead to a misguided notion that the patient is hostile and retaliatory. Open discussion of countertransference feelings becomes critical. Supervision should help staff members become aware of their own feelings in response to the patients' behaviors and aware of the feelings that patients can evoke. If they can analyze these feelings and discover ways to deal with them, this can become a part of their own treatment repertoire [54].

Denial and projection are common countertransferential defenses that can be activated by patients who have the capacity to be violent. When staff are guided by these defenses, risks of assaults and treatment failures are increased. Whenever a patient is believed to be assaultive, the staff should give careful attention to countertransferential feelings. Staff may also deny the risk of violence by working with a patient as if there were no reason for concern, using minimal precautions or give the patient much attention and many hospital privileges, believing that a patient who is content is unlikely to misbehave [55].

Conversely staff can project its own rageful impulses on a patient and exaggerate the patient's capacity for assaultive behavior. If this occurs before staff members have developed some positive feelings toward the patient, they will not emotionally accept the patient and this will adversely affect the quality of treatment. If projection occurs during the course of treatment, staff may reject and provoke the patient to violence. Staff may allow the patient to act disruptively and not report signs of decompensation to the team or psychiatrist in hope that the patient will later be transferred [55].

Staff Training to Prevent Assaults

A study in a Florida state hospital examined impact of staff training in aggression control on the incidence of patient assaults on staff and of assault-related injuries. The subjects were 96 unit staff and supervisors. Of the 65 untrained staff, 24 were assaulted. Of the 31 staff members who had received aggression control training, the single person who was assaulted was not hurt, yet 19 of the 24 untrained staff who were assaulted sustained an injury. Carmel and Hunter compared rates of staff injury from assaultive patients in two groups of wards in a forensic state mental hospital. Wards in which at least 60% of the staff complied with the training in the management of assaultive behavior experienced much lower rates of staff injury than wards in which less than 60% of staff complied with the training. Phillips and Rudestam compared didactic training, with didactic and physical skills training. During the two weeks afer training, those trained in physical and didactic skills were involved in 23% fewer assaults than those who received only didactic training and 20% fewer assaults than those who received no training. Those who were trained expressed significantly less fear and aggression. Moreover, subjects without physical competence in nonviolent defensive skills were significantly more aggressive than those who had been trained. Learning skills did not increase aggression; those who had been trained had reduced muscular tension, a lower pitched tone of voice and good eye contact in later role-playing demonstrations. [56–58].

Existing training programs provide staff with the skills and knowledge necessary for detecting and defusing potentially and imminently violent behaviors. These training programs, with their opportunities for practicing defensive and restraining techniques, presumably increase staff confidence. As a result they minimize the risk of injuries to both staff and patients, thereby reducing the costs resulting from such injuries.

VERBAL MANAGEMENT SKILLS

Verbal aggression is often less visible in its final effects. The treatment center also has a responsibility to help the staff deal with verbal aggression and threats. Inservice training can provide the staff with effective verbal management skills. Managing threats should be an important part of training. The team should legitimize anger and fear as very normal feelings so that the staff can share these feelings with each other. Maier and colleagues recommend that with training, the staff member should be able to develop an appropriate, "healthy social persona" with verbally threatening patients, so that they can be approached without focusing on the threat. Van Rybroek and colleagues warn that if the staff is not sufficently trained to deal with aggression, the conditions for good treatment are simply absent; countertransference (fear and anger) will then dominate staff decisions [59–60].

There are no guaranteed ways to prevent all violent behavior. The staff must remember the times on the unit when violence is not an issue and attempt to restore them. Rosenstock and McLaughlin have described a state they call dynamic homeostasis in which the therapeutic milieu can be most effective. Patients and staff share a mutually gratifying relationship in which patients are able not only to identify areas they need to improve but also to see and acknowledge progress. In this stage communication patterns are such that information is exchanged with minimal distortion and maximum effectiveness. Lines of authority are distinct. The atmosphere is one of optimism and security. The staff must recall these times when violence strikes the milieu [61].

References

1. Felthous AR. Preventing assaults on a psychiatric inpatient ward. Hospital & Community Psychiatry 1984 Dec;35(12):1223–6.
2. Engel F, Marsh S. Helping the employee victim of violence in hospitals. Hospital & Community Psychiatry 1986 Feb;37(2):159–62.
3. Convit A, Isay D, Volavka J. Characteristics of repeatedly assaultive psychiatric inpatients. Hospital & Community Psychiatry 1990 Oct;41(10):1112–5.
4. Durivage A. Assaultive behaviour: Before it happens. Canadian Journal of Psychiatry 1989;34:393–7.
5. Blomhoff S, Seim S, Friis S. Can prediction of violence among psychiatric patients be improved? Hospital & Community Psychiatry 1990 Jul;41(7):771–5.
6. Shah AK, Fineberg NA, James DV. Violence among psychiatric patients. Acta Psychiatrica Scandinavica 1991;84(4):305–9.
7. Binder RL, McNiel DE. Effects of diagnosis and context on dangerousness. American Journal of Psychiatry 1988 Jun;145(6):728–32.
8. Binder RL, McNiel DE. The relationship of gender to violent behavior in acutely disturbed psychiatric patients. Journal of Clinical Psychiatry 1990; 51(3):110–4.
9. Davis DL, Boster LH. The violent psychiatric patient. American Journal of Forensic Psychology 1986;4(3):3–17.
10. Werner PD, Yesavage JA, Becker JM, et al. Hostile words and assaultive behavior on an acute inpatient psychiatric unit. Journal of Nervous and Mental Disease 1983 Jun;171(6):385–87.

11. Morrison EF. A hierarchy of aggressive and violent behaviors among psychiatric inpatients. Hospital & Community Psychiatry 1992 May;43(5):505–6.
12. Garrison WT, Ecker B, Friedman MD, Davidoff MD, et al. Aggression and counteraggression during child psychiatric hospitalization. Journal American Academy of Child & Adolescent Psychiatry 1990;29(2):242–50.
13. Edwards JG, Jones F, Reid WH, Chu C-C. Physical asssaults in a psychiatric unit of general hospital. American Journal of Psychiatry 1988 Dec;145(12):1568–71.
14. Katz P, Kirkland FR. Violence and social structure on mental hospital wards. Psychiatry 1990 Aug;53:262–77.
15. Palmstierna T, Huitfeldt B, Wisted B. The relationship of crowding and aggressive behavior on a psychiatric intensive care unit. Hospital & Community 1992 Dec;42(12):1237–40.
16. See reference 4.
17. Fottrell E. A study of violent behaviour among patients in psychiatric hospitals. British Journal of Psychiatry 1980;136:216–22.
18. Armond AD. Violence in the semi-secure ward of a psychiatric hospital. Medicine, Science, & the Law 1982;22:203–9.
19. Quinsey VL, Varney GW. Characteristics of assaulters in a maximum security psychiatric unit. Crime and Justice 1977:212–20.
20. Conn L, Lion JR. Assaults within a university hospital. In: Lion JR, Reid WH, eds. Assaults within psychiatric facilities. New York: Grune & Stratton, 1983, 61–70.
21. See reference 9.
22. See reference 1.
23. Dubin WR. The violent patient: Emergency evaluation and treatment. Carrier Foundation Letter 1984; #96.
24. See reference 10.
25. Federn E. The therapeutic management of violence. Residential Treatment for Children & Youth 1989;7(2):5–15.
26. Boettcher EG. Preventing violent behavior: An integrated theoretical model for nursing. Perspectives in Psychiatric Care 1983;21:54–8.
27. Northrup G. The management of violence by personal relatedness: An interview with Karin Bar-Zeev. Milieu Therapy 1981;1(1):33–40.
28. See reference 20.
29. Carney FL. Treatments of the aggressive patient. In: Lion JR, Madden DJ, eds. Rage, hate, assault and other forms of Violence. New York: Spectrum, 1976, 223–248.
30. Brunstetter RW, Rackow D, Dillon K. Adolescents and violence. Psychiatric Annals 1988 Feb;18(2):118–26.
31. Marohn C. Management of the assaultive adolescent. Hospital & Community Psychiatry 1992 Jun;43(6):622–4.
32. See reference 9.
33. Patterson GR. A Social learning approach: coercive family processes. Eugene, OR: Castalia Press, 1982.
34. Morrison EF. Toward a better understanding of violence in psychiatric settings: debunking the myths. Archives of Psychiatric Nursing 1993;7(6):328–35.
35. Rumpler CH, Siegerman C. A behavior modification approach to dealing with violent behavior in an intensive care unit. Perspectives in Psychiatric Care 1978 Sept-Dec;16(5–6):107–9, 145.

36. See reference 23.
37. Lehmann LS, Padilla M, Clark S, Loucks S, et al. Training personnel in the prevention and management of violent behavior. Hospital & Community Psychiatry 1983 Jan;34(1):40–3.
38. See reference 1.
39. See reference 34.
40. Adler WN, Kreeger C, Ziegler P. Patient violence in a private psychiatric hospital. In: Lion JR, Reid WH, eds. Assaults within psychiatric facilities. New York: Grune and Stratton, 1983.
41. See reference 1.
42. See reference 3.
43. See reference 14.
44. Maier GJ, Stava LJ, Morrow B, Van Rybroek GJ et al. A model for understanding and managing cycles of aggression among psychiatric inpatients. Hospital & Community Psychiatry 1987;May 38(5):520–4.
45. See reference 3.
46. Tupin JP. The violent patient: A strategy for management and diagnosis. Hospital & Community Psychiatry 1983 Jan;34(1):37–40.
47. See reference 1.
48. See reference 44.
49. See reference 2.
50. Lanza ML. Nurses as patient assault victims: An update, synthesis and recommendations. Archives of Psychiatric Nursing 1992 Jun;6(3):163–71.
51. Storch DD. Starting an in-hospital support group for employee victims of violence in the psychiatric hospital. Psychiatric Hospital 1991;22(4):4–9.
52. See reference 17.
53. See reference 13.
54. Benalcazar-Schmid R, Berlin IN. Violence in the hospitalized adolescent: Some considerations on the management of aggression in the long term hospital unit. Bulletin Menninger Clinic 1986;50(5):430–90.
55. See reference 1.
56. Infantino JA, Musingo S. Assaults and injuries among staff with and without training in aggressive control techniques. Hospital & Community Psychiatry 1986 Dec;36(12):1312–4.
57. Carmel H, Hunter M. Compliance with training in managing assaultive behavior and injuries from inpatient violence. Hospital & Community Psychiatry 1990 May;41(5):558–60.
58. Phillips D, Rudestam KE. Effect of noniolent self-defense training on male psychiatric staff members' aggression and fear. Psychiatric Services 1995 Feb;46(2):164–8.
59. See reference 44.
60. Van Rybroek GJ, Robbins SI, Waters SJ. Safer psychiatric facilities. (Letter). Psychiatric Services 1995 May;46(5):516.
61. Rosenstock HA, McLaughlin M. On the primary prevention of critical mass: a systems strategy for adolescent units. Journal National Association of Psychiatric Hospitals 1982;13(1):9–11.

CHAPTER

VIII

Techniques for Milieu Management and Therapy

This chapter examines the techniques available for everyone who works in the psychiatric milieu. These are milieu techniques rather than techniques specific to a single profession. There are no instructions, for example, on how to conduct group or family therapy. These milieu techniques will supplement standard treatment, including psychopharmacology and psychotherapy. When techniques are formally organized with a theoretical foundation, they may form the nucleus of a treatment model. As an example, behavioral techniques, such as contracting, the token economy, time-out from reinforcement and a level system are all elements of a behavioral treatment program. Techniques for creating a positive peer culture constitute a model, not just a series of techniques.

Some techniques may have been omitted because there was no good literature about them. Others are not discussed because they are more a part of the person's interpersonal repertoire than a technique that can be taught. Empathy comes to mind. Psychologists can accurately describe the components of empathy but cannot really demonstrate its clinical application. Role modeling is in a similar category, but the presence of one helpful article argued for its inclusion. Many techniques, such as social skills training or psychoeducation are discussed only in passing. These are both very effective techniques, but they are precise and require special training. Some techniques, such as confrontation, are not discussed because they can be harmful if not used carefully. Other techniques that are discussed, such as humor, should be very carefully used.

One might distinguish between techniques that are just designed for the time the patient is in the milieu and those which may have a permanent or enduring effect. Some might be considered not as techniques, but as emergency measures, indicating a failure of other techniques. Seclusion is a good example. Restraint is not included; it would be going too far to consider it a technique.

1. Community Meetings

The English therapeutic communities during World War II were the first to explore the therapeutic potential of the large community meeting. It became the core of the therapeutic community. Now in most settings it is usually only a part of a multifaceted therapeutic effort, introducing community values and providing a forum for solving social and behavioral problems in the milieu. Zee defines the community as the patient and the meeting as the therapist who will examine, diagnose and treat its problems. The members examine how they are working together with the goal of creating a more gratifying environment. The lessons of the community meeting can be reinterpreted and applied to the unit meeting with beneficial results. The community meeting has endured despite theoretical and philosophical changes, reduced lengths of stay, the revival of the medical model and diminished investment in insight-oriented therapies. Community meetings help patients decrease their sense of isolation by identifying with the community and gaining strength from that identity. The emphasis on the value of cooperation helps to make up for the loss of freedom in the treatment setting. When trust develops in the community, patients will express their reactions to each other and staff can enter and influence this process [1–2].

Functions of the Community Meeting

The unit or community meeting becomes a mechanism for enculturation, which integrates new members, promotes the norms and ideology of the therapeutic culture, and decreases deviant behavior. Both new staff and patients learn what is expected of them and behave responsibly toward each other. The meeting can reinforce the unit's behavior norms and set the tone for each day. It can confront, analyze and help to comprehend the total experience of those who live and work in the milieu, functioning as a "social barometer." Not only is the atmosphere of the unit measured there, but what is accomplished in the meeting can also help to determine its climate [3–4].

Incorporating the Community Meeting in the Milieu

The staff must decide the function of the community meeting in the total treatment program and agree on its goals. Nonparticipating staff should regularly evaluate the meeting to see if goals are accomplished. Some goals are clear. The community meeting is always used as a means for exchanging information, a "cognitive map" of what is happening in the treatment center. It can be used as a way of introducing and establishing therapeutic values. At best, the meeting can discourage pathological behavior and encourage healthy behavior, using the staff as models [5–6].

Patients can begin to feel a sense of belonging and membership in the community. In a short-term unit the community meeting can help to encourage reality testing. The community meeting prevents the patient's problems from being seen as only intrapsychic. Baida recommends that group members confront behaviors so that residents can learn how they affect others and the unit living situation. However, the community meeting cannot exercise control over such behavior if attendance is not compulsory [7–9].

Community meetings are usually scheduled once a week for about 45 minutes, long enough to discuss prominent issues. If the goals of the community meeting include an attempt to control deviant behavior or share information, they should be more frequent. Most writers recommend a post-group staff review meeting where the staff can share observations about patients and the state of the milieu and discuss how to work together. Daniels and Rubin find that the "real action" takes place in this post-mortem meeting, where the staff can take the milieu temperature, analyze the manifest and latent content of the meetings, and plan therapeutic strategies. Goering recommends a discussion of process, rather than content, in these meetings and suggests that the staff focus on unexpressed feelings or the inhibitions that prevent people from speaking [10–11].

Structure in the Community Meeting

Structure in the community meeting is vital. There should be an agenda for each meeting, created and shared openly, so that all members will know what will be discussed. Failure to create an open agenda can lead to "secret agendas" not open to all members. The members should define the task of each meeting since only if the task is clearly understood can the meeting achieve its goals. Difficulties will arise if the participants and the leaders of the group have different ideas about the meeting's task. Seating can help to maintain structure in large community meetings [12].

Supportive beginnings and endings create a good climate for meetings. The leader should always welcome and introduce new members. If members are absent, the leader addresses or explains their absence. Each issue discussed should be brought to closure before moving on to another topic. Although discussion of one topic may not come to a logical end, the leader should still at some point indicate that discussion of one topic will cease and the community will move on to the next. It helps the group if the meeting can end with good news or in an upbeat fashion [13].

A question remains as to how structured the meeting should be. Milieu therapists now recognize how large meetings can stimulate regression and activate primitive processes such as projection and projective identification. If the meeting is loosely structured, members may feel confused or dissatisfied. Once a structure is chosen, it will allow the expression of certain content and process but prohibit others. Klein and Brown believe that an unstructured format that allows patients to bring up any topic often results in high anxiety, regressive thinking and less coherence. Their own view of the goal of the community meeting is to develop the patient's ability to plan ahead, negotiate with the staff, and make decisions in the community context, none of which they believe can be achieved in an unstructured format. They feel that when treatment is short term and the patients are severely disturbed, then the structured community meeting is the only option. Rubin studied two identical open wards and found that in one ward's highly structured meetings, a greater proportion of patients participated, with participation distributed in direct proportion to the relative numbers present. In the second ward, in the unstructured meetings, staff had greater participation. Rubin discusses these differences in terms of the ego functions of the patients involved, and believes that the structure in the community meetings compensated for these deficits. Rubin feels that participation in the community meeting can increase the patients' self worth, while minimal or no engagement will increase their sense of isolation [14–16].

Leadership in the community meeting is crucial, and once again the question of structure versus "flow" arises. The leader may have the choice of being directive (guiding the meeting from topic to topic) or nondirective (sitting back and seeing what happens). While directive leadership leads to more coherence, some believe that nondirective leadership stimulates the patient's pathology. Abramszuk reports that directive leadership keeps the patient closer to reality. The leader is in charge of both the community meeting and the post-mortem meeting that follows, helping the staff outline the goals and direction of the meeting and creating the format to achieve them. This requires the skills to mediate between the tasks in mind and the dynamics of the group. The leader is also responsible for establishing the group climate and norms that will enable goals to be accomplished. This will include promoting open and direct communication in a nonjudgmental atmosphere [17].

STAFF TRAINING

Unfortunately the purpose of the community meeting may not be clear to either patients or staff. Staff members usually do not receive formal instruction in techniques for participation, and most meetings do not realize their therapeutic potential. The leader should be responsible for incorporating new staff and training them for their roles in the community meeting. Direct care staff have primary data about the community which should be shared. The staff should promote reality testing during the meeting and be willing to confront and also evaluate projective distortions. The staff's reluctance to correct distortions will only reinforce psychopathology. Staff members should consider themselves as role models in these meetings, with the hope that the patients will come to internalize their behaviors [18].

Types of Community Meetings.

Swenson and Munich describe three types of community meetings: task-oriented, large group therapy, and those with an intergroup focus.

TASK-ORIENTED MEETINGS

The task-oriented meeting is found on short-term units where the goal is to quickly restore the patient's functioning. It introduces the unit's values and rules, provide social pressure to counteract deviance, and improve resocialization. These meetings may have required attendance, roll call, a formal agenda, and rules for speaking. Members may have the mandate to make decisions, even about the patients' status and privileges. There will be closure on each topic before moving on to the next agenda item. New patients are introduced and discharges announced. There are clear patient/staff boundaries in these meetings [19].

LARGE GROUP THERAPY MEETING

This meeting usually has no agenda and the group makes no decisions. The goal is to understand behavior of individual members and the group as a whole. The leader may point out conflicts, projections, and splitting. Here, too, there is a clear patient/staff differentiation, with the staff assuming a listening, analytic stance. The meeting examines patient/staff relationships. Units with long-term stays and a psychoanalytic orientation will find this type of meeting valuable [19].

THE INTERGROUP MEETING

The intergroup meeting has sociotherapeutic goals, integrating therapeutic and administrative work in the community. It provides an exchange of information and develops support for community plans. It is task and reality-oriented. Swenson and Munich find that these prototypes rarely exist in pure form, but that each reinforces the conditions of treatment and relieves the strain on individual members of both patient and staff groups [19].

Community Meetings in Day Treatment

Although reliance on the community meetings as a primary psychotherapeutic modality has declined in psychiatric hospitals, they are still essential to the day hospital. Rosie and Azim note that large group meetings usually reflect the major themes of day treatment. In addition to the large group, day treatment programs usually will have more focused community meetings dealing with patient government, personal relations, and daily living. They recommend that staff members be very active in such groups when there is a threat to the therapeutic alliance. Community meetings can also be organized with patient leadership, with the staff playing a resource role as facilitators [20].

The community meeting permits an observation of the milieu as a whole and helps to set its tone or climate. It establishes norms and values and helps in the acculturation of new patients. It can help the community prepare adequately for separations by announcing staff vacations and processing staff's separation and patient discharges. The meeting can serve as a forum for transferring information. The community meeting can often identify regressive countertherapeutic forces, clarify negative countertransference, assist with reality testing, help to solve problems and practical difficulties of living together. Whiteley describes the community meeting as "life speeded up." Community meetings are most successful when they can build staff and patient cohesiveness and develop a sense of community, cooperation, and caring. With a relatively stable population, there can be a progression from one meeting to the next, all of which will help to create a therapeutic culture [20–22].

References

1. Zee HJ. Reflections on the psychoanalytic hospital in the 1980s. Bulletin Menninger Clinic 1985;49(5):417–31.
2. Kisch J, Kroll J, Gross R, Carey K. In-patient community meetings: problems and purposes. British Journal of Medical Psychology 1981;54:35–40.
3. Trauer T. The relationship between large group meetings and patients' estimates of ward tension. British Journal of Medical Psychology 1979;2:205–13.
4. Klein RH, Brown SL. Large-group processes and the patient-staff community meeting. International Journal of Group Psychotherapy 1987;37(2):219–37.
5. Winer JA, Lewis L. Interpretive psychotherapy in the inpatient community meeting. Psychiatry 1984 Nov;47:333–41.
6. Edelson M. Sociotherapy and psychotherapy. Chicago: University of Chicago Press, 1970.

7. Russakoff LM, Oldham JM. The structure and technique of community meetings: the short-term unit. Psychiatry 1982;45:38–44.
8. Baida ED. Group-as-a-whole concepts and the therapeutic milieu on the inpatient psychiatric unit. Group 1989;18(3–4):179–86.
9. See reference 3.
10. Daniels DN, Rubin RS. The community meeting; an analytic study and a theoretical statement. Archives of General Psychiatry 1968;18:60–75.
11. Goering P. Training in large group therapy. Canadian Journal of Psychiatry 1981;26:53–6.
12. Arons DS. Effective use of community meetings on psychiatric treatment units. Hospital & Community Psychiatry 1982 Jun;33(6):480–3.
13. Russakoff LM, Oldham JM. Dynamic therapies on the inpatient unit. In: Sederer LI. Inpatient Psychiatry. 3rd ed. Baltimore: Williams & Wilkins, 1991, 227–97.
14. Firth ST. Regression in the hospital larger group: therapeutic implications. Psychiatric Journal of the University of Ottawa 1985 Jun;10:81–6.
15. See reference 4.
16. Rubin RS. The community meeting: a comparative study. American Journal of Psychiatry 1970 May;136(5): 708–12.
17. Abramszuk J. The type of leadership and the topics of discussion in a large open group: Observations on community meetings. International Journal of Social Psychiatry 1972;18(1):53–60.
18. Leeman CP. The therapeutic milieu. In: Sederer LI, ed. Inpatient psychiatry: Diagnosis and treatment. Baltimore: Williams & Wilkins, 1983, 222–34.
19. Swenson CR, Munich RL. Types of large-group meetings in the therapeutic community. Psychiatry 1989;52:437–55.
20. Rosie JS, Azim HFA. Large group psychotherapy in a day treatment program. International Journal of Group Psychotherapy 1990;40(3):305–21.
21. Whiteley JS. The large group as a medium for sociotherapy. In: Kreeger L, ed. The Large group: dynamics and therapy. London: Constable, 1974.
22. McLees E, Margo GM, Waterman S, Beeber MD. Group climate and group development in a community meeting on a short-term inpatient psychiatric unit. Group 1991 Spr;16(1):18–30.

2. Contracts

The admission of a patient to the psychiatric center signifies an agreement between the patient and staff to work together to alleviate symptoms and take the first steps toward restoring psychological health. A therapeutic contract will help to define their understanding and agreement. The contract should begin with a clear statement of the reason for treatment and, when possible, convey a psychodynamic understanding of the patient's behavior. It defines how the patient and staff perceive themselves, each other, and their mutual work. While patients often simply receive services, the contract allows them to become coadministrators and co-investigators of treatment. This fusion of purpose joins these two separate parties into a relationship that is "morally and psychologically compelling" [1–3].

Both the staff and patient will agree as to the nature of the problem, the goals of treatment, and the form it will take. The goals are not for the patient alone, but are shared by both patient and staff. Contracts structure the therapeutic relationship, but also change its nature, since patient and staff negotiate the contract as equals. Patients become consumers with rights, who are purchasing a service and making decisions about the treatment offered. When the patient begins to discuss problems and write a contract that will prepare to solve them, it is a first step toward mastery and a release from helplessness. Rosen describes it as frequently the major therapeutic event in the patient's treatment. Self-image and ability to function with others can change dramatically when the patient takes a consumer role. The goals should focus on what the person can realistically achieve during an inpatient stay as well as what the staff can and can't provide. The selection of treatment methods also selects the participating staff members, each of whom will work with the patient toward a specific goal. Treatment methods should review the anticipated outcome and possible complications. The contract outlines and explains the expected patient behavior and participation in each part of treatment [4].

Timing of the Contract

Contracts are usually written soon after admission, although some writers suggest that they not be written until the patient and staff have formed a trusting relationship. After the staff has examined the patient's history and can assess what can be gained from inpatient treatment, it can organize a contract conference with the patient [5].

Contracts for Specific Populations

Contracts can be effectively used with persons with manipulative behaviors, particularly for persons with eating disorders. Suicide prevention contracts have also been recommended, particularly because they decrease the person's sense of isolation and provide testimony that others care. Clinicians often recommend contracts for patients with borderline personality disorder. Making a contract conveys the message that the person is capable of exercising internal control over emotions, impulses, and behavior. The patient can experience the treatment team as there to bolster this self-control. Contracting stabilizes not only the patient but also the treatment team. It unites the team to become so that it will become less idiosyncratic in the patient's treatment. Contracts with this group of patients usually specify a discharge date, which helps to focus the treatment [5–7].

It is more realistic for patients to gradually discontinue maladaptive behaviors rather than for the staff to expect them to immediately cease. For the contract to be effective, the patient who has turned to destructive acts, such as wrist-cutting, to relieve psychological tension should be helped to find new mechanisms for coping. Despite its merits, the contract can't replace empathic, therapeutic relationships. It is still a supplement to the psychodynamically informed interactions that must continue to take place. The contract should never substitute for the patient and staff's dealing personally with each other. Nor should the staff feel so complacent as to believe that the contract is complete protection against destructive acts [8].

Patients who have contracted to report their self-destructive impulses may be reluctant to really do so, fearing the consequences if they do. If the consequences are not specified or if they seem too harsh, the patient is in a difficult and guilt-producing situation, either from reporting or not reporting. In such times contracting almost seems to work against open and trusting relationships. In addition, the impulsivity and instability of persons with borderline personality disorder may also make them easily overturn the contract [9].

The Contract as the Nucleus of Treatment

Berglas and Levendusky describe a therapeutic contract program that uses the contract as the core of the treatment program. The therapeutic contract program forms the structural milieu, while the individual contracts with each person provide the flexibility. This self-defined behavioral contracting allows the patient to define the treatment goals. Each long-term goal is broken down into a series of short-term goals to be worked on each week. The contracts specify weekly rewards for meeting the goals, such as a change in privilege levels. In addition, the patients receive support and social reinforcement for continuing toward their goals. By placing controls and goals in the patient's hands, the program works toward long-term effects. The patients continue to work on goals until their behaviors reach their own self-imposed standards. Their gradual resumption of responsibility for their own behavior changes and therapeutic gain can be carried over to their later lives in the community. Self-control training groups can also help them to do this [10].

In a later article on the therapeutic contracting program, Levendusky and colleagues relate some of the thinking behind therapeutic contracts to Bandura's theory of self-efficacy. Patients create their own motivation for goals and self-rewards for self-defined performance levels and create their own improvement criteria rather than depending on institutionally created criteria. Patients and staff write weekly contracts in this program. Staff members support the patient's increasingly positive views about their therapeutic progress and growing self-reliance. However, if the contract the patient drafts does not seem to be leading to therapeutic growth, the staff can make appropriate challenges. When completed, the personal contracts are placed on the community bulletin board for the week, where all staff and patients can consult them. A scheduled staff-patient talk reviews each day's accomplishments. The entire community meets at the end of the week for the contract evaluation group, which reinforces the patient's achievements. Patients read their contracts and explain how they reached their goals. The patients evaluate the week's accomplishments as well as their overall mood, using 10-point scales. Staff and patients give feedback about individual behaviors and progress [11–12].

Not all patients will successfully complete their weekly contracts. Negative sanctions can be implemented for community rule violations. One sanction that is applied in this program is a period of separation from the community—seclusion in a quiet room. Since community support is gratifying and provides social reinforcement for most of its members, they are usually quick to earn their way out of the quiet room to return to it [12].

The therapeutic contracting program does not overlook the power of the psychosocial milieu. Patients attend several groups daily and may have as many as 25–30 hours of group therapy each week. A core inpatient group is a lecture series that covers the basics of cognitive behavior therapy and helps project a future model of recovery. All lectures are summarized, typed, and given to patients in book form. Topics include cognitive distortions, relaxation and grounding techniques, cognitive resturcturing, impulse control/time delay techniques and time management. The training also includes identifying negative self-statements, irrational assumptions, and the tendency to catastrophize [12–13].

Formal written contracts can forge a therapeutic alliance, contain dangerous behavior, and insure treatment integrity. A signed contract becomes a living force in treatment and can be used in treatment planning conferences, staff meetings, and even in community meetings. Procedures for modifying the contract are included to allow more flexible treatment. Durrant, however, criticizes the use of contracts. Durrant finds that adolescents enter residential treatment with a self-image that expects failure. If they must sign a contract, this throws the fear of failure back in their face. He compares it to asking the adolescent to get well before it is a real possibility [14].

References

1. Miller LJ. The treatment contract in the inpatient management of borderline personality disorder. Hospital & Community Psychiatry 1990 Sep;41(9):985–7.
2. Cooklin AI. Exploration of the staff-patient "contract" in an acute female admission ward. British Journal of Medical Psychology 1974 Dec;47(4):321–35.
3. Bloom H, Rosenbluth M. The use of contracts in the inpatient treatment of the borderline personality disorder. Psychiatric Quarterly 1989 Win;60(4):317–27.

4. Rosen B. Written treatment contracts: their use in planning treatment programmes for in-patients. British Journal of Psychiatry 1978;133:410–5.
5. Lassig D, Schroeder K. Nursing in a therapeutic milieu. In: Wells LA, ed. A handbook of psychiatric nursing. St Louis: Warren Green, 1989, 319–52.
6. See reference 3.
7. Nurnberg HG, Suh R. Limits: Short-term treatment of borderline patients. Comprehensive Psychiatry 1980;21(1):70–88.
8. See reference 1.
9. See reference 5.
10. Berglas S, Levendusky PG. The therapeutic contract program: an individual-oriented psychological treatment community. Psychotherapy 1985;22(2):36–45.
11. Bandura A. Self-efficacy: toward a unifying theory of behavioral change. Psychological Review 1977;84:191–215.
12. Levendusky PG, Willis BS, Ghinassi FA. The therapeutic contracting program: a comprehensive continuum of care model. Psychiatric Quarterly 1994 Fall;65(3):189–220.
13. Meichenbaum DH. Cognitive Behavior Modification: An integrative approach. New York: Plenum, 1977.
14. Durrant M. Residential treatment: a cooperative, competency-based approach to therapy and program design. New York: Norton, 1993.

3. Family Involvement

We no longer need to ask whether the family should be involved in the patient's treatment, but only how this should be done. In many treatment centers, however, parents have few opportunities to help in treatment planning or play a role in treatment. A review by Collins and Collins in 1990 found that professional staff trace most of childhood symptomatology to parental influence and still do little more than provide information and offer family therapy. A 1991 survey of graduate programs in the core mental health disciplines revealed that 53% of all training programs still teach a theory of family causation of serious mental illness; in addition, 82% of these programs reported that they did not fully prepare their students to work with families of the mentally ill [1–2].

It is finally more helpful to take the position that the family is the patient's most important resource and can best provide the assistance that will be needed long after discharge. Working with the family will prepare for the patient's return to the community and prevent future rehospitalization. Because a child's separation from the home will create special problems for those who remain, the focus must be not on the child alone but on the family, to keep this system intact, by frequent participation and visits and by bringing the family together with other families who share their problems and will have similar work to do. When parents bring their child to treatment, they bring their own feelings of guilt, failure, and inadequacy. Their painful separation is accompanied by the fear that the child may never come back home. They are immediately deprived of their ability to provide nurturance and care and may seek to protect themselves from these painful feelings by emotionally withdrawing from the child and not wishing to participate in the services the treatment center provides. If treatment is going to be successful, the staff must make every effort to restore the parents' self-esteem. They must be able to empathize with the parent's sense of abandonment and acknowledge to the family that they have taken this courageous step because of the depth of their caring [3].

The staff should somehow convey the message that if one family member is in crisis, all members of the family will need help. Their immediate involvement will help to alleviate the patient's feelings of abandonment. If the family cannot establish a solid and supportive relationship with the treatment center, it, too, will feel abandoned. Family members must be respected and supported and find that hospitalization is a strong positive step toward their own family growth [4–6].

The treatment team must be vigilant in examining the subtle and not-so-subtle ways it may communicate that parents are responsible for their children's problems. Such outdated beliefs in simple linear causality still present the major obstacle in making an alliance with the family. Therapeutic relationships may need to be replaced by therapeutic systems. The traditional attempt to form an exclusive one-to-one relationship with the child needs to give way to a therapeutic system which includes the child, parent, and staff and the time in treatment must strengthen the bonds with all who will provide care in the future [7].

The family must begin to see itself as competent. When parents focus on their failures, they need to be reminded of some of their own parenting skills. Cooklin and colleagues describe a family day unit that organized treatment so that the family could discover and develop its own areas of competence. While in the beginning family members feel a disabling sense of failure and expect to be blamed, the staff must assure them that they can learn to work out their solutions. If the staff can validate the parents as the child's greatest resource, the family will be more willing to work [8].

The Therapeutic Alliance with Parents

The family needs support and acceptance, information, socialization, and structure. Stewart distinguishes between the family-institution alliance and a therapeutic alliance. While the former is the engagement of the family in a relationship that achieves understanding and support, the therapeutic alliance represents a commitment to change-oriented treatment for the entire family. The therapeutic alliance with the family becomes an absolute commitment to change. It is a relationship that builds mutual support and clear understanding, establishing acceptance and commitment to shared goals for the treatment of the individual patient and family. The parents must begin to feel needed by the staff and allowed to participate as fully as possible in treatment. The family will discuss discharge plans soon after admission [9–10].

The Family-Oriented Psychiatric Inpatient Unit

Family-oriented psychiatric treatment can be achieved in many ways: joint admission of the entire family, the use of the residential facility as a laboratory for family members, the inclusion of the family as a member of the interdisciplinary treatment team, and parent empowerment. Harbin describes such a unit in theoretical terms. The family-oriented psychiatric unit Harbin describes has fully integrated the principles of family therapy and theory into its structure, where it functions as a major component. The unit integrates families in many complementary ways: the family admission interview, conjoint family therapy sessions, multifamily groups, family-oriented therapeutic leaves of absence. and policies that integrate families into most aspects of unit life. There is an ongoing review of how the family is affecting the hospitalized patient's behavior and how the patient is affecting the family [11].

Admission

In the unit Harbin describes, staff members are trained not to direct their attention to the treatment of the single patient but to emphasize the family, even as they explain inpatient rules and regulations. They make it clear that they expect the family to participate during the hospitalization. Some families will be grateful to be included while others may not. Although many clinicians have advised against immediate use of family therapeutic approaches, experience in the unit that Harbin describes has demonstrated that the family and patient can benefit from early participation, and it may prove to be a crucial stage for change for the family system [11].

Engagement and the Therapeutic Contract

When the person who has caused anxiety in the family system is removed and placed in the hospital, the family may lose its potential for change. Family therapy must operate so as to not lose momentum—to keep the referred patient constantly involved with the family in order to increase its motivation for change and prevent its excluding the patient. Harbin writes that two of the major ways this can be done are the use of therapeutic leaves of absence and the threat of discharge from the hospital. Harbin recommends a therapeutic contract with the family. Since the family may view the reasons for hospitalization much differently from the patient or staff, all parties should negotiate an agreement on the problems requiring hospitalization. This may be the first time that the family has clearly communicated about the disturbing behavior that has brought about the hospitalization. If the early stages do not include the family, the staff will begin to take its place with the patient. All members of the treatment team repeatedly give the message that family members are essential to the treatment process. Families who decline to participate are told that the patient will have to leave the hospital if they cannot arrange to be there [11].

Family therapy focuses on symptoms and problems. The most common intervention is the assignment of tasks that will gather the forces in the family. This can usually be accomplished during therapeutic leaves of absence. The patient goes home with the family as soon as possible to allow time for the families to interact and to increase the pressure on family members to change the way they relate to each other and to the patient. This prevents the patient's exclusion from the family, decreases the family and patient's dependence on the hospital, and provides information about the possibility of discharge. Family therapy sessions focus on interactions during the leaves of absence [11].

Participation in the Treatment Team

Williams describes the integration of family members into the interdisciplinary treatment team in an adolescent psychiatric unit, an effort that has reduced the length of treatment. She believes that parents are willing to play an active role when the staff gives them an unequivocal message about the need for their participation. This participation counteracts one of the primary sources of family dissatisfaction, which has often centered on the lack of treatment information they have received. Williams reports that the integration of the family in the treatment team came after the adolescent patients' own successful participation in treatment. This began when a patient asked to attend a team meeting and was clearly able to articulate what she needed to do and how the staff could help her. The staff then invited the other adolescents to attend their team meetings. Even the less articulate patients demonstrated a good understanding of their own problems. Irrelevant material was eliminated and the goals for the patient became clearer and more realistic. This success then led to a decision to include the parents on the treatment team [12].

It was difficult to bring the adult parents into the "sacred" chamber of treatment planning, to reveal the staff's imperfections and uncertainties. Each family feared it was the cause of the adolescent's illness and anticipated a public blaming. These first treatment planning sessions required extensive staff preparation. Staff members were asked to empathize with the parent entering such a system, and reviewed systems theory with emphasis on interaction. They were encouraged to express their criticisms as well as their optimism for the new format [12].

The first parent meetings were unfortunately bland, sterile, and rigid, taking away the treatment team's earlier informal collegiality. The staff finally realized that in the beginning it needed to take the lead, to explore with parents their own expectations and fantasies of what might be happening daily on the unit. This gave them a more comfortable access to the treatment milieu and introduced the vocabulary of treatment planning. Staff became more comfortable and parents became more responsive. Although they began with questions, they were also able to share their own ways of working with the child. They were finally confident enough to offer suggestions and challenge the treatment plan. The families had joined the team! Evaluations for 6-1/2 years after that revealed no negative effects resulting from this arrangement. The adolescent's hospitalization was no longer a rupture in the family's attempt to solve its problems but became a time to continuously try new skills. The staff acknowledged from the beginning that the parents were the experts on their child and more important than the transient hospital staff could ever be. They actively sought the parents' advice and honestly admitted that their own efforts were dwarfed by the power the parents had in influencing their child. One parent, for example, offered to spend time in the unit showing some of her methods for working with her psychotic child. This was so successful that many other parents came to provide "consultations" in the unit. Another parent requested time in the milieu to learn new management techniques before the adolescent's first visit home. The parents' relation to the staff changed dramatically. Parents often made a strong bond with the nursing staff and were then able to forge a united front for the adolescent. The staff profited from a truly meaningful involvement with parents. The boundaries of the unit and the family system became permeable with a constructive flow between them [12].

Before the establishment of this procedure, length of stay had been between 15 to 29 months. For the five years after that, no patient stayed longer than 12 months. Williams concluded that treatment centers have often taken over family roles rather than building the family's own capacities, and without a planned procedure for teamwork, psychiatric hospitalization can complicate the very pathology that it had promised to alleviate [12].

Roles for the Milieu Staff and Child Care Workers

Most models of family intervention are now based on the belief that family problems do not reside within the parents or the child, but in their interactions. Now that surrogate parenting is no longer viable, child care workers must assume new roles as family intervention agents, as catalysts for family change. They no longer compete with parents but support and help to train them as they interact with their child. They may also serve as co-therapists in family groups so that they become familiar with family dynamics. In the model Garland describes, parents belong to parent education and family living groups that guide them in a variety of interactions with the children. They see many interactive techniques in practice as they observe child care workers and other families in varying contexts and relationships. The group living with parental participation is an ideal classroom, and the stronger parental ties moderate the children's' influence upon each other. Many of these parents had been isolated without a supportive social network to help them deal with parenting crises [13].

Collins suggests that child care workers can play a designated role in family-centered treatment as the child care family support worker. The family therapist, child care worker, and family support worker form a team that provides comprehensive care. The family therapist focuses on the family as a unit. The child care worker focuses on the child, and the family support worker focuses on the parent-child interaction, helping with parenting skills. The role of the family support worker is carefully distinguished from that of the family therapist. The family support worker focuses on consistency in parenting, working with actual interactions, events and problems as they occur in the home. All three participate in the family conferences conducted by the family therapist. The team meets after each conference to plan family involvement for the following weeks. The responsibility of each professional is clearly differentiated to avoid role conflicts [14].

The family support worker must be able to understand what the family needs and build a relationship. More formal practices will include setting goals and contracting, and implementing skills and strategies. The family support worker attempts to help structure family life so that it becomes therapeutic and produces growth for the family. The worker helps parents to acquire child management skills, manage daily life situations, communicate more effectively and learn to use community services. This process begins when the family support worker joins the family at home for several hours at a time [14].

Christ suggests that placing a milieu staff member in charge of the therapeutic care of the entire family unit helps to develop new attitudes toward the focus of residential treatment. If the staff includes parents in every major decision about their child in treatment, they will no longer feel taken over by professionals and will be able to continue to see the child as an integral part of the family [15].

Parent Empowerment

The staff that creates an environment that nourishes family relationships and competence must become comfortable with giving up total sovereignty over the child. The partnership begins soon after admission when both parents and staff meet in conference to define problems, formulate treatment goals, and develop a treatment contract. The staff learns to work through the family rather than take its place. Restoring parental authority, rather than replacing it, is most important for adolescents. Byalin believes that hospitalized adolescents are suffering from a breakdown in parental authority and the adolescent often dominates the family by threats of dangerous or strange behavior. Parents can no longer give them the protection or guidance they need. In many cases, restoring parental authority will permit the other treatment issues to be safely addressed in outpatient treatment.

Byalin describes a process of empowering parents that begin with the request for admission. Parents are told to visit and evaluate the program and the staff to decide whether it is appropriate for their adolescent, who is purposely excluded from this process. The staff empathizes with the parents' painful decision to hospitalize the adolescent and praises them for their courage to do it [16-17].

When the adolescent is admitted, the staff attempts the difficult task of relieving the parents' burden while continuing to empower them. The staff consults the parents on treatment decisions. Evening and weekend conferences make family participation convenient. The staff formulates treatment objectives by asking the parents what the child must do in order to live at home. These objectives also serve as criteria for discharge. Parents help develop strategies to achieve these necessary changes, although it is the clinical staff who will assume initial responsibility for trying them out. The adolescent unit functions temporarily as a parental agent, providing nurturing and discipline until the family is again able to meet those needs [17].

Every effort is made to create opportunities for parents to successfully exercise authority and gain confidence in their own power and competence. Within limits required for the operation of the unit as a therapeutic milieu, authority that might otherwise be assumed by staff is assigned to parents. Parents provided with information from the milieu, will be in charge of deciding when passes will be given. As soon as possible they resume active responsibility for implementing the treatment plan they developed in collaboration with the treatment team. Regularly scheduled group parent meetings provide peer support. The timing of discharge is also left to the parents. The authors report that this approach appears to have reduced the average inpatient stays from more than a year to less than four months. Families seem able to sustain the gains achieved [17].

Programs with Parental Milieu Participation

The ideal program for family involvement is full participation in the treatment milieu. Only a few treatment programs have made this commitment, but it is particularly helpful for younger patients.

Withersty and colleagues describe early attempts at treatment of the adolescent without family participation. Many families would bring their adolescent to the hospital for a "cure" and then refuse to be engaged in the treatment program. The young adolescent would then recreate the family dynamics in the unit, with staff members willingly taking on family roles and unconsciously repeating situations and conflicts from the past. Although the young person might learn new ways to deal with the family, it finally made more sense to have the family immediately participate in this learning. The program was changed so that all patients admitted to the unit were told that many behavior patterns are learned and that their patterns of relating to family members and others are no longer working.

They are told that they must accept responsibility for their own behaviors and are expected to learn new and more effective ways of operation [18].

The relearning process takes place in a milieu designed for full participation of the patient and family. The patient will be admitted only if the family agrees to stay for the first 25 to 48 hours and attend the therapy groups that are in session. However, during this time the contact with inpatient staff will be minimal, unless family members initiate it. The staff avoids attempts to get it to make decisions or take responsibility, with the hope of giving the family a vote of confidence that they can resolve crises on their own. This technique brings about productive family interactions. The staff then asks the family to bring its present conflicts and confrontations to the therapy group for arbitration. In the therapy group, staff and patients praise family members for their efforts in solving their problems and help them look at their effective and ineffective ways of interacting with each other. From the insights gained in group therapy sessions, they can begin to look at their relationships and practice new ways of relating to one another [18].

Lansky notes that a family-centered program provides a shift of emphasis from the way that milieu therapy is commonly done. The study of the family in action in the milieu focuses on the ways that families act that adversely affect patients and on the patient's role in stimulating such behavior. Lansky believes that the involvement of the family is almost never unrelated to the problems that brought the patient to the hospital. When the family joins the treatment, issues come to the fore to be played out in the milieu. The possibility of changing dysfunctional patterns in a family during hospitalization will lead to greater success after discharge [19].

Family participation corrects the staff's view of parents. Those who may have once felt that parents "caused" their children's illness are quickly disavowed of this belief after a period of working together. The staff comes to realize that these parents meant to do their best for the child. In the program Critchley and Berlin describe, weekly parental participation was part of the treatment contract written prior to admission. A staff member, serving as the parent liaison, plans the parent's participation with the milieu staff and the goals to be accomplished. This liaison provides assistance and serves as a role model for interaction with the children. Participation is never easy at first. There is a resistance to working together, anger when there are misunderstandings, impatience when changes in the child are so slow. Covert anger on both sides can be expected and parents will usually interpret it as being directed against them. As staff and parents continue to work together toward the same goal, these destructive feelings usually change. The parents are finally able to express some of their anger and fear of rejection by the staff. Staff members can come to realize that parents have long felt frustrated, helpless and inadequate. Staff and parents begin to develop trust as they experience working together [20].

When the staff member admits to making mistakes in working with the children, this will often bring about a change in parents. Both may find that trial and error in the milieu may be the only successful way to learn. The staff must be open to criticism from the parents and share their own failures as well as successes. Critchley and Berlin believe that difficult as it is, parental participation in the milieu is essential to the child's recovery. The staff should work to dissolve the barriers between the treatment center, the family, and community. If there is not a planned program for complete milieu participation, families should be invited to participate in daily activities, meals, assisting in the classroom, and helping the child get ready for bed. The opportunities for milieu participation are limited only by the staff's vision of how permeable the boundary should be. An activities group, for example, can be a low-key variety of family therapy [20].

The very structure of the inpatient unit helps parents to learn. Mansheim describes limit-setting which parents can observe on an inpatient unit. The mildest form of limit setting is the request for children to do something. If they don't respond, then they are told again. If they still don't do it, the staff member may offer some help. If this doesn't work the child may take a short time-out while sitting on a chair. If this is not successful, the child may go to a time-out room. The hierarchy of the procedures is important. Of equal significance, is the emotionally neutral fashion in which limits are set. They are set because they are necessary, not because the staff member is angry. Mansheim describes such observations for parents as "routine slices of life" [21].

Critchley and Berlin describe the stages of milieu participation in greater detail. Parents first participate in the milieu by observing how teachers and staff interact with children. Later they will join the children in activities. Parents seem to feel more comfortable and spontaneous when they can join in simple playful activities with staff and children. Parents of small children may benefit from playing games with their child in a room with a one-way mirror. A small earphone placed in the ear will allow them to hear suggestions from the staff about interactions which will increase the pleasure of play. This technique is recommended for parents of psychotic children who have become what Critchley and Berlin describe as "frozen" in their ability to play with their child. They have found, however, that leaving the parent alone to "talk" with the child seems not to promote greater understanding or help the parent deal more successfully with problem behaviors [22].

Staff members always have much to learn when working with parents. They discard their rescue fantasies, of wishes to whisk the child away from a troubled family. They begin to understand that the hostility they often encounter in parents defends against feelings of inadequacy and guilt. They find that there are no circumstances when it is helpful to criticize parents in front of their children. They learn to model effective ways of interacting and talking with child. Even parents who initially felt hostile or suspicious will find themselves trying out new ways of being with the child. When staff members are willing to share their own difficulties, the gap between the inadequate parent and the successful staff begins to disappear. Both staff and parents are surprised to learn that joining together in working with the child becomes a mutually gratifying activity [23].

Carlo describes family milieu participation as a process of weaving the parents into the everyday life of the residential milieu. The two main goals in the program he describes are parent education and socialization, providing both didactic and experiential learning. The experiential element includes field trips, exercise classes, holiday celebrations, meal preparations, conferences, and informal opportunities to observe how houseparents or child care workers manage children. Education is much more effective when accompanied by experiences. The experiential opportunities give parents the chance to change their feelings and attitudes. In order to provide the experiential component, child care staff meet frequently to review continuing problems and successes. Parents are invited to come and meet the staff. When comfort increases, they begin to participate in more structured activities, observing and then restoring their own parenting functions with the child [24].

Carlo describes interesting and optimistic results for parents. He finds that collaborative staff interaction between parents and staff members leads to great respect for what each is doing and allows the parent to become a valuable learning and working team member. When parents are finally deferred to as experts on their child, an interesting switch occurs. Staff are not simply teachers and role models; parents are no longer passive students. Parenting itself becomes worthy of study and the parent becomes a contributing member of the team. The staff's own confidence in the parents allows them to become much more confident in themselves and the children in turn are much less anxious and uncertain with their parents both in the milieu and during their time at home [24].

Stages in Family Involvement

Martone and colleagues describe the continuum of parental involvement in four stages: engagement, participation, empowerment and discharge. Issues arise within each stage which can affect all stages which follow. Participation allows the parents to absorb the structure of the therapeutic milieu, its routine and predictability. The process is described as similar to a job training for parents. The staff can nurture the parents while slowly moving them toward taking more responsibility. Delegation of responsibilities must be carefully orchestrated so that families who remain in the background can begin to make decisions [25].

Jones describes similar stages. The first stage is one of assessment and alliance, laying the groundwork for the family to feel safe to explore feelings. The second stage is devoted to education and socialization. Therapeutic attention is shifted to the interactional processes in the family and members are asked to make changes in the way they communicate and behave with each other. The information given is primary educational rather than emotional. It is an attempt to resocialize family members by showing them a different way to look at and understand their difficulties. This is a nonthreatening way to prepare them for change. The third stage has a focus on relationships and helping the family to then explore the meaning of their interactions. They will work in clarifying and strengthening boundaries between the parents and the child. The fourth stage is one of reintegration [26].

Joint Admission

The most complete family involvement would require admission of the whole family to the hospital. There have been a few experiments in admission of the whole family to the hospital, admission of mothers and babies during a postpartum illness, and admission of mothers and their children to chemical dependency residential treatment. Because of the high costs of hospitalization, admission of families will probably not occur frequently in the United States.

Admission of the Family

Abroms and Fellner published a preliminary report about the inpatient treatment of 100 patients and their families, and described the admission of whole families as a powerful therapeutic tool in itself. This policy required a new conception of the psychiatric hospital, as a learning laboratory with courses in basic psychosocial skills. The 100 index patients ranged in age from 18 to 64, and 137 of their family members entered the hospital with them. Most were spouses, but 16% were parents. The primary diagnosis for the index patients was personality disorder. Moreover, it was found that 70% of the family members also warranted a psychiatric diagnosis. The treatment design of the unit included a harmonious working together of group therapeutic modalities and personal interactions : unit meetings, staffings, sensitivity exercises and other group functions [27].

The treatment community required that the family members define their own problems, state their goals for the hospitalization, and explore the methods to achieve them. Although the family member might come to the hospital prepared to help a husband, wife or child, this commitment was redefined toward working on personal problems. This redefinition was the process by which each member began full participation in treatment, based on the understanding that each family member has difficulties that play a part in the family disturbance but that each has the task of differentiating the self from the family system. A daily family therapy session analyzed communication and relationship patterns and an individual psychotherapy session explored relationship difficulties against the background of the person's significant early relationships. In unit meetings and group therapy sessions, the community gave family members feedback on their current behavior. The authors conclude with the statement that having the whole family enter the hospital is a powerful act, both realistically and symbolically, which magnifies the therapeutic intensity and establishes control not possible in outpatient treatment [27].

Bandler describes a unit for up to eight families with 27 available beds. Although a child may be the index patient, the primary focus of treatment is on the parents. A therapist sees the parents individually. A child therapist works with the child. The nurse on the team works to increase the family's ability to carry out everyday tasks. The family interacts with many other staff. Bandler describes many of the daily emotions and events that staff who work intensively in the milieu with families will experience. The family brings many transferential responses that are irrational, primitive, and inappropriate. Families frequently experience the staff as if they are their parents or siblings or significant figures from their past or present. Under such pressure, staff can find themselves acting quite unpredictably, forgetting their own roles and feeling critical of colleagues. This could be very harmful if there were no arena for talking about reactions to the patients and to each other. These reactions will provide insight into the family's pathology and if understood, can help direct the treatment [28].

Bandler cautions against the staff's temptation to quickly try to manage these families and help relieve them of their inner struggle. Staff should resist this pressure and guide them toward thinking about their own feelings and actions. This is in contrast to many treatment programs for families described in this review, where staff members intervene in the lives of families with the hope of teaching parenting and life management to parents needing help. Bandler also warns staff members who work with these families not to try to act as therapists for each other, since these countertransference reactions should be related to the patient, not to the staff member's personal history. Many of the feelings that Bandler describes are also relevant to work with parents who participate in the milieu without admission to the hospital [28].

Dydyk and colleagues describe a program admitting whole families for short-term intensive assessment and treatment with the goal of either decreasing or circumventing a planned residential care for the children. These services (in Canada) are provided at costs comparable or less than that of traditional residential treatment, and results at six months indicated that 1/2 of the children referred with their families had not required further residential treatment. The theory of the intensive family therapy unit is that the child's behavior reflects dysfunction in the family and/or the larger system and that the complete therapeutic involvement of the family creates the best possibility for the amelioration of the symptoms of the referred patient. Families are admitted individually into a 4-bedroom living space in the children's treatment center. All family members must be free of the distraction of work or school. Before admission, all information has been provided and the team meets with the referral sources, who present the case.

Treatment techniques after admission include family sessions, overlapping interviews, individual sessions, task assignment, use of video feedback observation and practice solving daily family problems. The intensive family therapy unit provided an effective therapy to disturbed children and families with a shorter time and at a lower cost [29].

Despite current advice to include the family in all decisions, a survey of more than 200 staff members in three children's residential treatment centers indicated far more support for families as service recipients than as decision makers. In addition, those surveyed did not necessarily agree that family reunification was a realistic goal for the majority of their children [30].

References

1. Collins B, Collins T. Parent-professional relationships in the treatment of emotionally disturbed children and adolescents. Social Work 1990 Nov;35(6):523–7.
2. NAMI training matters. Newsletter of the NAMI Curriculum & Training Network 1991;1:2–3.
3. Braiman SG. The establishment of a therapeutic alliance with parents of psychiatrically ill hospitalized children. Social Work in Health Care 1977 Fall;3(2):20–8.
4. Maxmen JS, Tucker GJ, Lebow MD. Rational hospital psychiatry: the reactive environment. New York: Brunner-Mazel, 1974.
5. Hanrahan G. Beginning work with families of hospitalized adolescents. Family Process 1986;26:391–405.
6. Jones JM. Stages of family involvement in the residential treatment of adolescents. Journal of Marital & Family Therapy 1985 Oct;11(4):381–90.
7. Goren S. Clinical Forum: Practicing in partnership with families in the inpatient setting. Journal of Child & Adolescent Psychiatric Nursing 1992 Jul-Sep;5(3):43–6.
8. Cooklin A, Miller AC, McHugh B. An institution for change: Developing a family day unit. Family Process 1983;23(4):453–68.
9. See reference 5.
10. Stewart RP. Building an alliance between the family and the institution. Social Work 1984 Jan-Feb;30(4):396–8.
11. Harbin HT. A family-oriented psychiatric inpatient unit. Family Process 1979 Sep;19:281–91.
12. Williams BE. Parents and patients: Members of an interdisciplinary team on an adolescent inpatient unit. Clinical Social Work Journal 1988 Spr;17(1):78–91.
13. Garland DS. Residential care workers as primary agents of family intervention. Child & Youth Care Quarterly 1987 Spr;17(1):22–34.
14. Collins D. Child care workers and family therapists: Getting connected. Journal of Child & Youth Care 1989;4(3):24–31.
15. Christ AE, Wagner NN. Iatrogenic factors in residential treatment: A problem in staff training. American Journal of Orthopsychiatry 1965; 35:263–4.
16. Mansheim PA. Working with families on an inpatient unit: Hospital staff members are family therapists. Contemporary Family Therapy 1989 Win;11(4):267–75.

17. Byalin K. Patient empowerment: a treatment strategy for hospitalized adolescents. Hospital & Community Psychiatry 1990 Jan;41(1):89–90.
18. Withersty DJ, Porterfield PB, Spradlin WW. Treating the hospitalized adolescent: a family approach. Family Therapy 1975;2(2):129–35
19. Lansky MR. Establishing a family-oriented inpatient unit. Journal of Operational Psychiatry 1977;8:65–74.
20. Critchley DL, Berlin IN. Parent participation in milieu treatment of young psychotic children. American Journal of Orthopsychiatry 1981 Jan;51:149–55.
21. See reference 16.
22. See reference 20.
23. Berlin IN, Critchley DL, Rossman PG. Current concepts in milieu treatment of seriously disturbed children and adolescents. Psychotherapy 1984;22(1):119–31.
24. Carlo P. Implementing a parent involvement/parent education program in a children's residential treatment center. Child & Youth Care Quarterly 1988;18(3):205–17.
25. Martone WP, Kemp GF, Pearson SJ. The continuum of parental involvement in residential treatment. Residential Treatment for Children & Youth 1989;6(3):11–37.
26. See reference 6.
27. Abroms GM, Fellner CH, Whitaker CA. The family enters the hospital. American Journal of Psychiatry 1971 Oct;138(10):1463–70.
28. Bandler D. Working with other professionals in the in-patient setting. Journal of Child Psychotherapy 1987;14(2):81–9.
29. Dydyk BJ, French G, Gertsman C, Morrison N, et al. Admitting whole families: an alternative to residential care. Canadian Journal of Psychiatry 1989;34:694–8.
30. Baker BL, Heller TL, Blacher J, Pfeiffer SI. Staff attitudes toward family involvement in residential treatment centers for children. Psychiatric Services 1995 Jan;46(1):60–5.

4. Humor

Those who use humor as a technique in the treatment setting should do so with care. They must be aware of humor's masked messages. Although some masked messages may be therapeutic, others will not. Summers has written about the use of humor in addiction settings. Since substance use has been used by the residents to relieve stress, going through recovery usually causes frustration, anger, tension and anxiety. Humor can help to disrupt some of the irritations and can somehow free the recovering person from a burdensome frame of mind. It can bring about a change in perspective that lightens the threat of difficult situations. It can also help the person to temporarily step away from painful feelings and difficult situations [1].

Humor can also challenge nonproductive ruminative ways of thinking. If the person can learn to let go of self-concerns long enough to laugh, self-acceptance becomes easier. Summers writes that humor in the health care setting can not only decrease social distance but also provides an outlet for hostility and discontent. At the same time, humor can be used destructively when it is aggression disguised in a socially acceptable form [1].

Humor helps to build relationships, particularly with adolescents, since it gives a message of acceptance. It helps adolescents build relationships from a safe distance. It can be healing when it helps both children and adolescents relax and reduce stress. Zinger suggests that child care workers consider the use of cartoons and also remember that some of the funniest stories they will encounter are also true. Humor can also be used to reframe problem situations. Staff members can practice their own reframing when caught in difficult situations by allowing the way they see them to connect with the humorous side [2].

Brausa describes organizing a comedy club for a group of veterans with chronic psychiatric problems in day treatment. Each member is responsible for sharing something humorous during the 50-minute meeting—a joke or anecdote, something that happened to them or something they have read. Brausa believes that the therapeutic benefit comes for the members being able to change their behavior, despite their emotional state. Some of the members had to be instructed how to give a "polite chuckle" as a kind of a thank you for the joketeller. Laughing and applauding jokes seems to reduce stress, brighten emotions, and give a respite from problems that each member brings to the group. The comedy club gives a feeling of optimism that can carry over into other parts of the program [3].

Kuhlman describes how humor helps the staff relieve tension. He describes "gallows humor" in a maximum security setting for chronic assaultive patients. Gallows humor is a helpful response to the incongruity between idealized expectations and what can reasonably be achieved, the gap between one's efforts and their outcome. This gallows humor functions as a helpful response to dilemmas that will never be solved. It allows the staff to save face in defeat rather than adopting the usual macho attitudes that are displayed in most maximum security units that make the staff need to feel tougher than the patients [4].

References

1. Summers AD. Humor: Coping in recovery from addiction. Issues in Mental Health Nursing 1988;9:169–79.
2. Zinger DJ. Humor in child care: the double-edged sword. Child & Youth Care Quarterly 1988 Win;17(4):268–74.
3. Brausa R. The Comedy Club. Psychosocial Rehabilitation Journal 1991 Oct;17(2):189–92.
4. Kuhlman TL. Gallows humor for a scaffold setting: Managing aggressive patients on a maximum security forensics unit. Hospital & Community Psychiatry 1988 Oct;39(10):1085–9.

5. Impromptu Meetings or Groups

Extra or impromptu meetings can help to build a community, provide support, or solve milieu problems. O'Brien and colleagues describe an adolescent unit that allows any patient or staff member to call a meeting. Patients can use the meetings to make decisions, support each other, or even to make therapeutic changes. Any community member had the right to call a meeting. The adolescents often called meetings to support a friend or to settle disputes. The person who calls the meeting is the person who also must announce it. Everyone is expected to attend. The technique of extra meetings enhanced the therapeutic potential of the adolescent milieu by providing a forum for immediately solving difficulties and providing support. O'Brien and colleagues report that many adolescents took the technique home and found it helpful there [1].

Crabtree and Horowitz describe impromptu, single-session spontaneous groups. These groups met twice a week and responded to the actions and issues of community members. There were also theme-oriented impromptu groups that focused on such topics as becoming a patient or suicidal feelings. The network-oriented impromptu group formed around the natural relationships that were established in the unit. These group sessions often dealt with crises or changing conditions the group found destructive. Some of the groups that formed were known as the Elders of the Community, the AWOL group, and a group of patients helping each other to remain drug free. The impromptu groups could also center on one patient who had attracted community concern or feelings. Any patient could be selected by members of the community during the impromptu group. Here the interactions were high in emotions and sparked by confrontations.

Impromptu and extra groups place an effective treatment technique in the hands of patients. Problems are not solved simply by letting them age, and impromptu groups may be the secret of an active milieu. They can also serve as a training ground for deepening interpersonal experiences and increase the feeling of belonging to a community [2].

References

1. O'Brian C, Bruggen P, Dunn C. Extra meetings: a tool for decisions and therapy. Journal of Adolescence 1985 Sep;8(3):255–61.
2. Crabtree LH, Horowitz H. Impromptu group; beyond crisis intervention. Psychotherapy 1974;11(4):356–9.

6. Level Systems

The level system organizes privileges in a series of steps, allowing the person to move through varying levels in the treatment program, each of which allows increased freedom and privileges. A basic level system may have only three levels: an orientation level, middle level, and a predischarge level. A simple level system builds a structure that can contain and manage the child or adolescent patient [1].

Level systems that outline expectations and corresponding levels of privileges have worked as a behavior management tool. If levels can be changed rapidly in response to behaviors, this increases their efficacy. Colyar describes a daily level system that was extremely effective [2].

Level systems are also helpful in giving privileges according to their associated risks. They can be based on the patients' trustworthiness. For example, grounds privileges and off-grounds passes would be granted only to patients who had reached the highest level within the program. Level systems are organized so that improvements in target behaviors and increased responsibility are tied to increased privileges. Progression in a level system can increase the patient's sense of accomplishment and competence, even when all other improvements move slowly. Prosocial behaviors can be shaped and disruptive behaviors reduced as persons progress through a level system. Level systems seem generally acceptable in most residential programs [3].

References

1. Crabtree LH. Hospitalized adolescents who act out: a treatment approach. Psychiatry 1982 May;45(2):147–58.
2. Colyar DE. Residential care and treatment of youths with conduct disorders: conclusions of a conference of child care workers. Child & Youth Care Forum 1991 Jun;20(3):195–204.
3. See reference 1.

7. Life Space Interview

The life space interview makes use of the child's small daily experiences to work toward long-term therapeutic goals. Fritz Redl conceived of the technique when he realized that children often needed on-the-spot interventions and later found them to be as effective and meaningful as individual psychotherapy. This clinical exploitation of life events is helpful because children cannot always read the meaning of what is happening or will often misinterpret. Some children will not accept that they have done anything wrong, and the staff needs to keep providing evidence that their actions are causing trouble. Redl calls this "reality rub-in." When something upsetting occurs in the child's interaction with others, the staff member spends some time in private seeing the child through the "behavioral storm" and then, when appropriate, talking about it. It can help the child see the event as others see it, becoming more sensitive to the feelings of others and more capable of self-observation [1–2].

The staff member who does the life space interview should be a significant person in the child's daily life, who can provide brief therapy in the child's natural space in the child's natural moments. In his own colorful language Redl describes the therapeutic work that can be accomplished by the life space interview: "the reality rub-in," "massaging numb value areas," " manipulating the boundaries of the self," "emotional first aid on the spot." The life space interview can also help the child figure out new ways to solve problems or to handle difficulties with others. Redl calls this "new tool salesmanship" and writes that the life space interviewer can be quite specific in demonstrating the inadequacies of the present "tools" the child has chosen. For example, the child might learn to use "word tools" rather than physical aggression. This should eventually help the child find alternative ways of behaving and open up possibilities for more appropriate behaviors [1–2].

Pulling the child aside for the interview can help maintain the boundaries of the self. Redl notes that some children are extremely vulnerable to "group psychological suction." The interview helps the child resist group contagion and build up defenses against the negative influence of others. In addition, the establishment of boundaries will also help the child learn not to impose personal whims, prejudices and desires upon others without concern about their own rights and privileges. Wineman describes the phenomenon as invasions of a "foreign ego." When what Redl calls "group psychological suction" occurs, the person without boundaries is invaded by a foreign ego, which becomes part of the self. In another instance the foreign ego invades and presumes that the other person is now a part of the self, and will follow all orders and whims [1–2].

"Emotional First Aid on the Spot"

The life space interview is not always planned for long-term gain. There will be many times when the emotionally disturbed child simply cannot manage daily events in the environment. Redl calls this providing "emotional first aid on the spot." The staff member helps the child drain off frustration or manage panic, rage, or guilt. Emotions during such outbursts leave children out of control. Wineman describes this as "throwing support around the ego" when it retreats from relationships. Redl believes that the adult should stay right with the child, no matter how ferocious the temper tantrum or attack may become. The knowledge that the staff members are just as interested in protecting the child as they are in protecting others will be ego supportive. When the tantrum has come under control, the staff member can help the child put life back in focus and return to the events of the day recovered [1–2].

The interview can keep children communicating even at times when they are trying to shut the world out, Redl's "communication maintenance in moments of relationship decay." Emotional first aid can also accomplish what Redl calls "regulating social and behavioral traffic." Although children may know the rules, they often can't apply them to the task at hand or muster sufficient ego force to handle their impulsivity. The staff member is also called upon to provide umpire services, both for external and internal disputes [1–2].

Use of the Interview

Although there are many times during the day when an interview could be used, it should be used with care. The natural flow of the child's life should not be surrounded by too many outbursts exploiting life events. Rather, interviews should take place when actions are more relevant to the themes in the child's life or goals for therapy. The staff member should not jump into material that is deeply repressed. The life space interview can help the child look at what happened and why and provides the foundation for future changes in attitudes and behavior [1–2].

Standby

Farley describes "Standby," a technique based on the life space interview that is used in children's day treatment. "Standby" refers to the fact that a staff member is standing by to work in private with children who are verbally aggressive or in some way out of control. The teacher or staff member, rather than stopping the group process completely, calls for a Standby, who leaves with the child, helps the child to calm down, and when possible, conducts a 10- or 15-minute interview. When the problem is resolved, the child comes back to the classroom [3].

The Standby interviewer tries to uncover, understand, and help the child deal with the fears, feelings and thoughts that were preventing appropriate functioning in the classroom. A series of Standbys for a child can serve as periodic therapy sessions that will help to work through a problem. The child who is at first reluctant to acknowledge a repetitive pattern of behavior may eventually begin to see it when chronicled by a series of Standbys. The Standby interview may come closer and closer to the child's central conflicts. Standby sessions may later serve to explore the sources for the strong and upsetting emotions, and even touch upon the child's transference behavior. The interviewer may often be able to relate present difficulties and behaviors to past experiences and enable the child to sort out feelings about teachers that might have started with feelings about parents [3].

Soon after admission to day treatment, the staff tells the children about the Standby, the person who will be there to help them when they need it. They learn to see the Standby as a person who stands by to help, not to punish, and the staff encourages them to ask for a Standby whenever they need it. Treatment centers can lose their effectiveness when uncontrolled, aggressive behaviors take over. The Standby technique helps the children know that the staff is not afraid of them and that there is someone there at all times who can understand and manage their behavior [3].

Life Space Interview with the Group

Morse and Small used life space techniques with a group in response to aggressive behaviors, scapegoating, and breaking of rules. The staff leader can learn what's going on by observing the group interaction and makes "hygienic use of clinical authority." The group leader starts with a permissive opening, structures the current problem, and then asks for the group members' interpretation. The goal is more to find out how actions are perceived rather than to establish the facts of what happened. The final phase of the group interview is resolution, a clarification of what really happened and what it meant. There may need to be consequences for the behavior or the talking out process in the group interview may be sufficient [4].

The results of the life space interview group process are not predictable. The intervention may produce no changes but may at least drain off some hostility. Other group interviews may build compliance. Although the group members may recognize the rules, they won't seem to have the ego strength to obey them. Other interviews are more interpretative and accepting. If the group has a positive relationship with the adult leaders and feels their true concern, they may be able to connect their behavior in this setting with previous behavior and be able to talk about their earlier difficulties with peers or teachers. The ideal life space group interview creates what Morse and Small call "spontaneous therapeutic interaction." This happens when the group can move into a spontaneous discussion of significant life experiences. The whole atmosphere changes; the group members become intensely involved, reveal themselves with feeling and develop a sympathetic concern for each other [4].

There are few empirical tests of the life space interview. DeMagistris and Imber used it as an experimental intervention for six behaviorally disturbed students with data collected on target academic and social behaviors and results supported the interview technique. Sadler studied the effects of Standby in a psychoeducational setting. The life space interview remains a helpful technique. Both parents and treatment staff had probably used it instinctively at times but it took Redl to discover its varied uses. He later described the term as an unfortunate one, but he could think of no other way to describe the proximity of the interview to the child's actual life. Colyar describes the decline in treatment when child care staff begins to concentrate only upon controlling behavior and forget personal interaction. The life space interview uses difficult behaviors as "opportune events to build therapeutic relationships" [5–8].

The life space interview seems like such a natural human action that one might not describe it as a technique. What makes it a technique is that it requires thoughtful observation, theoretical conceptualization, carefully planned strategies and formulated solutions based on clinical experience [9].

References

1. Redl F. The life space interview: I. Strategy and techniques of the life space interview. American Journal of Orthopsychiatry 1959 Jan;29(1):1–18.
2. Wineman F. The Life-Space Interview. Social Work 1959 Jan;4:3–17.
3. Farley GK. Standby: A crisis intervention program. In: Farley GK, Zimet SG, eds. Day

treatment for children with emotional disorders. V. 1. A model in action. New York: Plenum Press, 1991, 51–61.
4. Morse WC, Small ER. Group life space interviewing in a therapeutic camp. American Journal of Orthopsychiatry 1959;29:27–44.
5. DeMagistris RJ, Imber SC. The effects of life space interviewing on academic and social performance of behaviorally disordered children. Behavioral Disorders 1980;6(10):12–25.
6. Sadler J, Blom GE. Standby: A clinical research study of child deviant behavior in a psychoeducational setting. Journal of Special Education 1970;4: 89–103.
7. Redl F. When we deal with children. New York: Free Press, 1966.
8. Colyar DE. Ten laws of residential treatment: What can go wrong when you're not looking. Child Care Quarterly 1983 Sum;12(2):136–43.
9. See reference 7.

8. Limit Setting

Limit setting clarifies therapeutic boundaries for the patient and spells out the consequences for breaking rules. It can include such techniques as verbal confrontation, change of privileges, time-out, closing the unit, or seclusion. Setting limits can provide security, gratification, contact and temporary ego boundaries for the patient. It will create a dependable but not dependent situation. The final goal is to help the patient gain control over destructive actions. An accurate estimate of the person's own ability to willfully exert controls is necessary before applying restrictions. Abroms describes the purpose of setting limits as stopping actions that are destructive to treatment. He finds the priorities for setting limits are to end destructive, disorganized, deviant, withdrawn and dependent behaviors [1–4].

Limit setting cannot take place without a clearly designated authority structure responsible for deciding what behaviors are inadmissible and what are the consequences if they occur. Although the staff has final responsibility, other patients can formally or informally contribute to limit setting. Patients nearing discharge are often part of the socialization process, telling new patients what behaviors are permitted or not allowed. Confrontation by peers about behavior is a valuable resource in creating appropriate therapeutic boundaries [5].

Limit setting should increase the patient's awareness of impact on others. Each staff member must also set personal limits. Limit setting is a process for the staff member of self-definition, defining what one can tolerate, and who one is as a real person. It can communicate true concern for the patient and is a crucial factor in day-to-day interaction. Some staff members have difficulty with firm limit setting because they can't distinguish between firmness and hostility. They may overidentify with the patient so that they unconsciously allow certain behaviors because of their own undeveloped controls. Limit setting then becomes laden with anxiety rather than providing an opportunity for growth. Hartmann believes that the patient with borderline personality disorder can learn to set limits by identification with the limit-setting ability of another person who has an emotional involvement, or stated more obscurely, when the patient is able to introject an object relationship with a limit-setting object. Limit setting can finally be effective only when the patient can come to understand that it will eventually contribute toward feeling better or to establish more gratifying relationships with others. If one can help the patient set limits on manipulative or impulsive behaviors, there will be more energy left for therapeutic efforts [6–9].

It is wise to set limits on acting out behavior in an anticipatory fashion, before it occurs. The staff will disagree about setting consistent limits, providing individualized treatment, and the need for flexibility. Large units with a lower staff-patient ratio will need firmer rules, while smaller units with active programs can allow individual limit setting and flexibility. Limit setting is never the only therapeutic technique employed. A good treatment plan outlines the wide variety of interventions the staff will use to help the patient work toward goals. By indicating what the staff can do for the patient, the treatment plan also can detail what the staff will not provide or tolerate. The family's own information about the patient's previous behaviors will help the staff to assess the limit setting that will be necessary for the patient. In turn, this should allow the patient to view the therapeutic boundaries as the result of concerns of everyone in the immediate environment, not merely hospital rules. The staff can help the family by modeling the distinctions between acceptable and nonacceptable behavior and how to respond to the latter [9–10].

LIMIT SETTING FOR IMPULSIVE BEHAVIORS

Patients with little impulse control engage in harmful behaviors such as wrist-cutting, bulimia, drug overdoses. The environment that surrounds them becomes unsafe, and treatment will depend on effective limit setting. The containment of impulsive behavior requires an incremental approach that will actively involve the patient. Green suggests that impulsive patients be told that impulsive feelings are not easily given up and may return in the hospital, despite its environmental support. They are then told about the difference between having impulses and acting upon them. Their goal will be to disconnect the link that was previously made between the impulse and the action. From these discussions, the patient and staff member can produce a written document together that defines behaviors that are unacceptable and outlines consequences for violating these therapeutic boundaries. Green suggests that this document be called a "safety plan," which should help to validate the patient's own sense of control and the collaborative nature of treatment. Working on this time lapse between impulse and action allows the investigation of other ways to cope with impulses. Since the patient was consulted on the safety plan, any consequences that result may be seen more as predictable consequences of an agreement rather than punishment [9–10].

Limit setting with dependent patients

Patients who are excessively dependent make many demands on the unit staff—for time, for attention, or by regression if discharge is planned. Limit setting for dependent patients should outline what the staff can and can't provide. Time spent with the patient is presented as directed toward a specific treatment goal. Then, when the staff refuses some requests, it is not seen as punishing but more as a part of the treatment plan. These patients may benefit from having their therapeutic time structured by the staff [10].

Limit setting with cognitively disorganized patients

Limit setting with cognitively disorganized patients should be established soon after admission since staff members will later find themselves reluctant to do so, and be left feeling frustrated and helpless. The consequences for undesirable behavior should be carefully explained. These patients will require daily structure, repeated orientation to the unit routine, and regular staff contact [10].

Noncompliant patients

These patients often use substance abuse as a way to sabotage treatment. Limits are most effective when set before noncompliant behavior happens. Patients known to abuse substances should be asked to sign a contract at admission specifying a visitor's policy and consequences for drug use. They should also be told that urine toxicology screens and breath analysis may be performed at any time. There are also patients who simply will not comply with treatment. For these patients the staff must negotiate treatment goals with the hope that some of the patient's own goals will intersect with that of the staff. Noncompliant patients will leave the staff feeling angry and helpless. Staff members must then adjust to what are realistic expectations for the patient and accept what is beyond their own control [10].

Lancee and colleagues examined nurses' limit-setting styles and the potential of each style for arousing anger. Scenarios using role playing of six limit-setting styles were used with 97 patients with varying diagnoses and with either high or low levels of impulsivity. They tested these limit-setting styles on anger in four common types of inpatient situations: when the patient wants something that can't be done, the patient refuses to participate in what is required, the patient demands instant gratification, or demands immediate emotional attention. Previous research with over 4,000 nurses had revealed six predominant interpersonal limit-setting styles: 1) belittlement and other responses causing the patient to defend a position; 2) platitudes or generic responses with a lack of attention to the specific situations of the individual patient, 3) presenting solutions without options; 4) presenting solutions with options; 5) affective involvement without options, and 6) affective involvement with options [11–12].

The study reveals that limit-setting styles exert a powerful influence on anger in limit setting situations, regardless of the patient's diagnosis or level of impulsivity. No one will be surprised to learn that belittlement brought about the most anger. Platitudes and offering solutions brought about less anger than belittlement but were not effective in setting limits witout generating anger. For those patients who were not impulsive, three limit-setting styles were effective: offering a solution and options, affective involvement without options, and affective involvement offering options. Only one limit-setting style kept anger at a low level for impulsive patients: affective involvement with options. Empathy alone could not contain anger; it needed to be combined with an offer of options. Limit-setting styles were affective in keeping anger down because attention was paid to the patient's subjective experience and responses were tailored to the individual, with useful suggestions, care and concern. Patients did not need to defend their positions or feel at the mercy of the hospital system [11–12].

The final act of limit setting, particularly for acting-out adolescents, may be suspension. Hazan and colleagues write that if the therapeutic dialogue fails, suspension can finally lead to the necessary clarification, confrontation, and interpretation. On an individual level, suspension will address the adolescent's own autonomy, responsibility and dependency [13].

Gabbard describes limit setting for borderline patients as a preinterpretive technique. An action has occurred, which gives a powerful message, but may only be interpreted later by a therapist. Limit setting at its best can convert acting-out behavior into an internalized experience. When a person acts out against the limits and is thwarted, there is an opportunity to step back and interpret the behavior. The staff's limit setting can also provide a model for patients, who can watch how the staff deals with the difficult behaviors of others. Those who find that limit setting has a permanent therapeutic effect believe that repeated confrontations with the external structure of the milieu can lead to the growth of an inner structure within the person [14–16].

References

1. Bloom H. The use of contracts in the inpatient treatment of the borderline personality disorder. Psychiatric Quarterly 1989 Win;60(4):317–27.
2. Cohen RE, Grinspoon L. Limit setting as a corrective ego experience. Archives of General Psychiatry 1963;8:74–9.
3. Pardes H, Bjork D, Van Putten T, Kaufman M. Failures on a therapeutic milieu. Psychiatric Quarterly 1971;46:29–48.
4. Abroms GL. Setting limits. Archives of General Psychiatry 1968 Jul;19:113–9.
5. Green SA, Goldberg RL, Goldstein DM, Leibenluft E. Limit setting in clinical practice. Washington, DC: American Psychiatric Press, 1988.
6. Lassig D, Shroeder K. Nursing in the therapeutic milieu. In: Wells LA, ed. A handbook of psychiatric nursing. St. Louis: Warren Green, 1989, 319–52.

7. Krug O. The application of principles of child psychotherapy in residential treatment. American Journal of Psychiatry 1952 Aug;10(8):695–700.
8. Hartmann J. Limit-setting as a group process. International Journal of Therapeutic Communities 1989;10(4):34–44.
9. Leibenluft E, Goldbert RL. Guidelines for short-term inpatient psychotherapy. Hospital & Community Psychiatry 1987 Jan;38(1):38–43.
10. See reference 5.
11. Lancee WJ, Gallop R, McCay E, Toner B. The relationship between nurses' limit-setting styles and anger in psychiatric inpatients. Psychiatric Services 1995 Jun;46(6):609–13.
12. Gallop R, Lancee WJ, Garfinkel PE. The expressed empathy of psychiatric nursing staff. Canadian Journal of Nursing Research 1990;22:7–18.
13. Hazan Y, Lerner Y, Subar R. Coping with acting-out in a psychoanalytically-oriented adolescent unit. British Journal of Psychotherapy 1992(Sum);8(4):359–73.
14. Gabbard GO. The therapeutic relationship in psychiatric hospital treatment. Bulletin Menninger Clinic 1992;56(1):4–19.
15. Marohn R. Assertiveness in the treatment of juvenile delinquents. Psychiatric Annals 1985 Oct;15(10):608–13.
16. See reference 6.

9. Patient Government

Patient government allows patients to learn how to govern themselves, to explore how representation, negotiation and social relationships work and to learn to create a congenial social atmosphere. It frees patients from some of the burdens of institutional rules made by others and they can work toward their own recovery by learning to take responsibility. Patient government requires the hospital administration to give up at least some of the decision-making power to provide a democratic sharing of authority with the patients. Each person can then have a part in the operation of the treatment program. Often the democratic process can encourage patients who are depressed or withdrawn to express themselves. Patient governments involving patients in their own care and in the care of others have good results, not because democracy alleviates mental illness but because it helps to restore the patients' highest functioning. The patients can make rules, change them, review the treatment center's privilege systems, and constructively examine one another's behavior [1–3].

The formation of a patient government can be therapeutic if it has effective patient leadership, clear definition of tasks, and definite authority. If the organization's work is trivial and with little meaning and if it has no authority, it will not be helpful. Staff representatives may also participate in patient government. Jacobs recommends that the representative be someone from the supervisory senior staff with no direct therapeutic or administrative responsibilities for the unit [4–5].

The senior staff member will give the government proper prestige and authority. If the staff member is not directly involved in the clinical treatment, then there will be no need to defend specific treatment regimens or administrative programs which patients may complain about. The patients must respect the representative as an effective advocate. The patient representatives can be responsible for thinking about the difficulties and problems in living together. They will also represent those patients who don't feel free to voice their complaints in public or can help them bring up difficult issues in patient government meetings. Representatives may extend their work by being in charge of welcoming new patients to the unit or publishing a weekly newsletter, which can help create a patient culture. They may also suggest, organize and carry out activities [4–5].

Patient governments may communicate by holding meetings with the staff or by sending a weekly written report to them. The staff then should bring about prompt corrective action or provide reasons why such actions cannot be taken. Depending on the authority structure of the hospital, the patient government may handle infractions by patients. If this is to be done, the group must have established an attitude of caring about each other and believe in learning from past errors, rather than simply punishing the guilty. It is more helpful to express concern and play down law and order [5].

Appelbaum and Munich find patient government essential to the rehabilitation model. A significant task of rehabilitation is to restore the ability to affect one's environment. They write that psychotherapy must be combined with successful exercises of power in order for rehabilitation to occur. In the program they describe, the unit treatment team meetings include all patients. Their meetings help them to understand their fellow patients' problems and devise management and treatment strategies to solve them. Patients make the primary decisions on behalf of each other and can be overruled only when the staff found their decisions to be in conflict with treatment strategy. They made real decisions and lived with the consequences until the next unit meeting. The unit administrative groups in this system had several functions. They represented the outside world within treatment. They also seemed to take on the functions of the family, providing socialization and integration into the community, as well as providing the opportunity to internalize adaptive values. The group also helped to guarantee each treatment plan, providing support for each person's rehabilitation goals and helping each member develop responsibility toward the group [6].

This representation can help patients prepare for later involvement in their communities. Each person who participates can develop feelings of concern and responsibility for others that will be of help in later life. Rather than being the passive recipients of the staff's therapy, patients can become agents of change. Psychiatric patients have been subject to strong imbalances in power relations. A reestablishment of power in patient government can also restore self-esteem, counteract passivity, and help patients to realize their considerable assets and ability to act [6].

References

1. Hyde RW, Solomon HC. Patient government: a new form of group therapy. Digest of Neurology & Psychiatry 1950;18:207–18.
2. Tucker GJ, Maxmen JS. The practice of hospital psychiatry: a formulation. American Journal of Psychiatry 1973 Aug;130(8):887–91.
3. Blase KA, Fixsen DL, Freehorn K, Jaeger D. The behavioral model. In: Lyman, Robert D, Prentice-Dunn S, Gabel S., eds. Residential and inpatient treatment of children and adolescents. New York: Plenum Press, 43–60.
4. Kernberg OF. Psychoanalytic object relations theory, group proceses, and administration: Toward an integrative theory of hospital treatment. Annual of Psychoanalysis 1973;1:363–88.
5. Jacobs MA. Promoting responsibility and mutual concern through a modified form of patient government. Journal of Psychosocial Nursing & Mental Health Services 1977 Feb;15(1):30–7.
6. Appelbaum AH, Munich RL. Reinventing moral treatment: the effects upon patients and staff members of a program of psychosocial rehabilitation. Psychiatric Hospital 1985;17(1):11–19.

10. Pets

The healthy effects of animal companions on the mentally ill was recorded as early as 1792 when English Quakers used small animals in their patients' courtyards. Pets can fulfill deep psychological needs, particularly the need to love and be loved, and their presence in the residential treatment setting can help to accomplish many therapeutic goals. What has been called PFP, pet-facilitated psychotherapy, has proved to be a helpful adjunct to treatment. Corson and colleagues find pets to be effective with adult patients. Pets were used with 50 hospitalized psychiatric patients, most of whom had not responded to conventional treatment. All but three of the patients became less withdrawn and more communicative. Patients experienced more self-respect, independence and responsibility when they began to take care of their dogs. The dogs seem to catalyze the interaction in the unit. Communication started with them but extended to others in the milieu. There were no ill effects or difficult experiences. Corson and colleagues worked with six breeds: border collies, beagles, a labrador retriever, a German shepherd, a husky hybrid and a wirehair fox terrier. Terriers were particularly helpful with extremely withdrawn patients, but the general mix of breeds with the potential for matching with personalities was also an advantage. Infection control is mandatory and should include health certificates, documentation of shots, fecal parasite analysis and blood tests in some instances [1–2].

Patients need to feel valued and some will accept the affection of a dog before they will accept it from others. Pets warm up the social interaction in the treatment environment and can start the process of communication with others. They can help children adjust to residential treatment after separation from home. By playing, petting, and walking with an animal, children can begin to relax and feel more trusting. Pets will often serve as intermediaries in communication with withdrawn children. They distract them from obsessive concerns about their own problems [2–3].

By taking some responsibility for a dog, the children gain a sense of competence. Work and play with the dog can develop responsibility, empathy, trust and affection. The process of training a dog provides some analogies for the child about human activities. Dogs must learn to obey instructions, learn to behave and be prevented from fighting, just as people must learn acceptable behaviors. Children in residential treatment can be withdrawn and depressed and lack trust in others, but the appearance of the "canine-therapist" may be the first step toward more trusting interactions with people. In a lighter vein, Loney writes that the inpatient staff with a canine therapist will have at least one member who is not concerned about status or getting ahead, who has no intellectual pretensions, and does not complain about being underpaid [3–4].

References

1. Hundley J. Pet project: the use of pet-facilitated therapy among the chronically mentally ill. Journal of Psychosocial Nursing & Mental Health Services 1991;29(6):23–6.
2. Corson SA, Corson E O'L, Gwynne H, Arnold LE. Pet dogs as nonverbal communication links in hospital psychiatry. Comprehensive Psychiatry 1977 Jan/Feb;18(1):61–72.
3. Gonski YA. The therapeutic utilization of canines in a child welfare setting. Child & Adolescent Social Work 1985;2(2):93–105.
4. Loney J. The canine therapist in a residential children's setting. Journal American Academy of Child Psychiatry 1973 Jul;10(3):518–23.

11. Post-Discharge Contacts

Post-discharge contacts provide communication between the staff and discharged patients. While some fear that these communications may keep the patient dependent, such contacts may actually help to sustain the person in the community. The therapeutic progress that the patient has made can be strengthened or weakened as a result of post-discharge contacts. Rather than letting such contact process informally, Austad and Shapiro recommend that they be considered as clinical events with therapeutic implications. The staff's response should give full attention to the nature of the therapeutic needs that are being expressed. Post-discharge contacts should be discussed in team meetings with attention given to the content of the patient's message and the patient's need for reassurance. Austad and Shapiro believe that the staff can learn a great deal from post-discharge contacts [1].

The treatment center should formulate a policy for handling post-discharge contacts. An appropriate and thoughtful response to discharged patients gives them the sustenance they need to stay in the community and may actually prevent readmission [1].

References

1. Austad CS, Shapiro RS. Treatment implications of the postdischarge contact. Hospital & Community Psychiatry 1986 Aug;37(8):839–40.

12. Reframing

Once techniques are found to be successful in the milieu, they will be used over and over again. The reliance on tested interventions can cause the staff to lose sight of other responses. Reframing as a technique can expand choices for both staff and patients. It can change the interpretation of a given situation, and the new interpretation can then change the behavioral response. The situation is placed within a new frame. It looks completely different, and it then commands a new response. Placing a situation in a wider frame allows consideration of an alternative explanation for the behavior. Is there a larger frame by which this behavior might have positive value or be useful? Is there a way to give the behavior a positive connotation [1]?

Reframing for staff members

Reframing can be an effective technique to help the staff work with difficult patients and with difficult situations. Shaffer and Pollack describe an adaptive reframing of the children's regression in the treatment center. The children's regression before school closes is a difficult phase for both the children and staff to endure. This regression is reframed as the children's attempt to ask if they will fall apart away from the treatment, and also as a way of asking the staff if they remember how they used to act and whether or not they haven't made a lot of progress. When this regression is reframed as the child's positive attempts to remember, review, and internalize, then the child can experience it as growth and not regression. The staff then sees this behavior not as a failure but as a way to symbolically work out the separation. Schaffer and Pollak find that adaptive reframing has the advantage of being concrete and rooted in the child's experience. It is useful when treatment alliances are weakened, and not only binds anxiety but improves self-esteem [2].

Reframing can be quite effective in helping the staff member to tolerate the frustration of working with manipulative patients. Reframing involves distinguishing intention from behavior. The manipulative patient may be behaving in such a way as to get attention or to meet dependency needs. If the meaning of an event can be changed, or the frame in which the person sees the event changed, the behavior can also change. So, in the face of a difficult behavior, the staff member must examine the needs that the behavior is expressing and how these needs could be met in more appropriate ways. In addition the staff member can also ask what beliefs the person might have that supports this behavior. This is not reframing for the patient but for the staff, reframing manipulative behavior itself. If staff members regard patient manipulation as a way to influence people, they may recognize that many patients need it for self-protection and to fulfill certain needs. A reframing of the manipulative patient as a masterful artist who can wield influence can help staff members to change their negative feelings, realize that at present they can't change the person, and achieve a more objective stance through this wider perspective [3].

REFRAMING WITH CHILDREN

Jessee and colleagues describe the ability of children to pull adults into power struggles. If adults can reframe these power struggles in positive terms, even if they don't share their interpretive reframing with the child, they can disengage from the struggle. If a child's difficulties can be reframed in a positive manner, it can improve the ability to consider both positive and negative attributes of all behaviors. Jessee writes about a depressed 12-year old who would withdraw in his room when he was urged to interact with peers. After all attempts to help him to interact were unsuccessful, the staff told him that they supported his retreating, that he probably wanted to stay in his room to get in touch with his sad feelings, and only after he did that for a long time would he be ready to interact with others. At first the 12-year old was confused, but after two days he started to spend all his time with peers, felt much better about himself and his ability to control his behavior [4].

When a child who had a history of conflicts with his mother continuously refused the female staff member's request to go to bed, he was finally told by the staff that he didn't go to bed because he wanted to feel close to this woman; the behavior was extinguished and he began to seek attention in more appropriate ways. These efforts at reframing were dramatically successful but may be risky in the hands of inexperienced staff members. Reframing has great promise, but it should be guided by experienced staff. Jessee and colleagues also describe a reframing of the group's behavior in response to peer conflict and scapegoating. After all other attempts had failed, fighting with peers was reframed as being an expression of affection and caring. The staff member pointed out that boys don't fight with boys that they don't care about. The boys denied this interpretation but they stopped fighting and allowed the scapegoated peer in the group. Later on, after the fighting had stopped, the child who had been a scapegoat found himself with a few new friends [4].

Jessee and colleagues find that children can change their behavior when its meaning is reframed. These efforts did not discourage the behavior the staff members wanted to stop. Instead, they prescribed it. These writers report that even when the person or group tries to refute a new interpretation, they can't ignore it. Even when they can verbally refute the new interpretation, they can no longer see their behavior in the same light. These techniques defuse the power struggle by altering the hierarchy of power. Children who won't change their behavior when the staff insists are exercising their own control. When staff members reframe the behavior, they regain control and change the hierarchy of the adult-child transactions. If the staff continues to demand that the children change their behavior, it confirms its powerlessness. The reframing makes the children's behavior legitimate but they then have no means of control. Reframing is a very interesting technique that redirects the no-win interaction. Jessee and colleagues believe that group reframing interventions are usually more successful than those with the individual [4].

Behavioral management of children has important therapeutic implications and what constitutes management for one therapist may be therapy for another. Reframing places little emphasis on insight, so if traditional psychodynamic approaches are central to the treatment setting, the use of reframing or paradoxical intention may result in conflicting approaches to patients. Jessee notes, however, that often reframing brings about self-awareness and interpersonal changes congruent with psychodynamic approaches [4].

Reframing a behavior can be a way of allowing the child to make sense of it. Reframing the behavior as positive will often allow the child to end it. In another article, Jessee and L'Abate write about reframing a little boy's inability to get to sleep as a demonstration of how much he loved his parents. The child was encouraged to stay up until he felt he had shown enough love for them. Reframing must always be done in manner that the child can understand [5].

Reframing of Symptoms

The effectiveness of dialectical-behavioral therapy relies in part on reframing the person's destructive behaviors as an habitual response to overwhelming emotions. This reframing of symptoms as habits then endows the patient with greater self-control. In residential treatment, Menses and Durrant reframe the adolescent's symptoms as "habits that have been pushing him and his family around" [6–7].

Reframing the Treatment Process

Treatment itself can be reframed. Menses and Durrant define the adolescent's placement in residential treatment as "practicing," as a time for information-gathering and experimentation. Residential treatment then is no longer about "fixing" the child or parents but helping them see themselves as competent and successful and able to build upon their strengths and resources. Reframing for its own sake which disregards the treatment plan or the relationship with the patient is irresponsible and may be harmful. Reframing is likely to be more successful if the staff member has a caring relationship with the child. Jessee and colleagues write that the benefits of positive reframing cannot be guaranteed to last after discharge [8–9].

References

1. Pesut DJ. The art, science, and techniques of reframing in psychiatric mental health nursing. Issues in Mental Health Nursing 1991;12:9–18.
2. Schaffer S, Pollack J. The interruption and resumption phases of milieu treatment with children and adolescents. Child & Adolescent Social Work Journal 1987;4(1):41–9.
3. Johnson GB, Werstlein PO. Reframing: a strategy to improve care of manipulative patients. Issues in Mental health Nursing 1990;11:237–41.
4. Jessee EH, Jurkovic GJ, Wilkie J, Chiglinsky M. Positive reframing with children: conceptual and clinical considerations. American Journal of Orthopsychiatry 1982;52(2): 314–22.
5. Jessee E, L'Abate L. The use of paradox with children in an inpatient treatment setting. Family Process 1980 Mar;19:59–64.
6. Gallop R. Self-destructive and impulsive behavior in the patient with a borderline personality disorder: rethinking hospital treatment and management. Archives of Psychiatric Nursing 1992;6(3):178–82.
7. Menses G, Durrant M. Contextual residential care: applying the principles of cybernetic therapy to the residential treatment of irresponsible adolescents and their families. Residential Treatment of Children & Youth 1990;7(3):11–32.
8. Durrant M. Residential treatment: a cooperative, competency-based approach to therapy and program design. New York: Norton, 1993.
9. See reference 4.

13. Religion

For many patients, religious needs are related to treatment, and information about patients' religious beliefs may be relevant to meeting their psychological needs. Guidelines developed by the American Psychiatric Association's Committee on Religion and Psychiatry advise that information be obtained about the patient's religious orientation and beliefs, that all religious beliefs be respected, and that religious beliefs should never be imposed on patients. Waldfogel and Wolpe write that the failure to learn about a patient's religious beliefs may result in an incomplete diagnostic assessment and neglect a significant means of intervention [1–2].

Religious beliefs and affiliation can provide the social support that patients so desperately need to maintain stability, decreases their isolation and give a sense of belonging. Church attendance, religious rituals, and prayer can be a great source of comfort for religious patients. In addition to the solace that is provided by religion, church affiliation can ease the patient's return to the community. The staff should continue to be respectful of the place of religion in the patient's search for meaning, and be careful not to challenge the patient's own religious convictions [2].

Gossett and colleagues, in an extensive follow-up of hospitalized adolescents, remark upon the attraction of former patients to charismatic or fundamentalist religions. They think that many patients were helped by such associations and found a feeling of belonging and stability not available elsewhere. The group included both chronically psychotic persons as well as those with severe personality disorders, who were able, with the help of religion, to establish impulse control [3].

Religious needs may be met by the inclusion of a chaplain on the staff or by a program of pastoral visits. In many hospitals the chaplain becomes an auxiliary member of the staff and will meet with each patient who requests a visit or consultation. The chaplain can meet with the patient either on a regular basis or upon request and may help to assess how the religious needs of the patient relate to treatment. The chaplain may also extend this individual work by consulting with staff or establishing religious discussion groups where spiritual concerns can be shared with others [4].

All efforts must be made, however, to stress that religion in hospital treatment is a service available at the request of the patient, and is not otherwise provided. There should never be a message that religious participation is in any way expected, nor should any member of the staff, including the chaplain, attempt to influence the vulnerable person's beliefs. There may be occasions when religious thought or practices have a problematic influence upon a patient's own psychological growth. This will be the time to assess the patient's religious beliefs to determine whether they strengthen a sense or reality or increase or decrease the person's self-esteem. When staff members are asked about personal religious beliefs, speaking about them is a personal choice. When the patient does not separate personal religious beliefs from all other areas of emotion and thought, then members of the team should not avoid talking about these beliefs with the patient [5–6].

The spiritual component of a person's life can provide a sense of purpose, a means of forgiveness, and a source of love and relatedness. There may be a need to learn whether the patient's religious beliefs help or harm the ability to feel forgiven or whether they increase or decrease the person's sense of freedom and responsibility. Religious support and affiliation can become a part of the psychological care of those patients whose religious beliefs and practices may be essential to understanding their symptoms and difficulties in living. The spiritual dimension may turn out to be one of their greatest personal resources for recovery [7–8].

References

1. American Psychiatric Association. Committee on Religion and Psychiatry. Guidelines regarding possible conflict between psychiatrists' religious commitments and psychiatric Practices. (Official Actions). American Journal of Psychiatry 1990;174:542
2. Waldfogel S, Wolpe, PR. Using awareness of religious factors to enhance interventions in consultation-liaison psychiatry. Hospital & Community Psychiatry 1993 May;44(5):473–7.
3. Gossett JT, Lewis JM, Barnhart FD. To find a way: the outcome of hospital treatment of disturbed adolescents. New York: Brunner-Mazel, 1983, 149.
4. Anderson RG, Young JL. The religious component of acute hospital treatment. Hospital & Community Psychiatry 1988 May;39(5):528–32.
5. Peterson EA, Nelson K. How to meet your clients' spiritual needs. Journal of Psychosocial Nursing & Mental Health Services 1987 May;25(5):34–9.
6. Pruyser P. Religion in the psychiatric hospital: a reassessment. Journal of Pastoral Care 1984;38:5–17.
7. See reference 5.
8. See reference 4.

14. Role Modeling

Role modeling brings about learning by imitation. Although it has always been a significant factor in residential treatment for children and adolescents, there is not much literature about how to use it as a technique in the milieu. Children have had contact with many role models before treatment, both positive and negative. They observe adults and imitate not what the adults intend to be, but what they see and hear. Placement in residential treatment controls the number and quality of role models available to the child. The staff member who takes role modeling seriously will try to clarify what the child might need to learn and what behaviors the child might imitate. Behaviors to be imitated usually involve good basic human qualities, not exceptional talents. For example, many staff members can easily model giving and receiving affection—toward the children, other staff members, or family. Staff members who repress these healthy expressions deprive the child of helpful modeling [1].

The child care worker must also consider what behaviors should be discouraged in the child and whether providing role models might also help with them. This might involve thinking about how to handle anger or disappointment, and sharing these reactions with the child. Planning behaviors to be modeled might also involve some thinking about how such behaviors can be rewarded. Rewards should be specifically related to the modeled behavior and attractive to the children. Role modeling can also be explicit. The child care worker can highlight desired behaviors and can demonstrate them to the child. Child care workers who share some of their own childhood experiences and problems can relate role modeling to the building of a relationship. When the child can identify with the staff member and find similarities, role modeling is a natural outcome. Children and adolescents will also benefit from role models nearer to their own age—Big Brothers or Big Sisters, or college student volunteers. Role modeling can also occur in groups or in community meetings. Staff members can reveal healthy aspects of themselves to patients and encourage use of healthy defenses or self-understanding [1–2].

Other patients may also be considered as role models, but the development of positive role models is possible only in long-term treatment. Patient role models are particularly effective in therapeutic communities for substance abuse. They can encourage the behaviors, attitudes and expectations of the community. Persons who use substances often lack a stable identity. Residents who have progressed in the program help to train newcomers on their way to a healthier identity. Their success in the program gives others hope and they are role models for the possibility of recovery. They can contrast their present and earlier behaviors. New residents change their behaviors by imitating and identifying with them. This also has a therapeutic effect on the role model, whose own behavior and attitude is reinforced when teaching others. Role models instill motivation and provide hope for change. The role model provides motivational cues, presents status and reinforcement. Teaching others reinforces the behavior and attitudes of the teacher [3].

There is not much literature on role modeling because so much of it occurs without specific planning. Staff members may modestly downplay their own importance as role models. Although there is a great difference between imitating and role modeling, pure imitation can be the first step toward learning new behaviors. Portnoy and colleagues advise that the child care worker can become a powerful therapeutic agent by channeling modeled behaviors into planned behavior modification [4].

References

1. Bertcher HJ. The child care worker as role model. Child Care Quarterly 1973;2(3):178–91.
2. Marcovitz RJ, Smith JE. An approach of time-limited dynamic inpatient psychotherapy. Small Group Behavior 1983;14(3):369–76.
3. DeLeon G. The therapeutic community and behavioral science. International Journal of Addictions 1990–91;25(21A):1537–57.
4. Portnoy SM, Biller HB, Davids A. The influence of the child care worker in residential treatment. American Journal of Orthopsychiatry 1972;42(4):719–22.

15. Seclusion

Seclusion may be described as closely monitored containment. It is never the treatment of choice, but there are times when it is needed to prevent harm to the patient or others. It can prevent serious disruption of the treatment environment and contain violent or uncontrollable behavior. It may also be used to remove a patient from destructive relationships or situations leading to paranoia, or to decrease sensory stimulation. Seclusion provides secure ego boundaries when needed, and can reassure the patient that control is available. The patient in seclusion is not locked in and ignored, but should have a schedule or growth-promoting activities and regular contact with staff. The treatment focus of seclusion is to allow the patient to gain control and monitor incoming stimuli. It is an acute management technique and usually has no long-term therapeutic function. Although staff members may find that seclusion restores the patient's control, having to place someone in seclusion is usually emotionally upsetting [1–4].

Precipitants of Seclusion

The most frequent reason for seclusion is escalating agitation, a behavior which can lead to violence or threatened violence. The behaviors that lead to seclusion are usually serious. Both milieu and patient factors influence seclusion. It may occur more frequently during unstructured patient time when staff are known to be in the building, but not with patients. Behavior leading to seclusion is also related to the stimulation provided by the presence of many staff members and other patients. The milieu culture and its acceptance of violence as an expected response to frustration, fear or anger will also affect the frequency of seclusion [5–7].

Procedures for Seclusion

Alternatives should be explored before a patient is secluded. Patients may be removed from conflict and talked to by staff members, or restricted from activities. There may also be varying degrees of seclusion. Open door seclusion with an in-out schedule may be appropriate for highly distractable patients who need decreased stimulation and structure. Locked door seclusion may be needed when the patient is too cognitively disorganized for an in-out schedule. What staff members do before and during seclusion can influence the patient's behavior and feelings about it. The staff member must clearly explain to the patient what behaviors led to seclusion as well as what behaviors will lead to release. Behavioral criteria for seclusion should be recorded. There should be contact, observation, and assessment of the patient every 15 minutes. These contacts should be documented and include assurance of safety as well as attention to treatment and daily living. The patient must not feel abandoned. Staff members should be accepting and reassuring. Although they should indicate that seclusion is the level of care the patient currently needs, they should stress that it is temporary. Communication should be kind and direct. It is not the time to discuss feelings, conflicts or ideas. Discussion of alternatives can be presented in a supportive and protective manner. When a patient is secluded, others in the milieu must be reassured about their own ability to control their impulses. They should also be prepared for the patient's return [8–12].

Phases of Seclusion

Seclusion may have three phases: initiation, reintegration, and reincorporation into the community. During the initiation phase containment, structure and support are provided. The seclusion room provides the external control for behavior and reality testing. A predictable schedule during seclusion provides the structure. The staff member attends to the patient's needs and attempts to re-establish a relationship that will give support. There should be a consistent staff member who can assess the patient's functioning, report on therapeutic issues and consult on clinical interventions. Once the patient feels safe and can cooperate with the external limits of seclusion, the reintegration phase can begin [13].

The Reintegration Phase

The goals of this phase are to help the patient regain control over thoughts and feelings, increase independence, and improve self-esteem. Attempts should be made to help restore the patient's identity, by frequently using the patient's name, bringing in personal belongings, and making personal choices. Reintegration is achieved when the patient has gained control of thoughts, feelings, and behavior. Before the patient returns there should be a debriefing to help alleviate the emotional impact of seclusion. This reviews the reasons for it, offers mutual feedback, and helps to restore self-esteem. Reincorporation involves a gradual return to milieu participation. The staff must be alert to the possibility that the end of seclusion can allow the behavior that precipitated it to return. Campbell and colleagues found that 74% of patients remained calm after seclusion [13–16].

Duration of Seclusion

Seclusion should last only as long as it takes to reestablish self-control. Little work has been done in measuring the differential effects of the duration of seclusion, but duration will be affected by the patient's characteristics, the precipitating incident, the unit's practices, as well as the ward atmosphere, including the mental state and behavior of other patients [17].

The Seclusion of Children

Seclusion for children has not been grounded in theory by those who prescribe it. If the treatment center uses seclusion, a decision-making process with parents and children about the future use of aversive procedures is recommended [18–19].

There is always a question whether the availability of the seclusion room can prevent the milieu staff from discovering more creative and less punitive interventions. However, Gair believes that this need for external controls for difficult patients is real and not a self-fulfilling prophecy created by the availability of a seclusion room [20–21].

Some have described seclusion as indicative of the failure of the treatment environment to meet the patient's needs, but seclusion may actually meet specific needs of the child and does not always indicate deficient treatment programs and policies. The treatment staff caring for ego-deficient children faces extreme stress. In the normal process of socialization, children have internalized controls through their attachment to parents, whose nurturant discipline has provided the nucleus for their development. This process did not work for psychiatrically hospitalized children. Seclusion for children is usually for briefer periods, but may also be more frequent than for adults. Cotton believes that if seclusion for children is not accompanied by a thorough understanding of its clinical rationale, it cannot play a curative role. She produces a careful argument for the role of seclusion in treatment that should be read by all who believe that it has no long term therapeutic effects [22].

Cotton examines the principle of developing inner controls and describes therapeutic management with children as having three phases: diminishing maladaptive behavior, developing adaptive, productive behavior, and rechanneling emotions and impulses into safe expression. Seclusion helps the child to gain control over behavior. It develops the habit of leaving situations that are overwhelming and helps to initiate rechanneling [22].

The frequency of seclusion is usually a sign of a child's distress rather than defects in the program. Cotton describes seclusion as the beginning of a disciplining process, an essential step in the process of learning control through the experience of control. Clear communication to the child about seclusion is vital. Seclusion introduces such coping skills as leaving the scene of conflict, finding quiet solace, thinking about a situation in private, delaying a reaction when frustrated, receiving consequences without creating a major problem and obtaining adult assistance before things get out of control [22].

Seclusion can allow a private release of emotions without loss of face with peers. The boundaries of the room can help the child restore personal boundaries. Seclusion must not psychologically separate the child from others for long. The child needs reassurance that seclusion is temporary and that it allows the staff to provide the external controls until the child can recover them. Cotton believes that if the seclusion room is cozy and safe, the seclusion process predictable, and the staff warm and caring, the child can experience the brief psychological separation, not as an abandonment, but as a caring response to impulsive behavior [22].

In summary, Cotton describes seclusion as part of a therapeutic process which supports and develops the child's internal controls. It is used consistently for clinically indicated predictable reasons, and is clearly explained to the child before and after its use. It is provided by a well-trained staff in a safe and comforting room, and monitored by professionals. Cotton describes what seems to be an ideal seclusion room, with plexiglass windows opening to a pleasant outdoor view and another looking into the director's office. The children can watch the director at work while in the process of trying to gain their own control. The physical features of a quiet room can influence the behavior of its occupants and the time it takes a patient to calm down [22–23].

Those who advise against seclusion for children must consider it against a background of other alternatives. Antoinette and colleagues studied the effect of an unlocked seclusion policy on three child psychiatric inpatient units. Unlocked seclusion was associated with increased use of tranquilizers. Their findings indicate that the appropriate use of locked seclusion may be clinically sound since it is preferable to the frequent use of tranquilizing medication or the patient's inflicting harm [24].

Seclusion remains a controversial intervention. Its effectiveness has no basis in research findings. Few treatments so frequently used for patients with widely different diagnoses are so deficient in information as to basic use and effectiveness. Garrison and colleagues found, for example, that the number of interpersonal conflicts did not change and usually remained stable throughout a patient's stay, indicating that neither seclusion or restraint show any permanent therapeutic effect. The milieu staff cannot usually justify seclusion as a treatment in itself. The problem of the patient's behavior is not solved by seclusion. Seclusion is a control technique that interferes with personal liberty and is ethically justified only under certain conditions, primarily to prevent physical harm [25–28].

Although staff members may feel that seclusion can preserve the unit's therapeutic environment by temporarily removing dangerous or disruptive patients, there are few patients who would describe it in positive terms. Chamberlin, an ex-patient, writing in response to an article on seclusion, notes that the person in emotional pain and stress yearns for human contact, not its denial by seclusion. Patients may also have delusional misinterpretations of their seclusion and it can also stimulate hallucinations. Patients who have been secluded describe the experience as making them feel confused, helpless, bored, angry, depressed, and safe. Seclusion continues in the absence of more effective and humane alternatives. A reduction in one intervention (such as seclusion) may lead only to an increase in another (such as restraint) [29–33].

The staff should frequently review seclusion policies. There should be a standardized form for recording the patient's behavior in seclusion, and the effects of the release should also be recorded.

Alternatives to Seclusion

ROOM RESTRICTION

Gentilin has found room restriction to be effective for adolescents in substance abuse programs. Room restriction can provide the external structure that helps adolescents develop internal controls. The adolescent in room restriction will usually stop the maladaptive behaviors that get attention, and while in the room can receive staff attention for appropriate reasons. Adolescents are told in advance what actions will result in room restrictions. The adolescent's ability to be in control through choosing behaviors is continuously reinforced. Ego strength is also reinforced when the adolescent learns over and over to accept the consequences of behavior. The room restriction is planned with the consultation of the adolescent who is aware of the reason for restriction and what will be expected. Treatment does not stop, and the adolescents can set up their own schedule during room restriction to accomplish certain tasks. Although outside stimulation is decreased, active treatment with the staff continues. The room restriction is not used to isolate but to allow the adolescent to work through anger and find new ways to handle feelings [34].

INTENSIVE CARE UNITS

Treatment innovations may often occur with changes in architecture or staffing patterns. Seclusion rooms may eventually be replaced by intensive care units. Intensive care is described as a solution to the isolation and banishment associated with seclusion. Craig, Ray, and Hix describe suites designed for intensive care with a room for the needs of the secluded patient, another for the patient requiring restraints, and another for a specially-trained intensive care staff who remain available to the patient at all times. The suites were recessed from the sound and sight of the unit environment to preserve patient privacy [35].

Musisi and colleagues describe a locked structure with eight beds, two quiet rooms, a TV room, bathroom and a nursing station which permitted ongoing treatment and evaluation of patients requiring constant observation. This consistent and controlled environment resulted in decreased patient or staff accidents and decreased nurse absenteeism [36].

Based on a questionnaire of 111 patients, Wise and colleagues report that those who had not been secluded had more negative feelings about seclusion than those who had. This suggests that it might be helpful to discuss the role of seclusion rooms during orientation to the unit. If patients become famiiar with them and how they are used, their fears will be reduced. Mann and colleagues interviewed 50 patients after their seclusion. Most reported that although seclusion was not described as restful, only a small number believed that there should not be seclusion rooms on a psychiatric unit [37–38].

References

1. Oldham JM, Russakoff LM. Prusnofsky L. Seclusion patterns and milieu. Journal of Nervous & Mental Disease 1983;17(11):645–9.
2. Gutheil TG. Observations on the theoretical basis for seclusion of the psychiatric patient. American Journal of Psychiatry 1978;135:325–8.
3. Stamm I. The hospital as a holding environment. International Journal of Therapeutic Communities 1985;6(4):219–29.
4. McCoy SM, Garritson J. Seclusion: the process of intervening. Journal of Psychosocial Nursing & Mental Health Services 1983;21(8):9–15.
5. See reference 1.
6. Phillips P, Nasr S. Seclusion and restraint and prediction of violence. American Journal of Psychiatry 1983 Feb;140(2):229–32.
7. Felthous AR. Preventing assaults on a psychiatric inpatient ward. Hospital & Community Psychiatry 1984 Dec;35(12):1223–6.
8. Gair DS. Limit-setting and seclusion in the psychiatric hospital. Psychiatric Opinion 1980;17:14–19.
9. Green SA, Goldberg RL, Goldstein DM, Leibenluft E. Limit setting in clinical practice. Washington, DC: American Psychiatric Press, 1988, 69–103.
10. Craig C, Ray F, Hix C. Seclusion and restraint. Journal of Psychosocial Nursing & Mental Health Services 1989 Jul;27(7):17–25.
11. Baradell J. Humanistic care of the patient in seclusion. Journal of Psychosocial Nursing & Mental Health Services 1985;23(2):9–14.
12. Hammill K, McEvoy JP, Koral H, Schneider N. Hospitalized schizophrenic patients view about seclusion. Journal of Clinical Psychiatry 1989;50(5):174–7.
13. See reference 11.
14. See reference 10.
15. Chu C-C, Ryan SJ. The role of seclusion in psychiatric hospital practice. Psychiatric Hospital 1987 Sum;18(3):121–5.
16. Campbell W, Shepherd H, Falconer R. The use of seclusion. Nursing Times 1982;27:1821–5.
17. Angold A. Seclusion. British Journal of Psychiatry 1989;154:437–44.
18. Fassler D, Cotton N. A national survey on the use of seclusion in the psychiatric treatment of children. Hospital & Community Psychiatry 1992 Apr;43(4):370–4.
19. Kazdin AE. Acceptability of aversive procedures and medication as treatment alternatives for deviant child behavior. Journal Abnormal Child Psychology 1984;12:289–302.
20. Tsemberis S, Sullivan C. Seclusion in context: introducing a seclusion room into a children's unit of a municipal hospital. American Journal of Orthopsychiatry 1988 Jul;58(3):462–5.
21. See reference 8.
22. Cotton NS. The developmental-clinical rationale for the use of seclusion in the psychiatric treatment of children. American Journal of Orthopsychiatry 1989; 59(3):442–50.
23. Glod CA, Teicher MH, Butler M, Savino M, et al. Modifying quiet room design enhances calming of children and adolescents. Journal American Academy of Child & Adolescent Psychiatry 1994 May;33(4):558–66.

24. Antoinette T, Iyengar S, Puig-Antich J. Is locked seclusion necesary for children under the age of 14? American Journal of Psychiatry 1990 Oct;147(10):1283–9.
25. See reference 4.
26. See reference 17.
27. Garrison WT, Ecker B, Friedman, MD, Davidoff R. Aggression and counteraggression during child psychiatric hospitalization. Journal American Academy of Child & Adolescent Psychiatry 1990;29(2):242–50.
28. See reference 15.
29. Brown JS, Tooke SK. On the seclusion of psychiatric patients. Social Science & Medicine 1992 Sep;35(5):711–21.
30. Chamberlin J. An ex-patient's response to Soliday. Journal of Nervous & Mental Disease 1985 May;173(5):288–9.
31. Norris MK, Kennedy, CW. The view from within: How patients perceive the seclusion process. Journal of Psychosocial Nursing & Mental Health Services 1992 Mar;30(3):7–13.
32. See reference 17.
33. See reference 2.
34. Gentilin J. Room restriction: a therapeutic prescription. Journal of Psychosocial Nursing & Mental Health Services 1987;25(7):13–16.
35. See reference 10.
36. Musisi SM, Wasylenki DA, Rapp MS. A psychiatric intensive care unit in a psychiatric hospital. Canadian Journal of Psychiatry 1989;34(3):200–4.
37. Wise TN, Mann LS, Leibenluft E, Goldberg RL. Isolated versus visible seclusion rooms: Attitudes of Psychiatric Patients. Psychiatric Quarterly 1989;Win 60(4):329–36.
38. Mann LS, Wise TN, Shay L. A prospective study of psychiatry patients attitudes toward the seclusion room experience. General Hospital Psychiatry 1993 May;15(3):177–82.

16. Therapeutic Alliance

The success of any therapeutic endeavor depends on the participants establishing an open, trusting collaborative relationship, or what has been referred to as a therapeutic or working alliance. The patient who does not form an alliance may be noncompliant, terminate treatment prematurely or show little progress. There is a prognostic value in assessing the alliance and identifying the patient, staff, and treatment characteristics that build it [1].

The concept was originally applied to the alliance made with the psychotherapist, but it can also be applied to the alliance that the patient makes with the milieu staff as well as its alliance with the patient. A treatment alliance is achieved in psychotherapy when the patient participates responsively in psychotherapy, is interested in understanding the illness, patterns of relationships with others, and will work to overcome problems and pursue therapeutic goals. The patient who establishes a therapeutic alliance usually believes that treatment will be helpful, and is not only willing to work with staff members, but has usually developed a mutually gratifying relationship with them. There are patients who are hospitalized after not being able to establish a treatment alliance in outpatient therapy. because of their own self-destructive or disruptive behaviors. The hospital can often help the patient develop the relationship necessary to continue treatment [1–3].

Johansen believes that the treatment alliance must be given highest priority, and that the staff should stress its importance in all interactions. He describes the alliance as the most respectful and egalitarian relationship available to help both patients and staff face the difficulties ahead. Johansen also writes about the problems in forging an alliance. The patient may not formulate the need for help in the same language of values as the hospital and may be left feeling puzzled and disillusioned. The patient's "resistance" will then frustrate the staff. The expectations of both parties rarely match. The staff's desire to help the patient adjust to hospital treatment usually means conforming to the staff's wishes, and the patient sees the staff as an intruder. The staff can also see the patient as an intruder into a previously well-ordered unit [4].

The Therapeutic Alliance with the Adolescent

The therapeutic alliance with the adolescent is even more difficult to achieve. Adolescents are usually brought to treatment by parents, not always voluntarily. This makes them distrust adults and retreat from relationships with them. They do not want to be dependent or even cooperative. They will undoubtedly feel that treatment is "done to" or "done by" the staff rather than "accomplished with" them. The therapeutic alliance with adolescents can begin to form when they finally can make an attachment. When the adolescent can begin to discuss symptoms with the treatment team, this may signal the beginning of a collaborative alliance. The adolescent and the staff can build an alliance by further collaboration in areas that are free of conflict. Adolescents who have begun to make an alliance and have invested in the treatment program often begin to recognize the part they played in their own difficulties with family and in school. Ideally, through the treatment alliance, they can come to collaboratively examine their lives. Adolescents can carefully disguise their growing interest in collaborating in treatment and some adolescent reach discharge without developing a successful alliance [5].

Alliance and Therapeutic Outcome

The therapeutic alliance is related to treatment outcome, but it is also an indication of the patient's level of functioning. The alliance is bound up with change, rather than predictive of it. Treatment difficulty, the therapeutic alliance and the severity of patient's problems are interrelated. Staff members have difficulties making a treatment alliance with patients who are psychologically inaccessible, self-destructive, angry and defiant, or who have cognitive and social impairments. The patient's "likability" as well as level of functioning will affect the alliance. As the patient's functioning improves, there will be more productive involvement in treatment. However, the treatment alliance can also deteriorate rather than improve [6–8].

DEVELOPING THE TREATMENT ALLIANCE

The therapeutic alliance can be built on the foundation of a collaborative agreement between the patient and the treatment team that allows the healthy part of the patient's ego to ally itself with the team's treatment objectives. If the patient as well as the clinical staff can jointly author the medical record, their communication will improve. They can settle down to mutual problem solving and negotiation about future actions. Establishing a therapeutic alliance often occurs in tandem with setting goals for hospitalization. Setting goals organizes the patient's thinking about the hospital stay. When the patient and the team set goals together, the team is trying to ally with the patient's observing ego, an alignment which should increase the patient's motivation to work with the staff on defined goals. Setting goals can develop the alliance by breaking down the patient's problems into manageable parts, making the hospital experience less threatening. Ideally, the goals should be framed in both interpersonal and behavioral language [9–11].

The therapeutic alliance is also achieved by building a positive connection with the treatment staff. When all goes well, the patient conceives of the staff person as someone who can help. The patient's ability to self-disclose and even to feel vulnerable helps to nurture this positive connection. This can result in a mutual investment, resulting in mutual trust and the security to take risks. The more the staff member feels valued by the patient the stronger the chance for an alliance [12].

References

1. Frank AE, Gunderson JG. The role of the therapeutic alliance in the treatment of schizophrenia. Archives of General Psychiatry 1990 Mar;47(3):228–36.
2. Stein EJ, Furedy RL. Patient access to medical records on a psychiatric inpatient unit. American Journal of Psychiatry 1979 Mar;136(5):327–9.
3. Zee HJ. Reflections on the psychoanalytic hospital in the 1980s. Bulletin Menninger Clinic 1985;49(5):417–31.
4. Johansen KH, Gossett JT. Therapeutic alliance versus "conversion" in hospital psychiatry. Journal National Association of Private Psychiatric Hospitals 1981 Spr;12(2):56–62.
5. O'Malley F. Developing a therapeutic alliance in the hospital treatment of disturbed adolescents. Bulletin Menninger Clinic 1990;54(1):13–24.
6. See reference 2.
7. Clarkin JF, Hurt SW, Crilly JL. Therapeutic alliance and hospital treatment outcome. Hospital & Community Psychiatry 1987 Aug;37(8):871–5.
8. Colson DB, Cornsweet C, Murphy T, O'Malley F, et al. Perceived treatment difficulty and therapeutic alliance on an adolescent psychiatric hospital unit. American Journal of Orthopsychiatry 1991;6(2):221–9.

9. Bloom H. The use of contracts in the inpatient treatment of the borderline personality disorder. Psychiatric Quartelry 1989 Win;60(4):317–27.
10. Barofsky J. Compliance, adherence and the therapeutic alliance. Social Science & Medicine 1976 Sep;12(5A):369–76.
11. Leibenluft E, Goldbert RJ. Guidelines for short-term inpatient psychotherapy. Hospital & Community Psychiatry 1987 Jan;38(1):38–43.
12. Heifner C. Positive connectedness in the psychiatric nurse-patient relationship. Archives of Psychiatric Nursing 1993;Feb:7(1):11–5.

17. "Time-Out" from Reinforcement

Time-out is usually referred to as time-out from reinforcement, a behavioral intervention that deprives the person of desired reinforcement because of maladaptive behavior. Its purpose is to reduce the behavior's frequency, duration, or intensity. Time-out is often the treatment of choice for child and adolescent behavior problems. Time-outs have some similarities to seclusion in that the person is placed in temporary isolation following a disruptive behavior. Since the time-out is defined as time out from reinforcement, there must obviously be a significant difference between the time-in and time-out environments. There are many variations on time-out: removing all sources of reinforcement while the child remains seated; removing the child from the site with continued opportunities to observe it; placement in a contained area of the room where observation is not possible; and placement in a "time-out room," "seclusionary time-out" [1].

The child should be given a warning if time-out is to be used, and told that if the disruptive behavior doesn't stop, consequences will follow. The child then has an opportunity to stop the behavior, and the warning gives the child more control to stop before a time-out is imposed. Verbally telling the child the reason for time-out provides important instruction. Describing the behavior which brings about the time-out and describing the appropriate alternative behavior is recommended [2].

One of the most serious difficulties with this technique is that the staff member may have to use physical force to take the child to time-out. Every effort should be made to teach appropriate responses to bring about compliance. Removing the child physically escalates the emotional level and lets other children know that there are times when physical aggression is all right to use. One alternative is to have the child remain in the same location with a staff member and have the adults and other children removed. When possible, nonexclusionary alternatives such as having the child sit alone at another table are preferred. These alternatives give more control to the child and provide opportunities to learn from observing others. Although some research has indicated that longer time-outs are more successful, there are some studies which indicate that tine-outs as brief as five minutes can be effective. After the time-out is completed, instructions about the child's inappropriate behavior and more appropriate alternatives should be discussed. This debriefing is an instructional component of the time-out and brings the procedure closer to a cognitive technique. [3–7].

THE QUESTION OF SECLUSIONARY TIME-OUT

Seclusionary time-out may be necessary to prevent harm to the child or other persons when other controls have not worked and to prevent disruption to the physical environment. Seclusionary time-out can also be used as part of ongoing behavior therapy when the benefits are clear and not merely for the staff's convenience. Time-outs may also be used to decrease overwhelming stimulation or to comply with a child's request [8–9].

Adult involvement in time-out is determined by the characteristics of the child. Self-injurious behaviors, such as headbanging will call for full adult participation. Children who become disoriented if left alone or have no ability to calm themselves will require an adult presence. Gallagher and colleagues describe various levels, even in seclusionary time-out. The child can be inside a time-out room with the door ajar and an adult outside the room, with an adult inside the room with the door closed and unlocked, inside the time-out room, with an unlocked door and observation by an adult outside, and inside the time-out room with an adult, who must provide physical restraint until the child is calm [9].

POLICIES FOR TIME-OUT

The treatment center should have a written treatment plan for time-outs for each resident who requires them. In addition, for each resident there should be a written statement which describes previously attempted, less restrictive techniques, a plan to provide positive reinforcement for appropriate behaviors as well as the time-out procedure that will be used. Once written, the plan should include written parental approval. It should also indicate that staff will be trained and supervised to assure competence in designing and implementing management plans that include seclusionary time-out. All staff members should be aware that whenever children are removed from their peers, this may be characterized as seclusion, which can result in a series of legal considerations which could be overlooked by clinical staff [9–10].

References

1. Gast DL, Nelson CM. Legal and ethical considerations for the use of time-out in special education settings. Journal of Special Education 1977;11:457–67.
2. Scarboro ME, Forehand R. Effects of two types of response-contingent time-out on compliances and oppositional behavior of children. Journal of Experimental Child Psychology 1975;19:22–64.
3. Porterfield JK, Herbert-Jackson E, Risley TR. Contingent observation: An effective and

acceptable procedure for reducing disruptive behavior of young children in a group setting. Journal of Applied Behavior Analysis 1976;9:55–64.
4. Foxx RM, Shapiro ST. The timeout ribbon: A nonseclusionary timeout procedure. Journal of Applied Behavior Analysis 1978;9:471–82.
5. Wilson DR, Lyman RD. Time-out in the treatment of childhood behavior problems: Implementation and research issues. Child & Family Behavior Therapy 1982 Spr;41(8):5–20.
6. Burchard JD, Barrera F. An analysis of time-out and response cost in a programmed environment. Journal of Applied Behavior Analysis 1972;5:271–82.
7. White GD, Nielson G, Johnson SM. Time-out duration and the suppression of deviant behavior in children. Journal of Applied Behavior Analysis 1972;5:114–20.
8. Gutheil TG, Tardiff K. Indications and contrindications for seclusion and restraint. In: Tardiff K, ed. The psychiatric uses of seclusion and restraint. Washington, DC: American Psychiatric Press, 1984, 11–18.
9. Gallagher MM, Mittlestadt PA, Slater BR. Establishing time-out procedures in a day treatment facility for young children. Residential Treatment for Children & Youth 1988;5(4):59–68.
10. Landau RJ, MacLeish R. When does time-out become seclusion and what happens when the line is crossed? Residential Treatment for Children & Youth 1988; 6:33–8.

18. The Token Economy

Token economy methods have been described as one of the most well-validated nonmedical treatments for serious psychiatric illness. Token economies use operant learning principles to influence patient functioning. They help to decrease inappropriate and harmful behaviors and strengthen desirable behaviors. Tokens are provided as positive reinforcement for appropriate behaviors. They may be withheld or even taken away for inappropriate behaviors. (Taking them away is called response cost.) The tokens then can be used to buy various rewards the patients desire, such as snacks, passes to leave the grounds, later bedtimes, extra television privileges, or weekend passes. (These are called back-up reinforcers.) Tokens are usually given soon after they are earned, resulting in more rapid learning. An effective token economy requires planning and establishment of behavioral contingencies that are logical, predictable and consistently delivered. This constitutes treatment integrity [1–4].

Most components of the token economy are applied for the entire unit so that everyone will have the same rules and the same consequences. The procedures must be consistently applied to all patients in the program. In addition, the individual treatment program can target patients' specific problems by awarding tokens for the behaviors that they need to correct. A patient, for example, who is withdrawn and isolated might be awarded ten extra tokens for each day spent socializing in the lounge. The token economy is usually put into operation for each patient after the orientation is complete. There should be a period before the patient joins the token economy, so that there can be a collection of baseline data which will permit future evaluation of its influence. As patients continue in the token economy program they can save tokens for more expensive rewards such as weekend passes. Being able to save tokens helps patients learn to delay gratification and learn to plan.

VALIDATION OF THE TOKEN ECONOMY

The token economy has been a part of many effective psychiatric programs, including all of those based on the Achievement Place or Teaching Family Model. Paul and Lentz provided definitive validation of its effectiveness for patients with chronic schizophrenic disorders. They assigned 84 long-term state hospital patients with schizophrenia to one of three programs: conventional custodial care, milieu therapy, and social learning. The social learning group used a well-planned token economy program as well as many hours of educational activities. The milieu program, designed with a therapeutic community structure, also included academic and living skills classes. The purpose of the therapeutic community structure was to identify individual and community problems and use peer group pressure to influence growth and change. Formal treatment was scheduled for 85% of the time in all programs. Careful assessment revealed that the social learning group needed to spend less time in the hospital, achieved higher discharge rates, required less psychotropic medication and were able to remain longer in the community than the other two groups. Although the study was completed in the late 1970s it was so carefully done that no group that currently plans treatment can afford to forget it. Glynn notes that although interest in the token economy has declined, this modality has been shown to improve the quality of life of those afflicted with schizophrenia and other disabling psychiatric illness. However, the token economy does not work for all and still requires a careful selection of patients [5–7].

The need for brief treatments with rapid discharge has also restricted the use of the token economy. Token economies can take many months to achieve results. There is usually a baseline phase, then a series of progressive levels that require greater responsibility as well as a higher potential for reinforcement, followed by a maintenance and generalization phase where the token reinforcement can be gradually removed to test the patient's own motivation and learning. Many token economies are designed to continue until discharge by progression through levels of the program. As the patient progresses through the levels, the treatment team continues to assess the appropriateness of discharge. Short-term treatments may no longer allow this natural progression or allow discharge to be based exclusively on clinical judgment [8].

COMPLIANCE WITH THE TOKEN ECONOMY

There will always be patients who do not respond to the token economy, but this may have something to do with how the program is administered. Rewards might need to be made more attractive or residents might be allowed to save for more attractive prizes. Changes in the program should be considered before assuming that the program won't work for the individual patient. Other treatment failures may be avoided by careful investigation of effective reinforcers for each patient, establishing treatment integrity and designing the economy to reduce inflation. Giving the residents a voice in designing the program and suggesting rewards can increase compliance [9].

Involving Peers in the Program

The token economy program can become more effective when combined with peer influence. In some programs, peers share in the rewards or consequences given to the resident. The most effective system in the Achievement Place program had an elected peer manager who had the authority both to give and take away points. When patients give tokens to reinforce each other's behavior, it extends social interaction among a larger number of residents. A combined milieu therapy/social learning approach can also produce a group incentive program, which rewards the group's performance. This can increase peer interaction and generalize to other settings [9–11].

Staff Training

Although the principles of the token economy seem simple, intensive staff effort is required. The behaviors and their rewards must be carefully defined. The data must be continuously collected and summarized. None of this can be accomplished without complete staff support and enthusiasm for the token economy system. However, it requires such extensive staff monitoring and supervision that staff resistance can be extreme. This monitoring of treatment is necessary to insure that the program is being carried out as planned. Not only must patient-staff interactions be monitored but staff members should receive corrective feedback (both positive and negative) about the way they administer the token economy. Despite these requirements, studies have indicated that staff members working in token economies have more positive attitudes toward both the treatment and patients than in conventional units and that the social climate in token economy units has many positive dimensions [12–15].

An ideal training program for the token economy will include detailed instructions in procedures, usually with a published treatment manual for training and reference. Since the treatment procedures focus on difficult clinical problems, they must continuously be updated in the treatment manual. The token economy requires a highly trained person to supervise and coordinate it, the treatment plans, and the staff who will carry them out. Without such a person with the authority to carry out the day-to-day details, the token economy will lose its effectiveness. VanderVen criticizes the token economy because of the training it requires. He feels that the staff continually have to refer to manuals in order to administer it, and the time involved usually takes away from more significant treatment such as activities or nurturing routines or casual time with adults. VanderVen feels that token economies rob programs of real content and make them boring, leaving workers with less time to interact with children [16].

TOKEN ECONOMIES WITH CHILDREN AND ADOLESCENTS

Token economies have been extremely effective for adolescents, and this has been well demonstrated in the Achievement Place programs. Crabtree describes a token economy program for adolescents that allows them to start with a clean slate every day so that success or failure can be experienced daily, rather than leaving some adolescents with nothing left to lose [17].

Token economies for children should be consistent; children in treatment have previously experienced so many unpredictable and erratic responses to their behavior, that this should not be replicated in treatment. Titus and colleagues believe that a token economy can be more effective than a level system for latency-age children, since a treatment program needs to address all age-specific developmental problems with wide individual differences. The token economy program allowed individual targeting of behaviors for specific rewards. In addition, the program developed trust and predictability as well as valuable staff-child interactions. Staff members were able to sit down with the children often during the day to let them know what they did right. These immediate and meaningful consequences kept their interest and motivation alive [18–19].

Children were able to understand the token economy better than a level system. It also appealed to their sense of play, since poker chips and play money allowed them to win prizes and feel a sense of accomplishment. Tokens were awarded three times each day in group meetings. Children were able to get immediate recognition as well as quickly learn what behaviors brought rewards. The third group in the day was devoted more to talking about individual concerns. Right after the groups let out, the children can go to buy prizes with the points they earn. Snacks were successfully used for prizes for children with short attention spans who needed frequent prizes for their behaviors. Children also enjoyed exchanging tokens in order to ride the unit bike or use the unit Walkman, or go on outings [19].

A system of deposits helped to reduce problem behaviors. Agreements were made at the beginning of each week that if a child chooses an antisocial behavior, it will cost money. Each resident had a deposit at the beginning of the week, and money was deducted for any problem behaviors. The deposit earned interest. Not only did this system avoid fines but it also framed the child's behavior as a choice. The decision, for example, to have a temper tantrum sometime during the week is treated as a choice paid for in advance, rather than as an uncontrollable behavior. Titus and colleagues describe the token economy as empowering for the children, as they experienced actually being in charge of what happens and knowing that their behavior has consequences and meaning [19].

VanderVen finds both the token economy and the level system undesirable for adolescents or children. He believes that point systems take everything pleasurable that is a part of normal living and makes it a privilege attached to earning points. VanderVen feels that giving points create rather than reduce crises since the child will protest about the number of points or get very angry when points are taken away [20].

LONG-TERM EFFECTS

The success of the token economy will bring up the question of whether it is simply a good technique to manage patients while in the hospital or whether the learning that takes place will last after discharge. The treatment environment is certainly much different from the patient's usual living situation. Although it may be more realistic to assume that little transfer of learning is guaranteed, the change in behavior is not inevitably lost. The use of such techniques in school programs have provided some lasting effects. Paul and Lentz found that the social learning program retained its effectiveness for as long as 1.5 to 5 years after discharge. There are ways to test whether behaviors will be maintained without reinforcement. Reinforcement can be less frequent and delayed. Increasing peer reinforcement or ways to self-reward for residents may allow prosocial behaviors to become a normal part of the person's character. Natural reinforcers, such as praise, can be tried instead of tokens. Vanderven points out that children should not be expected to develop internal responsibility when artificial, not natural reinforcers are used [20–22].

Token economies can greatly improve inpatient functioning and can change behaviors in many, but not all patients. The token economy program can have an immediately beneficial effect on the functioning of many persons with schizophrenia and serious psychiatric illness. Yet most of the important research on the token economy was written before the 1980s. Shorter inpatient stays, fiscal constraints, and community-based treatment have made this technique less predominant. There have always been legal and ethical concerns, which have required assurance that patients are not deprived of necessities. One may have retrospective shudders when remembering that cigarettes were once given to reinforce behaviors. The token economy principles have been incorporated into inpatient settings in the form of privilege or level systems which are easier to implement and receive very little criticism, even in psychoanalytic settings.

References

1. Glynn SM. Token economy approaches for psychiatric patients: Progress and pitfalls over 25 years. Behavior Modification 1990 Oct;14(4):383–407.
2. Ayllon T, Azrin NH. The token economy: A motivational system for therapy and rehabilitation. New York: Appleton-Century-Crofts, 1968.

3. Lavigne V, Novak J. Insights from behavior therapy: A case study combining behavioral and psychoanalytic therapies. Psychotherapy 1981;18(1): 74–9.
4. Pizzelli L, Beitmayer BJ. Evaluation of treatment integrity on a child psychiatric unit: An illustration. Journal of Child & Adolescent Psychiatric Nursing 1993 Jul-Sept;6(3):15–22.
5. Paul GL, Lentz RJ. Psychosocial treatment of chronic mental patients. Cambridge: Harvard University Press, 1977.
6. See reference 1.
7. Hall J, Baker R. Token economy systems: breakdown and control. Behaviour Research & Therapy 1973;11:253–63.
8. Woods PA, Higson PJ, Tannahill MM. Token economy programmes with chronic psychiatric patients: The importance of direct measurement and objective evaluation for long-term maintenance. Behaviour Research & Therapy 1984;22:41–51.
9. Kazdin AE. Failure of persons to respond to the token economy. In: Fox EB, Emmelkamp P, eds. Failures in behavior therapy. New York: Wiley, 1983.
10. Crabtree LH. Hospitalized adolescents who act out: a treatment approach. Psychiatry 1982 May;45(2):147–58.
11. Greenberg DJ, Scott SB, Pisa A, Friesen DD. Beyond the token economy: a comparison of two contingency programs. Journal of Consulting & Clinical Psychology 1975; 43(4):498–503.
12. See reference 1.
13. McReynolds WT, Coleman J. Token economy: Patient and staff changes. Behavior Research & Therapy 1972;10:29–34.
14. Wilkinson L, Reppucci ND. Perception of social climate among participants in token economy and non-token economy cottages in a juvenile correctional institution. American Journal of Community Psychology 1973;4:23–40
15. Milby JB, Pendergrass PE, Clarke CJ. Token economy versus control ward: a comparison of staff and patient attitudes toward ward environment. Behavior Therapy 1975 Jan;6(1):22–9.
16. VanderVen K. Views from the field: The case against behavior program point and level systems. Journal of Child & Youth Care 1991;7(3):97–9.
17. See reference 10.
18. See reference 4.
19. Titus S, Savage MA, Krebs F, Aquino D, et al. The process of changing from a level system in a token economy. Residential Treatment for Children & Youth 1990;7(3):75–84.
20. See reference 16.
21. See reference 5.
22. See reference 16.

19. Treatment Planning

Treatment planning transforms clinical information into planned interventions, moving from diagnostic understanding into action. The treatment plan becomes a therapeutic contract with the patient, outlining the goals of hospitalization and the ways to achieve them. It specifies the problems that will be addressed during inpatient treatment, designating goals and objectives for each problem. The staff then formulates the most effective strategies for each goal. Treatment plans should include a progress rating scale that will allow objective monitoring of treatment [1–2].

The treatment plan should represent a multidisciplinary approach. The team that constructs the plan together can learn from each other, share a treatment strategy and build a consistent approach. Although the milieu staff carries out much of the treatment, it is not always included in the treatment planning. Kennedy warns that if the milieu staff disagrees with the plan, it is doomed to fail [3].

Inclusion of Patients in Treatment Planning.

Patients should be directly involved in treatment planning, particularly because staff and patients often differ on treatment goals. Their participation in formulating the goals will increase their later involvement and keep them from being passive recipients of treatment [4].

Using the Patient's Strengths in Planning Treatment

If the treatment plan concentrates exclusively on problems, the patient's strengths will not be considered in planning therapeutic strategies. Even when the treatment plan lists the patient's assets, they are frequently not used as a basis for planning treatment. Lehnhoff recommends that goals be formulated in terms of the development of coping behaviors. In order to formulate these short-term goals, the patient might be asked, for example, what would be different after things got better, or how would the staff notice improvement. Questions can focus on the patient's coping abilities and how they can be developed as a force against illness. Patients need to become more aware of these coping strengths and how they might be used [5].

Treatment Planning in Residential Treatment

Dahms recommends that treatment planning in residential treatment conceptualize change as a progression of tasks that are begun and completed on specific target dates. The plan should be written in such a way that the resident, staff, and parents can think about what they are doing and what they are experiencing. When residents see their treatment plans they can clarify where they have been, where they are, and where they are going. Successful completion of these tasks will help to build confidence. Yet completion of each task should be regarded as a process rather than a finished act. Treatment plans should be written in a language that residents, their parents, and the staff can understand. The plan should translate into methods and goals for the direct care staff and the criteria for achieving the goal should be clear [6].

TREATMENT PLANNING FOR CHILDREN

Children in psychiatric hospitalization usually present with a multitude of problems, so there will always be a question of what problems to attack first. Problems that are immediately threatening require urgent interventions. However, in instances when one problem is more serious than another, clinicians may realize that the child and family is not really ready to work on it. The formation of an alliance to work on a less serious problem may restore the family's confidence and the more serious problem can then be approached. The child's diagnoses do not necessarily determine the treatment plan, since children with the same diagnoses but at different developmental stages will require different treatment approaches [7].

There are strong ethical reasons for continuously refining the treatment plan for children, since they usually will have few opportunities to complain if it isn't working. The child psychiatrist must stand firmly as the child's advocate, selecting treatment approaches, based neither on narrow ideological commitments nor on pressure from those who pay for treatment and try to manage how the clinician will carry it out [7].

Treatment Planning for Brief Hospitalization

Brief hospitalization requires a change in treatment planning with exclusive concentration only on the problem which brought about the patient's hospitalization. The purpose of brief hospitalization is to stabilize this problem so that treatment can proceed at a less restrictive level of care. Treatment planning for brief hospitalization focuses on what Nurcombe calls the pivotal problems. The pivotal problems are formulated by simply asking what needs to change so that the patient can be safely discharged from the hospital. This would include examining the changes required in the patient's emotions, behaviors, symptoms or dysfunctions. Nurcombe further defines pivotal problems as those biopsychosocial factors that cause vulnerability, perpetuate the patient's disorder. The clinician must ask which of the patient's physical, psychological or social issues are central to the disorder, as well as which can be altered and are feasible to address, given the time and resources available [8–9].

Treatment planning also examines the patient's own strengths and resources that can be called on to compensate for the disability. Nurcombe calls these strengths "potentials." These pivotal problems and potentials are formulated into stabilization goals. This goal-directed planning still begins with a biopsychosocial diagnosis with a selection of therapies appropriate to each stabilization goal. The planning should include a target date and a way of evaluating progress in order to monitor the plan. It should allow for revision if progress does not occur. The plan should be shared with the patient and family so that they can contribute to it and modify it, with the hope of building a therapeutic alliance. A discharge plan should be made at this time [8].

Goals represent what the staff plans to do to help the patient. Objectives are the end points the patient will reach. There should be clear objectives for the goal. Nurcombe distinguishes goals from objectives by indicating that goals are what the team is trying to achieve and objectives describe the patient's behaviors when treatment succeeds, or the end point the patient will reach. For example, in addressing the problem of suicidal impulses, while the goal should be to eliminate suicidal impulses, the objective would describe the patient at the time of discharge as 1) expressing no suicidal ideation and 2) having a plan for telling others about suicidal feelings if they occur [8–9].

Nurcombe writes about the language of treatment planning, suggesting that stabilization or reconstructive goals should be written by applying to pivotal problems such verbs or verb phrases as eliminate, eradicate, counteract, remedy, restore, resolve, alleviate, or reduce. Compensatory goals are introduced by such verbs as enhance, promote, foster, improve, or facilitate.

Nurcombe summarized the process clearly in an article on goal-directed treatment planning and outlines the following steps:

1. Abstract pivotal problems from the diagnostic formulation.
2. Restate the problems as goals.
3. Select appropriate therapies for each goal.
4. Choose target dates for goal attainment.
5. Stipulate specific objectives.
6. Select methods of evaluation based on the objectives
7. Implement the plan.
8. Monitor progress as stipulated in the evaluation.
9. Review and revise the plan if progress is too slow, if there are complications, or if the patient regresses.
10. Terminate treatment when goals and objectives have been obtained.

These principles were fleshed out with even greater clarity in another article, providing a detailed case example of a emotionally disturbed adolescent [10].

Harper criticizes the belief that "more is better" in treatment planning and recommends that inpatient treatment be organized around the single crucial problem that brought the patient to the hospital—the focal problem. Harper emphasizes that hospital treatment can no longer be definitive and focus in treatment planning begins by asking what changes must occur before the patient can be discharged. The focal problem may be tested by asking where most patients with this problem are located. If they are not in the hospital, then the problem is not written specifically enough [11].

Harper stresses that treatment planning be written in clear language sympathetic to the patient and family. This will help to build the treatment alliance between the staff, family and patient. He recommends that the patient's voice be heard in the treatment plan and that the plan conveys the sense of the patient as a person. Harper also agrees that the plan be built around the patient's strengths and introduces another term in the treatment planning lexicon: factors. Factors are the elements that have helped to create or perpetuate the focal problem. They might be biomedical, familial, or social features of the patient's environment. Factors are more concentrated than a narrative psychodynamic formulation and relate specifically to the focal problems. Although both Harper and Nurcombe's articles on treatment planning began by work with children and adolescents, they should be relevant to work with any patient [11].

PROTOCOLS IN TREATMENT PLANNING

Kiser and colleagues describe the development of treatment protocols for the various psychiatric conditions of children and adolescents. The use of protocols can validate treatment effectiveness. These protocols were written by multidisciplinary groups and based on the current literature on specific disorders, case reviews, and clinical experience. They were written to be used for the psychiatric dysfunctions found in patients in day treatment: encopresis, enuresis, impulsivity, hyperactivity, learning disabilities, pervasive developmental disorders, anxiety and personality disorders. Each protocol defines the treatment options to be considered and develops a multimodal systems approach to interventions [12].

The clinician with long experience in treatment planning may sometimes find that the plan becomes one that may be carried from patient to patient, when the patients share symptoms and diagnoses. There is often a fear that the process will become automatic, somehow done to get something down on paper, rather than making real plans that will be carried out for helping the patient. Harper's advice to "hear the patient speaking in the plan" is extremely helpful. Kiser and colleagues' work with treatment protocols is inspiring, satisfying the need for specific answers to problems. It builds on an accretion of knowledge in the field as well as on the staff's accumulated clinical wisdom and case reviews. It is informed treatment in the true sense of the word. The protocol becomes a hypothesis that has been tested with many patients and will continue to be tested with many others. Experience is not lost. It carries the same sense of solid confidence that can be found in the American Psychiatric Association's *Treatments of Mental Disorders* or in the current guidelines for the treatment of psychiatric conditions begun in the 1990s in the American Journal of Psychiatry. These efforts will undoubtedly be criticized as "cookbook" approaches that do not allow for clinical judgment. However, all of them are exceptionally trustworthy [12–14].

Yet no one believes that treatment planning has progressed sufficiently to constitute a scientific technology. Treatment is often an intuitive process for the skilled clinician, who, like the artist, cannot always describe what happens between the beginning and the end of a creative act. When the clinician is skilled in some modalities and not in others, this affects the matching of treatment problems with treatment modalities. Yet it is rare that all problems necessarily warrant a specific treatment [15].

Although many clinicians object to short-term behavioral goals, Allen and colleagues believe that these goals can be incorporated into a broader conceptual framework that reflects a psychodynamic approach, with reference to ego psychology, object relations theory, self psychology, and family systems approaches [16].

Treatment planning is an optimistic act which can build confidence in the milieu staff—to say, here is the problem, here is the way we plan to solve it, and here is what each of us will do. Harper and Nurcombe's work meets the challenge that short-term hospitalization imposes on planning treatment and forces us all to face the inevitable conclusion that inpatient treatment can no longer be definitive.

References

1. Lewis JM. Early treatment planning for hospitalized severe borderline patients. Occupational Therapy in Mental Health 1983;3(3):67–81.
2. Green SA, Goldberg RL, Goldstein DM, Leibenluft E. Limit setting in clinical practice. Washington, DC: American Psychiatric Press, 1988, 69–103.
3. Kennedy JA. Fundamentals of psychiatric treatment planning. Washington, DC: American Psychiatric Press, 1992.
4. Evans HM. Increasing patient involvement with therapy goals. Journal of Clinical Psychology 1984; 40(3): 728–33.
5. Lehnhoff J. Assessment and utilization of patient strengths in acute care treatment planning. Psychiatric Hospital 1991;22(1):11–15.
6. Dahms WR. A task-centered approach to treatment planning. Child Care Quarterly 1977 Fall; 6(3):196–203.
7. Looney JG. Treatment planning in child psychiatry. Journal American Academy of Child Psychiatry 1984;23:529–36.
8. Nurcombe B. Goal-directed treatment planning and the principles of brief hospitalization. Journal of the American Academy of Child & Adolescent Psychiatry 1989;28(1):26–30.
9. Nurcombe B. Diagnostic reasoning and treatment planning. II. Treatment. Australian & New Zealand Journal of Psychiatry 1987 Dec; 41(3):483–90.
10. Nurcombe B. Diagnostic reasoning and treatment planning: III. A case example. Australian and New Zealand Journal of Psychiatry 1987 Dec; 41(3):490–9.
11. Harper, G. Focal inpatient treatment planning. Journal of the American Academy of Child & Adolescent Psychiatry 1989;28(1):31–7.
12. Kiser LJ, Heston JD, Millsap PA, Pruitt DB. Treatment protocols in child and adolescent day treatment. Hospital & Community Psychiatry 1991 Jul;42(7):597–600.
13. See reference 11.

14. American Psychiatric Association Task Force on Treatment of Psychiatric Disorders. Treatments of psychiatric disorders. 3 v. Washington, DC: American Psychiatric Press, 1989.
15. See reference 7.
16. Allen JG, Buskirk JB, Sebastian LM. A psychodynamic approach to the master treatment plan. Bulletin Menninger Clinic 1991 Fall;56(4): 487–510.

20. The Unit Freeze

The unit freeze is a technique to promote prosocial behavior among group members and develop their responsibility for each other. A unit freeze stops normal unit activities and may include the loss of group privileges and activities. The community must then focus its attention on resolving the problems that brought about the freeze [1].

References

1. Zaozirney J. Separation in the adolescent community. Journal of Psychosocial Nursing & Mental Health Services 1988 Jan;2611):20–27.

21. Techniques for Waking Children Up and Putting them to Bed

Writings about getting up and going to bed in the treatment center are usually about children, although waking up is usually difficult for both children and adults. For children, waking up means the end of the warm security of the bed and protection from the external world. The coming day does not always hold promise. If this vulnerable time is not managed with care, it may affect the rest of the day. Disturbed children need an auxiliary ego to structure their reentry into the more complex reality of morning. This is only in the beginning until the child can take over. Hughes describes the waking up process as taking place in three phases: the engagement, supportive, and task phase. In the engagement phase, the staff member approaches with full recognition of the child's reluctance to get up. In the supportive phase, the staff member structures the situation so that the child can begin to meet the demands of the day. In the task phase, tasks such as dressing and making the bed are broken down into manageable units [1–2].

Bettelheim writes that the staff tried to arrange the world the child meets on awakening in such a way that by leaving the world of bed to a world of activity, the child will get greater pleasure without running serious risks. Redl describes the process in detail. About 10 minutes before it is time to wake the children, the staff member would enter the bedroom, much as a mother might do for a child.

As the children awaken, the staff member can reassure them that they still have plenty of time and can stay in bed with their eyes closed for a while until the staff member comes back [3–4].

Redl suggests that sufficient time should be available for argument as well as compromises about getting up in the morning. Although the waking up process is time-consuming and inefficient, giving it proper attention creates the right psychological set for the day. Whittaker writes that certain rules must be part of the morning routine, such as, not disturbing other children, staying in the room until dressed, speaking in a low voice [4–5].

The staff member can help the child begin the day by communicating both verbally and nonverbally. Nonverbal forms of engagement include such actions as opening the curtains, putting clothes away, or picking up toys. Conversation should be light, some comments about the weather or clothes to wear or about what the child had accomplished in the previous day. Bettelheim says that after one child is awake, a quiet conversation can do the rest. Bettelheim believes that it's not wise to describe events of the day with too much cheer, particularly if the child is depressed. Understanding and empathy are better. A quiet conversation helps the child to focus on the staff member, providing some leverage for the rest of the morning routine. Quietness is the key. Every way should be found to avoid rushing or pushing. A dependence on the routine of the morning will help to carry the child through to the demands of the day. Each child must find time and a way to reenter the waking world and if the staff tries to speed it up, many difficulties can occur [5–6].

Bedtime.

At bedtime, when the child is tired there is a danger of a temporary weakening of controls. All of the children's needs become urgent. Pleasant activities must end, and for some children, going to bed is an unpleasant and frightening event. The children have to finally stop what they are doing and leave the world they share with adults. When separation anxieties increase, the disturbed child can become more disorganized. This situation leaves the child with many frustrations and opportunities for aggression. Bettelheim writes that as bedtime approaches, the staff must slowly help the children to quiet down. He recommends quiet games after bathtimes and a snack time together. He describes bedtime as one of the most difficult periods of the day for disturbed children. Not only do they fear the dark and their own nightmares, they may also be frightened that they won't awake in the morning or fear the next day. Children need assurance to fall asleep. They feel that the person that they trust most will not be physically present. They will need time and reassurance so they can put their anxieties into words so that they are amenable to verbal intervention. Children must also be allowed to perform those rituals which reassure them at night—counting their stuffed animals and being tucked in in special ways. Some children will need to get rid of their angry feelings by talking about the events of the day before bedtime with an understanding adult [6–8].

Delaney describes an evening routine "punctuated by individual bedtime plans" that teaches children how to use staff members appropriately to cope with the challenges of bedtime. This transition to bedtime hours should begin in the early evening with stimulation kept at a tranquil range and child and staff interactions setting a pleasant and positive tones. The schedule becomes even more centered upon the children and keeping them content. Delaney describes strategic pacing with a mix of somewhat demanding followed by rewarding tasks. After the children have their showers, they are given a rewarding evening snack. As the evening progresses, activities are shortened to 15- to 30-minute blocks of time and continue to be less demanding. This predictable routine decreases stimulation and helps the children feel less anxious [8].

Children go to their room and the unit begins to quiet down, but staff members always anticipate that there will be a flurry of requests before bedtime. They willingly fulfill them, setting a comforting tone for bedtime and teaching children how they can use adults appropriately to deal with separation anxiety. The children can sit in their doorways, observing staff members go about the unit. This provides a calm, reassuring presence and decreases the children's need to act out to get adult attention. Some children will need special attention to go to sleep. Bedtime stories and back rubs are available. Some will need staff members to be present outside the door. Delaney writes that what is consistent is the staff's attempt to translate the message of the child's bedtime behaviors so that the environment can meet the child's psychological needs sufficiently for relaxation and sleep [8].

Bedtime stories can create a group pressure for quietness since the children themselves will make it quiet enough so that everyone can hear the story. When the group is doing the same thing together, they are getting equal time from the staff and there is little need to compete for attention. The bedtime stories should be simple and not frightening. While children listen to stories, they move around less and it is easier to establish contact [8].

Delaney believes that giving staff members great freedom to design bedtime routines that are special for each child will help them focus on how they are meeting the children's needs. Other staff members may want to invest in other aspects of the bedtime program, such as structuring free time with quiet games or choosing music or comforting stories [8].

References

1. Whittaker JK. Managing wake-up behavior. In: Treischman AE, Whittaker J, Brendtro L, eds. The other 23 hours. Chicago: Aldine Publishing, 1969, 120–35.
2. Hughes DS. Supporting the child during wake-up time. Child Care Quarterly 1973;2(4):277–81.

3. Bettelheim B. Love is not enough. Glencoe, IL, Free Press, 1950.
4. Redl F, Wineman D. Children who hate. Glencoe IL: Free Press, 1951.
5. See reference 1.
6. See reference 3.
7. Treischman A. Managing bedtime behavior. In: Treischman AE, Whittaker J, Brendtro L, eds. The other 23 hours. Chicago: Aldine Publishing, 1969, 150–79.
8. Delaney KR. Clinical Forum: Putting the unit to bed. Journal of Child & Adolescent Psychiatric Nursing 1992 Oct-Dec;5(4):52–6.

22. Work Programs

The mere employment of a patient is not by definition "work therapy," but work can help the patient learn about behavior and interpersonal relations in a natural setting. Work programs are most effective when they are part of the total treatment program and relate to a diagnostic understanding of the patient. The work should be consistent and related to the goals of treatment. A therapeutic work program would include a plan to incrementally increase the difficulty of work assignments and responsibility so that the person can develop skills as well as a sense of growing competence. Work assignments should later include appropriate amounts of pressure and stress, so that the person's reactions and abilities to respond to the normal stress of a workplace can be assessed and considered while still in treatment [1–3]

There is a question of whether the person should be assigned work in the community or within the treatment center. This will often depend on the person's own abilities and previous experience. If the work program is located at the treatment center, it should not consist of household tasks that all patients would be expected to perform. Jacobs and Schweitzer write about a work program designed for delinquent boys in residential treatment. The first attempts to employ the boys in the community failed because they simply "exported their delinquency "to the job. They were late or frequently absent from work, and there were reports of theft. When the work program was transferred to the treatment center, the experience of being connected to the facility through one's own work created a stronger attachment to the program and a feeling of belonging. Relocating it within the treatment program provided it with a container and a structure [4].

It goes without saying that patients should be paid for work performed. Bell and colleagues found that pay was a factor in the patient's motivation to continue in a work program. Even if patients had other sources of income, they continued in the program if they were paid. If patients can be paid soon after completion of their work, cash in hand can be a strong incentive to stay with the program. If the work program is going to be helpful, it should include a periodic objective evaluation of job performance which addresses the person's initiative, attitude, and ability to get along with fellow workers [5–7].

The person involved in the work program has a real-life situation for learning and testing the ability to function and take responsibility. Wholesome and natural relationships can develop with fellow workers and emotional difficulties do not necessarily play a part. A work program will be much more successful if administered by a staff member who serves as the work therapy counselor. The counselor can work with the patient on adjusting to work and solving problems. Patients will often need help solving problems in situations that arise in their work, and many respond well when their learning can be put to immediate practical use [8].

DeLeon describes the work program as central to rehabilitation in therapeutic communities for substance abusers. In the therapeutic community work assignments are progressive. The person moves through a series of jobs, learning about every part of the community. It allows and confirms upward mobility. Job assignments begin with the most menial tasks but can lead to management levels. In contrast to most programs, residents in therapeutic communities can come as patients and leave as staff. Job mobility is an effective therapeutic tool, providing a measure of the resident's growth and further incentives for change. In this setting mobility is not based only on work performance but also on how well the resident assimilates the community's teaching. Each job level represents a broadly defined behavioral repertoire that indicates competence. DeLeon notes that progression in work assignments resembles mobility in the real world, but in the therapeutic community the resident can fail safely and be able to try again [9].

WORK PROGRAMS IN ACTION

Some work programs become so successful that they eventually come to form the nucleus of successful treatment programs. Harris and colleagues describe a work program in residential treatment as central to the rehabilitation of many of the adolescents. Productive adults and hard-working peers served as models for these adolescents. And for many, an internalization of the work ethic took place. The ability to work became a major source of strength as the adolescents confronted their own social and personal problems. They found that work was an antidote to idleness, antisocial activity and aggressive activity. It gave the adolescents a new arena for personality growth. It helped their self-esteem and self-concept. The concept of one's self as a worker was able to replace a self-concept as a "stupid," failing, or criminal person. The work situation helped build new relationships with both adults and peers [10].

Stead and colleagues write about the SHARP Carwash, a work program started by patients in a veteran's substance abuse recovery program. The program provided financial support as well as helping many former addicts start to interact productively with others. It became a prosperous weekend business; patients who participated usually made from 60 to 110 dollars each weekend. The carwash taught patients how to deal with the public, handle money, and divide up earnings. There were many chances to learn to be assertive and take responsibility, to accept constructive criticism and to confront peers when they weren't doing their job. Conflicts that arose between peers at work were then discussed and settled within patient groups before work began again. The participants learned how to compromise and negotiate [11].

Evaluation of the SHARP program revealed that most patients considered it to be the most helpful part of the recovery program. They were able to become independent members of the community and learned to interact with people both in and out of the workplace. The carwash became an institution that introduced patients to the community and relationships developed primarily because the quality of the carwash service was respected. This participation reduced the patients' feeling of isolation and eased them back into community [11].

Kennedy writes about a "cottage industry" program in residential treatment that provided business training by giving the residents the actual experience of starting and running a small business. They learned marketing, accounting, and other aspects of business. The patient group at first studied the market, found a product that people would buy, produced and sold it. They sold shares in the company, usually to staff members. Arts and crafts can also be integrated into a work program [12].

References

1. Morrice JKW. A day hospital's function in a mental health service. British Journal of Psychiatry 1973;122:307–14.
2. Bond RJ. Work as a therapeutic medium in the treatment of delinquents. American Journal of Orthopsychiatry 1962;32:846–50.
3. Gralnick A. The socially-oriented psychiatric hospital. International Journal of Social Psychiatry 1987;33(3):218–33.
4. Jacobs BJ, Schweitzer R. Conceptualizing structure in a day treatment program for delinquent adolescents. American Journal of Orthopsychiatry 1979 Apr;49(2):246–51.
5. Bell MD, Milstein RM, Lysaker PH. Pay as an incentive in work participation by patients with severe mental illness. Hospital & Community Psychiatry 1993 Jul;44(7):684–6.
6. Howe MC, Weaver CT, Dulay J. The development of a work-oriented day center program. American Journal of Occupational Therapy 1981;35:711–8.
7. See reference 2.
8. See reference 1.
9. DeLeon G. The therapeutic community and behavioral science. International Journal of the Addictions 1990–91;25:1537–57
10. Harris DP, Cote JE, Vipond EM. Residential treatment of disturbed delinquents: description of a centre and identification of therapeutic factors. Canadian Journal of Psychiatry 1987;32:579–83.
11. Stead P, Roszynko V, Berman S. The SHARP Carwash: A community-oriented work program for substance abuse patients. Social Work 1990;35(1):79–80.
12. Kennedy R. Residential treatment of adolescents: A treatment model. Canadian Journal of Psychiatry 1985;30:18–21.

for thought, room for trying out ideas on the way to theory, and places to reflect upon the emotional aspects of working with psychiatric patients.

The literature of milieu management is by no means an exclusively American contribution. We are blessed with many journals in English from other countries and thereby protected from a parochial view. In order to remain current, one may consult the following journals, which represent psychiatry in many nations: *Acta Psychiatrica Scandinavica, Australian and New Zealand Journal of Psychiatry, British Journal of Psychiatry, the Canadian Journal of Psychiatry, Indian Journal of Psychiatry, Irish Journal of Psychiatry, Israel Journal of Psychiatry and Related Sciences,* and the *Japanese Journal of Psychiatry & Neurology.* All of these journals have articles in English.

In addition to Canadian and British sources which will be discussed in the following pages, other journals from Europe also contribute toward the literature of milieu management and therapy: the *European Journal of Psychiatry, Acta Paedopsychiatrica, Nordisk Tiddskrift, Psychopathology,* and *Psychotherapy and Psychosomatics. Acta Paedopsychiatrica* is an international journal of child and adolescent psychiatry, with articles in English and German. *Psychotherapy and Psychosomatics,* an excellent source for articles on psychosomatic illness, is published in Switzerland and provides access to European thinking,

Abstracts, Indexes, and Databases

This book may be updated by thoughtful browsing, but abstracts, indexes and computerized databases are the best solution to finding literature on specific topics. Although there are many abstracts and databases, the most inclusive are MEDLINE and PSYCINFO, which will provide complete coverage on the literature of milieu management.

MEDLINE is the predominant bibliographic database produced by the U.S. National Library of Medicine and contains all publications in biomedicine from 1966 to the present. MEDLINE contains citations of journal articles in *Index Medicus,* the printed source, and provides abstracts.

Psychological Abstracts is extremely useful and covers the residential treatment literature as well. Readers who want to stay current with the literature of milieu management may consult the section on Health and Mental Health Treatment and Prevention (most specifically Inpatient and Health Services, Nursing Home and Residential Care, and Drug and Alcohol Rehabilitation) in *Psychological Abstracts,* which appears monthly in printed form. Both *Psychological Abstracts* and its database, PSYCINFO (1972 to the present) are published by the American Psychological Association and contain abstracts of the worldwide literature of psychology and the behavioral sciences. Beginning in 1980, the database includes more citations than the printed publication. This database provides access to the international literature in psychology and related behavioral and social sciences, including psychology, psychiatry, sociology, anthropology and education, and also includes dissertations. The *Thesaurus of Psychological Terms* will help the reader plan searches and strategies.

The periodical literature is reviewed in several categories, the journals for inpatient psychiatry, residential treatment, psychiatric nursing, and journals covering the fields of substance abuse treatment, behavioral treatment and social work. Following this, other helpful journals are listed and briefly discussed. These are in alphabetical order.

1. Journals which Frequently Cover Topics on Inpatient Psychiatry

Psychiatric Services. Formerly called *Hospital & Community Psychiatry,* with a title change in January, 1995. *Psychiatric Services* is the ultimate source for information on inpatient treatment. It has the great advantage of not being addressed exclusively to a specific professional group, so that all who work in the mental health field will find timely articles related to their own professional contributions and interest. All topics pertinent to milieu management quickly find their way here.

Psychiatric Hospital. Published by the National Association of Private Psychiatric Hospitals, and previously known as the *Journal of the National Association of Psychiatric Hospitals,* this journal ceased publication in 1993. This represents a serious loss to all who work in inpatient treatment. *Psychiatric Hospital* was multidisciplinary, with articles of great interest to all who worked in psychiatric hospitals. It covered topics on the architecture of hospitals, for example, that would not have been appropriate for other publications. An article by Steinmeyer (1991) on treatment of patients with multiple personality disorder is worthy of attention.

General Hospital Psychiatry. This journal is valuable for translating milieu management principles into short-term treatment. Although written specifically for those who work in psychiatric units in hospitals, there are often valuable articles for other settings. Contents are not always predictable and there are many nice surprises. The article by Bartels (1987) on the aftermath of suicide is a fine example.

International Journal of Partial Hospitalization. This journal translates milieu management principles into day treatment settings. It consistently makes a strong case for what can be accomplished in partial hospitalization. Perconte's article on post-traumatic stress disorder (1986) and Forbes and Maddron's article on systems therapy (1988) are strong contributions to the literature.

Bulletin of the Menninger Clinic. The *Bulletin of the Menninger Clinic* offers a psychodynamic perspective on milieu management and therapy. This quarterly, peer-reviewed journal for all branches of the mental health profession has been published since 1936 by the Menninger Clinic, an international psychiatric center for treatment, prevention, education, and research. The Bulletin routinely features articles and topical issues on various facets of hospital treatment. Outstanding topical issues include an issue on "Psychoanalytic Hospital Treatment in the 1980s" published in 1985, which featured articles on the theoretical basis for psychoanalytic hospital treatment and specific treatment issues such as countertransference, nursing in the therapeutic milieu, and the patients' experience of hospitalization. The Winter 1990 issue focused on "Hospitalization in the Psychiatric Treatment of Children and Adolescents," addressing such topics as the severely disturbed adolescent, the therapeutic alliance, family therapy, assessment of treatment difficulties, and the future of mental health services for children and adolescents. More recently, the Bulletin has published articles on such subjects as the effects of extended hospitalization, the therapeutic relationship in psychiatric hospital treatment, short-term hospitalization, nursing interventions for children with attention deficit disorder, hospital treatment for borderline patients, management of aggressive and dangerous patients, family treatment for families of patients with multiple personality disorder, and nursing care of self-mutilating patients.

International Journal for Therapeutic & Supportive Organizations, previously *International Journal of Therapeutic Communities*. This journal, published in England, has a truly international flavor and produces the kind of psychoanalytic writing that has disappeared from American journals on milieu treatment. Reading the titles from this journal stirs up deep longings for what has been lost. Edgar's article on Rose's creation of myth at Peper Harow (1985) is an outstanding example.

The following journals are included in recognition of their early work on milieu therapy and management. Although they are not journals that concentrate specifically on inpatient treatment, the significant articles which built the foundation for the psychiatric milieu appeared in the following journals.

Psychiatry strives for an integration of both interpersonal and biological perspectives in psychiatry and mental health. Prior to 1986, *Psychiatry* was particularly successful in cross-disciplinary research and writing in anthropology, sociology, and psychiatry. The principles of milieu therapy were hammered out in this journal by pioneering sociologists and psychiatrists. *Psychiatry* often focused on the inner experiences of psychiatric patients as well as their social relationships. Since the 1980s, *Psychiatry* has published fewer articles on inpatient psychiatry, but those that have been published are simply outstanding. In contrast to the development of many journals in the psychiatric field, *Psychiatry* has somehow not skimmed off interesting clinical details in the name of empiricism. The eclectic attitude has been expressed as a "respect for different ways of knowing reality, with case histories, historical analyses, theoretical syntheses, as well as empirical studies placed side by side in a single journal." The editorial board of *Psychiatry* has refused to believe that clinical wisdom can be summarized by research reports and acknowledges that it is also built from an accretion of personal and clinical experience. The journal often publishes a section, Intensive Clinical Studies, centered around a particular problem, diagnosis or therapeutic technique. Case histories have maintained a place in the journal when they can be integrated into the development of significant psychiatric concepts. Since 1986 *Psychiatry* has more conscientiously integrated the findings of biological psychiatry, but without sacrificing its original interest in interpersonal psychiatry. There will be fewer articles on milieu therapy than there were in the earlier golden age and golden pages of this journal, but those that will appear will be extremely valuable. Katz and Kirkland's 1990 article on violence and social structure in hospitals and Yank and colleagues' 1992 article on treatment teams are fine examples. The journal has not abandoned milieu management, but its careful selection guarantees the high currency of the articles that will appear.

American Journal of Orthopsychiatry. The purpose of the *American Journal of Orthopsychiatry* was to unite and provide a common meeting ground for those engaged in the study and treatment of problems of human behavior. Its mission as an interdisciplinary journal for psychiatrists, psychologists and social workers remains unique. Articles are often authored conjointly by members of these three professions, with no single viewpoint predominating. The journal originated in the child guidance movement, with the focus of inquiry the child's interpersonal relationships and environment. Articles by Bettelheim and Redl established this journal as the pioneer in milieu management and therapy. The classic articles on residential treatment appeared in this journal and are still helpful today. The journal has an annotated index for volumes 1–50, 1930–80, with very helpful short abstracts that provide a rich historical recording of the growth of the field. The increasing gravity of social problems in American society have eclipsed the journal's special interest in residential treatment. Recent articles of distinction include Cotton's 1989 article on the rationale for seclusion of children as well as helpful articles for work with parents in inpatient treatment and with the multicultural population.

Psychiatric Quarterly is a publication with an illustrious history in the field of inpatient psychiatry. Some of the fundamentals of milieu therapy were created in this journal. Gutheil's articles on clinical administration first appeared here in 1977 and 1982. Rinsley's writings, one of the first applications of object relations theory to residential treatment, appeared in 1965 and 1968. Recent work of value includes work on specific psychiatric populations: patients with dual diagnoses, borderline personality disorders, and the young adult population.

Psychiatric Services. See *Hospital and Community Psychiatry*

2. The Psychiatric Nursing Journals.

Archives of Psychiatric Nursing. This journal allows time for theory and reflection which brings a scholarly approach to psychiatric nursing. This is a reliable journal to consult for cutting-edge topics in the field. Some invaluable articles include Gallop's 1992 article on rethinking hospital management for patients with borderline personality disorders and Morrison's work on violence (1987, 1993). This scholarly but adventurous journal is poised to reexamine the conventional wisdom in psychiatric treatment.

Issues in Mental Health Nursing. This journal provides an excellent integration of research findings with practical applications. Tuck and Keel's 1992 review of milieu therapy is a significant contribution. Articles on the concept of reframing were the first to introduce this technique to the periodical literature on milieu management. Rosenthal and McGuinness's 1986 article on delusional patients provides helpful guidance not available elsewhere in the milieu literature.

Journal of Child & Adolescent Psychiatric Nursing focuses on the psychosocial care of children, adolescents, and their families. Its short publishing history has been characterized by extremely relevant articles examining such contemporary issues as multiculturalism and sexual abuse as well as returning to such basic problems as putting the unit to bed. The writings in the "Clinical Forum" section are always helpful. This journal quickly challenged a belief that there was no longer room for another publication in the field.

Journal of Psychosocial Nursing & Mental Health Services, previously titled *Journal of Psychiatric Nursing & Mental Health Services,* and originally known as the *Journal of Psychiatric Nursing.* This journal provides excellent coverage of all significant subject matter in the field. It publishes timely articles on staff matters and patient care that are absolutely vital and not previously found elsewhere. Field's article on hallucinations (1985) and Chitty and Maynard's work on manipulation (1986) are strong examples. Coltrane and Pugh's (1978) article on staff/patient relations is a detailed and practical examination of the need for boundaries.

Perspectives in Psychiatric Care. Although this is a nursing journal, the title invites all in the mental health field. This is a welcome invitation since the psychiatric nursing literature is such a excellent source for all who work in inpatient treatment. Early articles on taking care of depressed and suicidal patients have been very helpful. Several valuable articles translate psychoanalytic concepts into practical applications. Kerr's 1992 interview with Gabbard is an outstanding example.

3. The Child Care and Residential Treatment Journals.

Child & Youth Care Forum. This journal was previously titled *Child Care Quarterly*, then *Child & Youth Care Quarterly.* The last title revision reflected a change to bimonthly publication. The profession of child care work in residential treatment has been lovingly carved out in the pages of this journal. It includes material on practice, selection, training, theory and research, as well as professional issues. The next generation of thinkers in residential treatment will all appear here. Early articles provide the theoretical and practical background for the peer culture model, acquaintance with the Teaching Family Model and the training of the educateur. Colyar's articles on the treatment of conduct disorder (1991), child care workers (1992), and residential treatment (1983) illustrate the value of this journal to milieu literature.

Residential Treatment of Children & Youth. This journal, previously titled *Residential Group Care & Treatment,* concentrates exclusively on residential treatment and therefore is a predominant source to consult. It was the first residential treatment journal to introduce the contextual model of treatment to America (1990) and the first to publish Melvyn Rose's extraordinary writing on the symbolic environment. Recent volumes on the work of Bettelheim (1993) and Redl (1991) by those who knew them summarize the special qualities not found in other work. The journal has attracted a stable of authors who produce sensitive writing about the milieu culture and emotional ups and downs of residential treatment.

Journal of Child & Youth Care is published in Canada and was previously called the *Journal of Child Care.* This journal has consistently made room for tributes to the real meaning of the work in residential treatment and carefully delineates the changing roles of the child care worker. New writing in this journal on institutional abuse (1990) provides an exciting new intellectual direction in its coverage. Keliher's work on the interdisciplinary team (1993) provided contemporary scrutiny of the team concept from the child care worker's perspective, and used a new word "transdisciplinary," to replace the description of multidisciplinary teams. Oles' 1991 article on treatment for victims of child abuse was a groundbreaking article for treatment of this population in the milieu.

4. The Substance Abuse Treatment Journals.

To the uninitiated, these journals often seem to resemble each other and are therefore more difficult to characterize.

Alcohol Health & Research World. Presents current research findings and contains articles on the prevention and treatment of alcoholism. This journal will be of value primarily in providing research findings which can finally be translated into inpatient treatment. McCready's 1991 article on promising but underutilized approaches to alcoholism treatment is a prime example.

Alcoholism Treatment Quarterly. This journal is geared toward the needs of clinicians who work with alcoholic clients and their families and will only occasionally have writing on inpatient treatment. An article by Attia, Wallace and Weiner on dual diagnosis (1988) and Carroll's 1988 article on AIDS/ARC clients were early contributions on subjects where literature was slow in coming.

International Journal of the Addictions. Although not singularly devoted to inpatient treatment, this journal has published a wide variety of interesting and helpful articles. DeLeon's article on behavioral science and the therapeutic community (1990–91) is an outstanding work. Dean's 1982 article on the treatment facility as co-alcoholic was a valuable article that extended beyond the daily realities of inpatient treatment toward a larger view.

Journal of Chemical Dependency Treatment addresses the specific needs of all professionals who provide direct clinical services to drug dependent clients and their families. Thematic issues take an in-depth look at a treatment problem and usually provide practical approaches to addressing that concern. While the journal emphasizes clinical technique and method, theory and research are integrated to support clinical experience. The journal provides a forum for the exchange of methods, concepts and ideas in the field of chemical dependency treatment. Articles on residential treatment for HIV-positive clients and countertransference toward this population in a 1991 issue devoted to that theme are examples of important work not easily found in the other professional journals on inpatient psychiatry.

Journal of Child & Adolescent Substance Abuse. This journal provides realistic and usable strategies for the chemically dependent adolescent.

Journal of Psychoactive Drugs, formerly the *Journal of Psychedelic Drugs,* has been the source of many helpful articles, particular about serving the multicultural population (1992, 1993), 12-Step principles (1987) and adolescent dual diagnosis (1989).

Journal of Substance Abuse Treatment. This journal is particularly valuable for comprehensive descriptions of exemplary inpatient programs, usually described in an "In the Spotlight" section. These problems are not mere advertisements for programs but provide valuable ideas. O'Farrell and Langenbucher's 1987 article on inpatient behavioral treatment of alcoholism was a valuable contribution to the literature.

5. The Behavioral Therapy Journals.

These journals may become an important testing ground for new techniques in inpatient treatment.

Behavior Modification describes assessment and modification techniques for problems in psychiatric, clinical, educational and rehabilitational settings.

Behavioral Residential Treatment is concerned with the application of behavioral techniques in residential treatment settings. Vandereycken's 1988 article on a leading European program for anorexia nervosa is a significant contribution.

Behavior Therapy. This international journal is devoted to the application of behavioral and cognitive sciences to clinical problems. This journal may be consulted for evaluations of procedures for solving various problems in the milieu with full knowledge that those who carry them out will need special training. For this volume, the journal was helpful in discussing research on cognitive self-instruction (1979) and various techniques for controlling delusions (1990), as well as treatment of childhood firesetting (1991).

Behaviour Research & Therapy focuses on the application of existing modern learning theory to psychiatric and social problems, relating learning to maladaptive behavior. For example, in 1993, there were articles on changes during treatment for bulimia nervosa, a comparison of three psychological treatments of obsessive compulsive disorder, an interesting article about putting stress into words, and the healthful effects of doing so, and a cognitive approach to measuring and modifying delusions.

Child & Family Behavior Therapy may be of occasional help for the transfer of successful behavioral techniques to the milieu. An article by Jones and colleagues on level systems in a child inpatient setting (1992) was of particular interest.

Journal of Applied Behavior Analysis often features special sections devoted to selected topical areas, such as applications of behavior analysis to school psychology. It might be consulted about various helpful techniques in the milieu, such as time-out from reinforcement.

6. The Sociology and Social Work Journals.

Sociology and social work journals have made only minimal contributions to the literature of milieu management, even in the early days. This might be explained by the fact that social workers sought psychiatric journals for publication instead, or often appeared as the collaborator or third author in articles that appeared in psychiatric journals. The contribution of these journals to this volume centered on the organization of treatment, particularly teams, and family participation in inpatient treatment. Some social work journals are excellent and should be scrutinized for possible application in inpatient treatment, specifically:

Child & Adolescent Social Work Journal

Child Welfare, although not specifically a social work journal, has provided some excellent information on institutional abuse (1992), firesetting (1991), and team treatment (1987).

Clinical Social Work Journal

Progress in Behavioral Social Work

Social Work

Social Work and Human Sexuality

Social Work in Groups

Social Work in Health Care

Sociology of Health and Illness.

If it is true that a major contribution to inpatient treatment may be made from the theories of family therapy, certain family therapy journals will be of heightened value:

Family Process has provided some excellent literature on family participation in inpatient treatment (1979, 1983, 1986) and paradoxical intervention (1980).

Marital and Family Therapy should also be consulted for articles on family participation and family therapy techniques that can be applied to the milieu.

7. Other Journals.

The journals which remain are arranged in alphabetical order, not by subject, and are discussed only when more explanation would be of help.

Administration & Policy in Mental Health, previously titled, *Administration in Mental Health,* publishes articles helpful for hospital administrators, on such topics as organizing psychiatric care in general hospitals or "turnaround" management in psychiatric hospitals. The journal also publishes reports which are commentaries, observations and/or opinions that are briefer and less research-oriented than the articles. Brent's article on how systems resemble their clients, published in this journal in 1983, is an example of the illuminating analysis that often graces its pages.

Adolescence is helpful as a source for practical and theoretical information about residential treatment for adolescents. If the journal had produced only two articles in its long history, Zimmerman's article on the history of adolescent inpatient treatment (1990) and the article by Miskimims on the theoretical model of adolescent treatment (1990), it would justify years of subscribing. *Adolescence* covers the "physiological, psychological, psychiatric, sociological aspects of the second decade of life."

American Journal of Psychotherapy. Although this journal does not specifically publish milieu topics, it often publishes articles about therapeutic techniques that can be applied to the milieu. Huszonek's 1987 article on making therapeutic contact with schizophrenic patients is an example.

British Journal of Medical Psychology. The combination of medicine and psychology somehow liberates both fields. This journal is consistently valuable for insights into milieu management and therapy. It is an adventurous journal full of eclectic, delightful surprises.

Comprehensive Psychiatry

Diseases of the Nervous System. See *Journal of Clinical Psychiatry.*

Human Organization

Human Relations integrates work from such fields as psychology, sociology. anthropology, politics and economics as they apply to organizations in the workplace, home and community. The journal has published many articles that are helpful in providing the tools for analyzing organizational or hospital cultures.

International Annals of Adolescent Psychiatry, formerly *Adolescent Psychiatry.* This journal explores the issues and problems concerning adolescents and the professionals who serve them. It provides a forum for international and interdisciplinary research in adolescent psychiatry.

International Journal of Group Psychotherapy contributed significantly to the literature on community meetings, and often provides some delightfully relevant surprises, such as a 1993 article by Kemker and colleagues on inducting new professional in the recovery movement, very helpful for the milieu treatment of dual diagnoses.

International Journal of Offender Therapy and Comparative Criminology. This journal provides some pleasant surprises in the wealth of subjects covered.

International Journal of Social Psychiatry. This journal provides a European slant and opinion to social psychiatry, with a group of writers from many countries. Social Psychiatry examines the life experiences, social causes and consequences of mental disorder, social treatments, and the organization and evaluation of services. This journal is distinguished by editors representing various fields: art therapies, community nursing, cross-cultural psychiatry, developing countries, and European studies.

Journal of Adolescence is of interest because of its early roots in the United Kingdom. It therefore publishes articles about residential treatment with a new outlook.

Journal of Consulting & Clinical Psychology publishes work on the development, validity, and use of techniques of diagnosis and treatment and studies of populations of clinical interest. Although articles helpful for practical application in the milieu will be rare, this journal should be consulted to examine techniques that have been used successfully with various psychiatric populations. Hanson and colleagues' 1993 article on recidivism of child molesters, for example, was very helpful.

Journal of Nervous and Mental Disease

New Directions for Mental Health Services provides practical discussions of new treatment techniques, models and approaches, as well as guidelines for planning effective services.

Psychiatric Annals. Each issue of this journal covers a single theme. When a psychiatric diagnosis or particular population is written about, there may be helpful information on milieu management and treatment. Bremeer's article on juvenile sex offenders, Favazza's article on self-mutilation, and Brunstetter's article on adolescent violence (all published in 1992) are outstanding example of *Psychiatric Annals'* helpful and informative work.

Psychiatric Clinics of North America. Each issue is devoted to a single subject, and examination of a particular diagnosis or population or problem. Each issue is truly authoritative, comprehensive, and written by the recognized experts in the field. The issue on multiple personality disorders in 1991 was an example of the journal at its most helpful.

Psychotherapy covers milieu topics from time to time, and publishes articles than can be effectively translated to milieu use.

Schizophrenia Bulletin. Although current issues of this journal published by the U.S. government are usually restricted to research, its coverage of all issues concerning schizophrenia is exemplary. First-person accounts by persons with schizophrenia in this journal have long provided guidance for work with this population.

Books

Although the periodical literature provides answers more quickly, books covering inpatient psychiatric treatment will be of value. This book depended on some of the inspirational classics of milieu therapy: Bruno Bettelheim's *Love is not enough* (Glencoe, IL: Free Press, 1950) and *Home for the heart* (New York: Knopf, 1974), all of Fritz Redl's books—*Children who hate* (Glencoe IL: Free Press, 1951), *Controls from within* (New York: Free Press, 1952), and *When we deal with children* (New York: Free Press, 1966). The early sociological works are still interesting reading today, particularly Alfred Stanton and Morris Schwartz, *The mental hospital* (New York: Basic Books, 1954), and Erving Goffman's *Asylums* (Chicago: Aldine, 1962). Alfred Treischman's edited volume, *The other 23 hours* (Chicago:

Aldine, 1969) still contributes residential treatment. Lloyd Sederer's editions of *Inpatient Psychiatry* (Baltimore: Williams & Wilkins, 1986, 1991) were indeed an inspiration for *Informed Treatment* and will remain a basic source to be consulted for all who work in the milieu. While the emphasis in Sederer's work is primarily psychiatric, *Informed Treatment* extends the literature to include residential treatment. Short-term hospitalization and the decline of milieu therapy have not stopped the publication of good books which cover the subject. Some books published in the late 1980s and 1990s have continued to give comprehensive information on residential treatment for children and adolescents, particularly:

R. Lyman, S. Prentice-Dunn, and S. Gabel. *Residential and inpatient treatment of children and adolescents* (New York: Plenum Press, 1989).

R. L. Hendren and I. N. Berlin. *Psychiatric inpatient care of children and adolescents: A multicultural approach* (New York: John Wiley, 1991).

Ellen Leibenluft and her colleagues recognized that inpatient treatment needed to make drastic changes and produced a multiauthored volume. While *Informed Treatment* is the tortoise, their book is the hare, and covers many of the same topics.

E. Leibenluft, A. Taxman, and S. A. Green. *Less time to do more: Psychotherapy on the short-term inpatient unit* (Washington, DC: American Psychiatric Press, 1993).

To continue to update the chapter on specific populations, the reader will wish to consult books which cover these populations in depth, such as:

American Psychiatric Press Textbook of Substance Abuse Treatment—edited by M. Galanter and H. D. Kleber (Washington, DC: American Psychiatric Press, 1994).

The Juvenile Sex offender—edited by Howard E. Barbaree, William L Marshall, and Stephen M. Hudson (New York: Guilford Press, 1993).

N. S. Cotton, *Lessons from the lion's den: Therapeutic management of children in psychiatric hospitals and treatment centers.* (San Francisco: Jossey Bass, 1993).

Readers who wish to remain current may also become familiar with the Library of Congress headings to search for recent books in the library. For books on residential treatment, the reader should use the Library of Congress headings: Adolescent Psychotherapy-Residential Treatment or Child Psychotherapy-Residential Treatment. For books more specifically on patients, see Psychiatric Hospital Patients. The heading Psychiatric Hospitals will usually include most works on milieu management. Therapeutic Communities will be a helpful heading for this special form of treatment. To read about professionals working in the milieu (in addition to psychiatrists, social workers, and psychologists) the Library of Congress headings Psychiatric Nursing, Psychiatric Nurses, Psychiatric Aides, and Allied Health Personnel cover the field sufficiently. In addition there are more specific Library of Congress headings, such as Adolescent Psychiatric Nursing and Child Psychiatric Nursing.

Index

About the Author

Nancy Soth has worked in psychiatric hospitals for nearly 20 years, in a variety of positions, including director of research, director of admissions, family services coordinator, and coordinator of internships. A mental health librarian by profession, she has studied at the New School of Social Research, received an M.A. from New York University, and an M.L.S. from the University of Minnesota. Soth is currently an administrator at Carleton College, Northfield, Minnesota.